MW01463161

THE ESSENTIALS OF
BELGIAN CUISINE

An Imprint of EtViola
5120 MacAurthur Blvd NorthWest
Washington, DC 20016

First publication in the United States of America by EtViola

Copyright © 2023, 2024 Et Viola
Photography by: Jay Snap, Washington, DC
Book Designed by: Shubham Prasad Soni, India

LIBRARY OF CONGRESS CATALOGING-INPUBLICATION DATA

Pirollo, Claudio
Malaise, Alex
Martell, Nevin

The Et Voila! Cookbook: The Essentials of Belgian Cuisine

pages in
Includes index

ISBN: 979-8-218-96851-9

Printed in China by: Guangzhou Galant Package Printing Co., Ltd

While the author has made every effort to provide accurate measurements and information, quality of product used and different source of products can vary results. Neither the publisher nor the author assumes any responsibility for errors, or for changes that occur in quality and taste of the ingredients or the recipe to not produce the desired result.

Cheers!

For those who inspired me. You know who you are.

Content

Introduction **06**

The Belgian Pantry **14**

Kitchen Equipment **15**

Eggs **16**

Bread **26**

Waffles **36**

Pasta **46**

Potatoes **56**

Asparagus **62**

Baby Spinach **72**

Belgian Endive **82**

Gray Shrimp **94**

Mussels **106**

Beef **118**

Pork **128**

Rabbit **140**

Beer **150**

Chocolate **160**

Pâte à Choux **176**

Speculoos **186**

Building Block Recipes **202**

Acknowledgments **220**

About the Co-Author **222**

Introduction

Being a chef is neither an easy nor a glamorous job. Shifts are long and the work grueling, exacting an increasing toll on the body. Some crucial piece of equipment inevitably breaks at the worst possible moment, leaving you scrambling to fix it or figure out a workaround. Staff call in sick when you're totally slammed. There is always a long to-do list and never enough time to accomplish everything on it. And on Easter and Father's Day, you're at your restaurant helping your guests have a perfect holiday instead of being at home celebrating with your wife and children.

I'm not complaining. I find cooking and owning a restaurant to be gratifying to my core. There's nothing else I'd rather be doing. I love building something from the ground up, whether that's a dish, the business, or my team. I trace my passion for food and work ethic back to my parents, who have always been an inspiration to me.

I'm not complaining. I find cooking and owning a restaurant to be gratifying to my core. There's nothing else I'd rather be doing. I love building something from the ground up, whether that's a dish, the business, or my team. I trace my passion for food and work ethic back to my parents, who have always been an inspiration to me.

Though it is rich in so many ways, it's difficult to make a living in Cassino. So, following a cousin and the promise of a construction work, my father moved to Belgium in 1962 when he turned 18 years old. It wasn't an easy life; he still had to scrape by. After long days of doing masonry and carpentry, the two cousins walked home five miles or more to save the bus fare. They lived in a cramped attic, the only space they could afford. I still remember him telling me how they owned a single fork. One would eat, the other would wait.

My father would always go to the market on Sundays. There he befriended a vendor selling Italian foods out of a truck. At some point in his mid-twenties, my father ended up buying the business, which he renamed Da Pirollo, for $500 US. Every Tuesday through Sunday, he would wake up at 3:00 a.m., load up the truck, and drive it to markets, where he would hawk all things Italian—from wine and cheese to dry pastas and freshly sliced salumi.

Belgian market culture is close knit and deeply interactive. Customers and vendors have longstanding relationships often spanning generations. When browsing, customers will closely inspect whatever they are considering buying—touching, smelling, and taking a nibble. There's nonstop comparison shopping to make sure the best, the freshest, the most economical choice is being made. Haggling is an art, one that's often loudly practiced with lots of gesticulation and more drama than a production of Les Misérables. The constant back and forth between those in front of the stalls and those staffing them all adds up to a joyful buzz that's unlike anything else I've experienced.

While he was getting his career at the market off the ground, my father and mother were dating long distance. Ultimately, they were married on August 31, 1966. I was born in 1974 in Etterbeek, Belgium, one of the 19 municipalities that make the up the country's capital region. My brother, Tiziano, had preceded me by two years. Romina, my sister, followed me six years later.

Our house had three floors. My brother and I d in the attic, while my mother and father occupied the middle level with my baby sister. On the first floor we had a tenant, Mami, who doubled as our nanny. She would make us traditional Belgian food, like chicon (endive) gratin and mussels marinière. Wednesdays were my favorite, because we got out of school at noon and she would whip up crêpes loaded up with cassonade sugar (an unrefined brown sugar) as a treat. For dinner, she'd often make a meaty main dish with frites accompanied by plenty of mayonnaise for dunking—and there was almost always chocolate mousse for dessert.

To help tamp down the constant sibling rivalry, one of us kids would always go with my father to the markets on the weekend or whenever we had a school holiday. I was always really motivated to help, because I loved the whole experience—working with my hands, reveling in all the market's scents, and spending one-on-one time with my father, which I didn't get otherwise.

He woke me up well before sunrise, but I fell asleep again as soon as I got in the truck for the ride. When we arrived at the market, I drank a cup of hot chocolate or coffee from the thermos my mother filled for us, and my father gave me money to go buy a freshly baked croissant. I'd take as much time as I could to scope out all the other stalls, each one boasting a different specialty. I can still remember the fishmonger who gutted eels with a casual, practiced ease. There was a Sicilian produce guy who erected a giant tent, as if he was putting on a circus. And the Greek vendor, who roasted chickens to sell alongside 6 feta and olives, had a young son my age with whom I walked around the market and played games of foosball in a nearby café.

My parents worked constantly, but Sunday afternoon offered a moment's pause. Nicandro and Concetta, my godparents, came over to the house with their three children. All the kids ran rampant playing hide and go seek. The husbands watched the soccer game, while the women started cooking a big dinner that we ate later in the evening. My favorite part was always the tarts my godmother brought, sometimes vanilla custard with Chantilly cream and candied hazelnuts, sometimes topped with glistening strawberries.

My mother worked as a housekeeper for a Belgian family. They taught her how to make the food of her adopted homeland—fluffy waffles, steamed mussels, and filet Américain (known in the States as steak tartare). Through this tutelage, some Belgian dishes made their way onto our table. Carbonnade à la Flamande, a thick beef stew, was popular in the wintertime (page 122). Every Tuesday after we came home from school, she made us crêpes schmeared with strawberry jam or sprinkled with cassonade brown sugar. Sometimes she would make Brussels waffles (page 38) as a treat. Golden and crispy on the outside with a fluffy, featherweight interior, they were best enjoyed slathered with as much Nutella or chocolate sauce as my mother would allow. No matter what she was cooking, my mother did everything by hand. Even washing the dishes. My parents still don't own a dishwasher

For the most part, though, my mother still cooked Italian at home, which is the only way my father would have it. Pasta is his lifeblood. He can eat it for breakfast, lunch, and dinner. Many days my mother would fill his thermos with freshly made bucatini, rigatoni, or penne rigate, so he could enjoy a hot meal during his lunch break at the market.v

In the winters, she braised lamb shoulder with tomato and plenty of garlic, until the meat was so tender you didn't need a knife to cut it. She ladled the rich stew over a tumble of tubular rigatoni. It has always been my favorite dish; I still insist she make it whenever I go home.

When I was 10, we moved to a new home in Kraainem, another town outside of Brussels but in the Flanders province. On the property there was a warehouse where my father's goods could be stored properly, and he bought a larger Bedford truck to do market visits. Cream colored with a brown racing stripe, it was essentially a grocery store on wheels. There was terraced shelving out front where we displayed all the wine. The truck had three meat slicers and a cheese slicer in the back. Shelving was packed with dry goods and canned goods. Meats and cheeses hung from the ceiling. There were barrels full of fresh mozzarella bobbing in milky water. He didn't offer prepared foods, except for one panino, his favorite: mortadella with shaved pecorino from Auricchio.

In 1987, my father opened Traiteur Giordani grocer in Woluwe-Saint-Lambert, one of the city's most high-end neighborhoods. He still sold Italian and Belgian goods, and began offering house-made prepared foods as well, such as tortellini, eel with seven herb sauce, waterzooi (a fish or chicken stew), sandwiches, fish lasagna, eggplant parmesan, deep-fried mozzarella, and cheese croquettes.

I began working there as a dishwasher when I was 13, and soon transitioned to helping with the prep work. I loved being in the middle of the action. The kitchen was alive with scents that still take me back: yeasty waffles getting griddled golden on the iron, perfectly ripe melons bursting with honeyed sweetness, and fish so fresh they still smelled like the ocean.

Though I enjoyed school, especially math, I got the most satisfaction from hands-on work. A teacher urged me to follow a professional track and undertake culinary training. Given my father's business and the joy I derived from being in the kitchen, I began an apprenticeship with a customer of my father's, a French chef, Dominique Gaudemer, who headed up Le Ledrus, a fine-dining restaurant in Brussels.

There I worked under Roland DeBuyst, a 25-year-old chef who was already making a name for himself. Now he's a big deal. He owns a series of restaurants throughout Belgium and helps train culinary students who compete in the Bocuse d'Or, the biennial world chef championship.

DeBuyst pushed me hard, but I never resented it. He wanted me to be successful, so he was always a patient explainer and took my apprenticeship very seriously. I worked as his chef garde manger, doing all the prep, and ultimately moved up to the saucier position. Even after I left that job, I would occasionally work for him on the side. Throughout my career, he has been one of my most important mentors.

The same year I started culinary school we moved again, to a house in the nearby neighborhood of Sterrebeek. My brother moved out to live with his wife, which meant I finally had a bedroom all to myself. I covered the walls with posters. There were some of cars, but most were of cuts of meats and extravagant Italian pastries—signs of things to come.

I graduated when I was 17, which was a little awkward, because I needed to be 18 to officially work. I continued working for DeBuyst until my birthday, when I obtained a job at the Michelin one-star Maison du Boeuf in the Brussels Hilton. It was massive in every aspect. The giant kitchen was powered by a sprawling brigade organized by a strict hierarchy. At the top, there were two chefs de cuisine. One or both worked the pass, depending on how busy we were. Beneath them were the sous chef, saucier (sauce chef), chef de partie (station head), cuisinier (line cook), and commis (assistant and prep cooks).

The brigade can be a harsh, unforgiving system, but it was the best way for me to earn an education. I learned the value of leadership, the necessity of timeliness and cleanliness, and why you need to be serious and consistent in your work. There was an officers-eat-last mentality. You took care of everyone working below you before you took a moment for yourself.

At Maison du Boeuf, I began working at the hot station for banquets overseeing meats, fishes, and sauces (a position even below the hierarchy of the brigade) before being promoted to commis. Basically, I did everything no one else wanted to do. Prepping endless vegetables. Running errands. Cleaning up whatever was dirty. I still remember some of the recipes we did there—côte de boeuf baked in salt crust, beef consommé, lobster ravioli, gray shrimp croquettes. It was hard labor, but I loved it. Each new challenge was a new opportunity to learn. I worked at the hotel for three years, slowly working my way up. By the time I left, I was balancing three jobs: demi chef de partie (lesser station head), saucier, and the fish and then meat stations.

While I was working there, I met another young chef, Alex Malaise, through a mutual friend. On Mondays, we'd all play indoor soccer, which was inevitably followed by a few rounds of beer. Alex and I became friends, often hanging out in the afternoon between double shifts to play badminton, ping-pong, and paintball. I didn't know it then, but our friendship would be a cornerstone of my success at Et Voila! many years later.

The other highlight of this period was taking part in a national cooking competition, where I was a finalist for Best Young Chef in Belgium. My mother was very proud. I'm sure she still has my certificate somewhere.

When I was 21, I transferred to Geneva, Switzerland to work as a demi chef de partie at Noga Hilton's Michelin two-star Maison du Cygne under the watch of chef Philippe Jourdain. He referred to my previous job as an assembly line. "This is not a factory," he said. "We are a two-star Michelin restaurant."

This was be a very traditional, refined experience. No microwaves. No leftovers used meal to meal. No shortcuts. I learned the true meaning of à la minute cooking, done quickly and served immediately. It felt like perfection to me.

After three years under Jourdain, I returned home to Belgium, but then soon departed for a job opportunity in the United States. My friend Christophe was working at Le Figaro, a small French restaurant in Greenwich, 9, Connecticut. When I arrived, I felt like my potential was limitless and I was going to make it big in no time.

I quickly realized the fact I didn't speak English was a massive roadblock. My brilliant visions of the future were dimmed, but not extinguished. After all, America is the land of hope and dreams.

I flew back across the Atlantic for a job at the Lausanne Palace in Lausanne, Switzerland, and I ended up getting my friend Alex a job there, too. For the first six months, I worked on the menu for their spa, so I learned a lot about nutrition and diet food. When the hotel's fine-dining concept, La Table, opened under chef Eric Rédolat, I began working there as a junior sous chef. A year later, we received a Michelin star.

Ultimately, I returned to America in 1998. I was following a girl who was interning as a housekeeping manager at the Four Seasons in DC. My first job in the District was at Lavandou in Cleveland Park, which has since closed after an impressive two-decade run. It wasn't a good fit for me; I only lasted there three weeks.

One night after shift I went to Georgetown Station (sadly, it, too, has closed) for a drink while I mulled over what the hell I was doing in DC. As I was sipping my beer, I heard someone down the bar speaking French with a Belgian accent. It was Paul Fourier, a fellow countryman from Bruges who was the personal chef of the Belgian ambassador. Over the course of a few beers, we figured out we had friends in common and quickly formed a friendship of our own.

Not long afterwards, Paul found out the Irish ambassador, Sean O'Huiginn, was looking for a personal chef. His last one had been from Belgium and he'd loved him. I finagled an interview, which didn't go as well as possible because my English was still not very good. However, in a stroke of luck, O'Huiginn used to dine at Maison du Cygne, so he thought I was up to the job.

A few days later, I flew back home to Brussels to get a visa and within a week I was the executive chef of the Irish ambassador's residence. I oversaw all kinds of events—St. Patrick's celebrations for 700 guests, lavish meals for dignitaries, and epic state dinners—and I cooked for the O'Huiginn and his family.

It was a great opportunity, but my then-girlfriend got a job offer in Paris, so I once again moved to be with her. I wound up at Alain Ducasse's La Cour Jardin. He got such great products—the most beautiful leeks I've ever seen in my life, the tomatoes smelled of summer, and the fish was always fresh from the depths. There was a military structure to the kitchen, which helped me refine my leadership skills further.

Though my girlfriend ended up leaving, I stayed in Paris, ultimately taking a job at Le Meridien Hotel, at L'Orenoc by Michel Rostang. I worked as a sous chef but left less than a year later.

Ultimately, I ended up back in DC where I took a sous chef position at Restaurant Montmartre on Capitol Hill. I was there for a year and a half before I once again became the executive chef for the Irish ambassador, who was now Noel Fahey. On the side, I did catering gigs for other embassies in the city. This work helped me save up for my own restaurant, a dream that had always been percolating in the back of my mind, but I had never done anything concrete to make it a reality. Over the next six years, I worked hard and saved relentlessly.

I started looking for a restaurant space in 2006, a hunt that continued into the next year. My main requirement was very simple: the kitchen had to be big enough to handle the needs of both the restaurant and my catering company.

I looked at dozens of locations before I finally found one at the end of 2007 that met all my needs. Tucked into the south side of MacArthur Boulevard in the Palisades neighborhood, it was a tiny place—but the price was right. Not only that, but I loved the idea of being set at the heart of this warm neighborhood whose residents were fiercely loyal to their local spots.

I didn't have the money for an architect, so I drew an outline of the kitchen by hand and got to work. We did everything we could ourselves—ripped down the walls, pulled up the floor, and cleaned out the place. After we stripped it down to its bones, we called in a contractor to help with the construction. Originally, there was just a tiny patio, a cozy four-seat bar in the front and a 55-seat dining room, including a high-top chef's table in the back right by the kitchen.

As homage to my roots, I hung Matisse prints and outsized covers from Hergé's Tintin graphic novels on the walls, and put out a miniature statue of the Atomium, the giant replica of an iron unit cell that is one of Brussels's most iconic landmarks.

My opening menu hewed traditionalist. I wanted to offer guests familiar Franco-Belgian favorites, many of which are still on the menu today and can be found in this cookbook, including Classic Brussels Waffles (page 38), Croque Monsieur (page 26), and Flemish Beef Stew (Carbonnade à la Flamande) (page 122). I kept the dishes straightforward, because I wanted to make sure I could do everything well. I didn't start getting playful with my dishes until two years later, after I built a strong team and developed my own self-confidence. Then I began adding items, like Our Famous Mussel Burger (page 110) and Roast Squab with Blackcurrant Beer Sauce and Celery Root Puree (page 150).

I considered lots of names for the restaurant. None seemed to capture the magic I was hoping to create. Then one day I was watching a cooking show—maybe it was Emeril, though I honestly don't remember. When the chef was finished making the dish, he held it out to the camera and said, "Et voilà!" Everything about the phrase was perfect, including the exclamation point. My quest for a name was over.

Opening a restaurant never takes as much time as you think—it always takes so much longer. Ultimately, we spent four months getting the space just right. We pushed back the opening several times, because we were overwhelmed with our catering business. I thought that was going to be our biggest moneymaker. Boy, was I wrong!

Our opening team was tiny. It was just me and a dishwasher in the back. Up front we had a pair of waiters, a busser, and a single manager. We welcomed our first guests on May 6, 2008 for dinner. We started lunch a week later and began offering brunch a week after that.

My expectations for my little bistro were modest. If we served 20 diners at lunch and another 60 for dinner, I would have been happy. But from the first day, we had a hard time keeping up. The neighborhood had clearly been waiting for a new restaurant, as our happy guests kept telling us over and over. Then Tom Sietsema from the Washington Post gave us a glowing review, calling us a "hot ticket" and noting, "The eyes feast first at Et Voila!, where every dish gets the beauty treatment."

That piece took Et Voila! to a whole new level by introducing us to a broader clientele. Many nights, there was a line out the door and down the block. For the first five years, we regularly turned away.

It was the first big notice we got in the press, but it was just the beginning. Washingtonian magazine named us one of the 100 very best restaurants a number of times, while the Washington Post honored us with call-outs for the best crêpes and French fries in town. In 2012, the Restaurant Association of Metropolitan Washington nominated me for a Rising Culinary Star of the Year RAMMY Award, while the restaurant nabbed a Neighborhood Gathering Place of the Year nomination. This led to me cooking a dinner at the celebrated James Beard House in New York City, truly a dream come true.

It wasn't long after we opened that notable guests began dining with us. Former President Bill Clinton and Hillary Clinton caused quite a stir when they came in. Everyone was taking pictures; I'm still kicking myself for not getting a photo with them. All night, kept stopping by their table. I'm surprised they were able to finish their meal.

They aren't the only political powerhouses who graced our dining room. Nancy Pelosi, John Kerry, Susan Rice, Rod Rosenstein and first lady Jill Biden have all been here. Sports world stars, such as Tim Howard, goalkeeper for the US men's national soccer team, and former NFL commissioner Paul Tagliabue, have eaten with us. Et Voila! even made its way into Daniel Silva's riveting spy thriller and number one New York Times best seller, The Other Woman. He calls the restaurant Brussels Midi, but we know it's us.

There is almost always a well-known chef or two in the dining room, sometimes still clad in their whites. Over the years, we've fed big names—the legendary Alain Ducasse, the late, great Michel Richard, and chef turned TV-host Pati Jinich, who hosts the James Beard Award–winning PBS show Pati's Mexican Table—alongside some of the most talented chefs in DC whom I am proud to call my friends: Fabio Trabocchi (Fiola), Vikram Sunderam (Rasika), Nick Stefanelli (Masseria), Amy Brandwein (Centrolina), David Deshaies (Unconventional Diner), Cedric Maupillier (Mintwood Place), Frank Ruta (Annabelle), Yannick Cam (Bistro Provence), and Roberto Donna (Al Dente). I'm sure I'm forgetting a few ; I hope they forgive me.

Honestly though, I love our regulars from the neighborhood the most. Some of them came in the first week we were open and still dine with us regularly. I've watched couples turn into families, met their babies, and then followed along in amazement as the children grow up. We've toasted their high points and comforted them during their downswings. Our lives are intertwined with theirs on a deep level. They're not just customers to us. They're like an extended family, and I know many of them feel the same way about us.

My own family has been an important part of this journey. In 2009, I took my first vacation in four years and went to Costa Rica. I met Mariella on the first night. She was bartending at an establishment in San Antonio, a district northwest of the capital city San José. I ended up coming back night after night. After I left, we dated long distance for nearly two years. She came to see me in the States, and I visited her in her home country of Nicaragua. We were married in 2011 and now have two children, John and Clara.

Mariella works at the restaurant, doing some of the admin, completing the paperwork, running around town to pick up ingredients if we run out. John likes working at the front of the house; he's got the right personality for it. Clara is beginning to show an interest in cooking, but for now she's mostly just an adventurous eater.

In 2014, my old friend Alex called to tell me he was closing Flaneries Gourmandes, his fine-dining FrancoBelgian restaurant in Brussels.

He wanted to get some distance from the venture and take advantage of the downtime by coming to visit. I was losing some staff, so I invited him to come stay with me and help out at the restaurant while he was here. He graciously agreed and soon enough we were back in the kitchen together again. It was a wonderful reunion—like no time had passed. There is a comfort and confidence in the way we work together, because we know each other so well and we have such similar backgrounds.

After a month, I convinced him to stay on permanently to take charge of the pastry program, which he took to the next level, and work as chef garde manger. I'm lucky to have Alex at my side. He's one of those chefs who combines technical precision with unfettered creativity. Every time he steps into the kitchen, he wants to learn something new and push himself beyond his own boundaries. Nothing gives him more pleasure than surprising guests with unexpected flavors and interesting techniques. To get a sense of his creativity and expertise, make the Raspberry Beer Tart (page 153), Eggs à la Coque with Potato Puree, Smoked Eel and Caviar (page 20), or Speculoos Tiramisu (page 192)—he played an outsized role in creating all of them.

The restaurant expanded into the space next door in 2017. It was a godsend. With more than 1,000 extra square feet, we doubled the size of the bar, opened a second dining room, and debuted a charming little market where we sell gourmet dry goods, chocolates, baguettes, and more. It's like a very miniature version of my father's market back home. In the back by the kitchen, I packed a set of bookshelves with the cookbooks that inspired me, which I frequently flip open to spark my creative process —from foundational texts, like The Escoffier Cookbook and Le Répertoire de la Cuisine, to contemporary French classics from Daniel Boulud and Alain Ducasse, to forward-thinking tomes such as Hervé This's Molecular Gastronomy and Salt Fat Acid Heat by Samin Nosrat.

I was just talking to Alex the other night about how I couldn't believe Et Voila! had sailed past its tenth anniversary in 2018. It seems like just yesterday we opened the doors for the first time. It all happened so fast. We still continue to receive plaudits from the critics. At the start of 2019, Tom Sietsema named Et Voila! one of his favorite places to eat. He raved about our "superlative steamed mussels," called our fries "the best around," and gushed about our hamburger.

Getting great press is always nice, but as a chef, the biggest compliment I can get is an empty plate coming back from a satisfied diner. Over the years, there have been more than I can count. I got into this business because I love to make happy with my cooking, so I'm lucky I get to do that dozens of times every service.

I've come a long way from my father's market business and traiteur. Every day I push myself to try new things, refine my craft, and create a dining experience that helps my guests transcend the troubles of their day or celebrate a special moment in their lives. It's my hope that the recipes I'm sharing in this cookbook will help Et Voila!'s fans create that joy at home when I don't have the honor of cooking for them myself

The Belgian Pantry

Most of the ingredients you need to craft the dishes in this cookbook are found in a well-stocked American pantry. However, these oft-used specialty ingredients are essential for anyone who wants to regularly cook Belgian cuisine, so consider stocking up on them.

Espelette pepper—Smoky, slightly citrusy, and smoothly spicy, it is the perfect accent seasoning. Biperduna offers an excellent option imported from France; it is available on Amazon and at specialty food stores.

00 flour—With an almost silky feeling, this finely milled Italian flour is perfect for pasta and pizza dough. I prefer Caputo, which you can find online and at Italian import stores.

Semolina flour—Though it looks similar to cornmeal, this coarse yellow flour is made from wheat. The texture makes it ideal for use in pasta and pizza dough. Caputo is my go-to brand; purchase it at Italian import stores and online.

Keros Extra Virgin Olive Oil—Cold-pressed and unfiltered, this single-origin olive oil is buttery rich with peppery pep. Use it to finish dishes, poach fish, or marinate meats. Purchase it online at ancientfoods.com—or at Et Voila! if you happen to be in the neighborhood.

Sirop de Liège—Despite the name, the jammy condiment is closer to fruit compote. It brings balance to foie gras, adds sweetness to goat cheese salads, or works simply schmeared on toast. Siroperie Meurens is the best-known manufacturer and, in my opinion, the best. Their products are available at belgianshop.com and at specialty food stores.

Dijon mustard—A good one is necessary to forge the foundation of an exemplary sauce, marinade, or vinaigrette. My favorite is made by Edmond Fallot, which is easy to find online and in specialty food stores.

An important note about salt: I cook with Diamond Crystal kosher salt at the restaurant, and it's what I used to test these recipes. All the kosher salt measurements in the book are based on the conversion of roughly 14 grams per tablespoon and approximately 5 grams per teaspoon. If you use another type or brand, please doublecheck the conversions if measuring by teaspoons and tablespoons.

Kitchen Equipment

In an effort to make this cookbook as approachable as possible, most recipes don't require any specialized equipment to complete. However, there are a few pieces of kitchenware I call for repeatedly, which are either necessities or will make your life much easier.

Stand mixer—Every serious home cook should own one, because it will save you a lot of time and energy. The best brand is undoubtedly KitchenAid; make sure to purchase the pasta roller attachment.

Waffle iron—You don't need to spend a fortune to get a good one. Cuisinart's classic model works nicely. Countertop fryer—These minimize mess and make it easy to precisely control the oil temperature. Waring, AllClad, and Delonghi all make excellent models.

Ice cream maker—Cuisinart makes reasonably priced, efficient models that work well.

Immersion blender—These small, but mighty, handheld blenders are great for making sauces, whipping cream, and quickly combining liquid ingredients. KitchenAid and Waring make excellent options.

Digital instant-read thermometer—You'll use it to check on the doneness of any meat you're cooking. There are plenty of reasonable options available online for less than $20.

Fine-mesh strainer—Use this to sift dry ingredients, strain sauces, and even wash herbs. You don't need to buy an expensive one and they're easy to find (your local grocery store probably carries them).

Dutch oven—A sturdy workhorse with myriad uses, it's perfect for braising, stewing, and even deep-frying. Staub is my preferred brand. They can be expensive, but they're a worthy investment.

Stew pot—You should own at least one of these heavyweight pots, which are great for making soups, stews, and stocks. Staub and Le Creuset offer the best options.

Brazier pan—Sometimes also referred to as brasiers, these wide, shallower pans live up to their name by working well for braises. No need to buy an expensive enameled cast iron model; a far more reasonably priced stainless steel one will work just as well.

Cocotte—Similar to Dutch ovens, these enameled castiron cooking pots have multiple uses. Whether you need miniature ones for individual portions or a larger 10-inch model to make a batch of something, Staub makes the best options.

9-inch (23 cm) tart mold with removable bottom—There's no need to seek out a particular brand; whatever you can pick up at a cookware shop or big box store, like Target, will do the trick.

PAGE 16

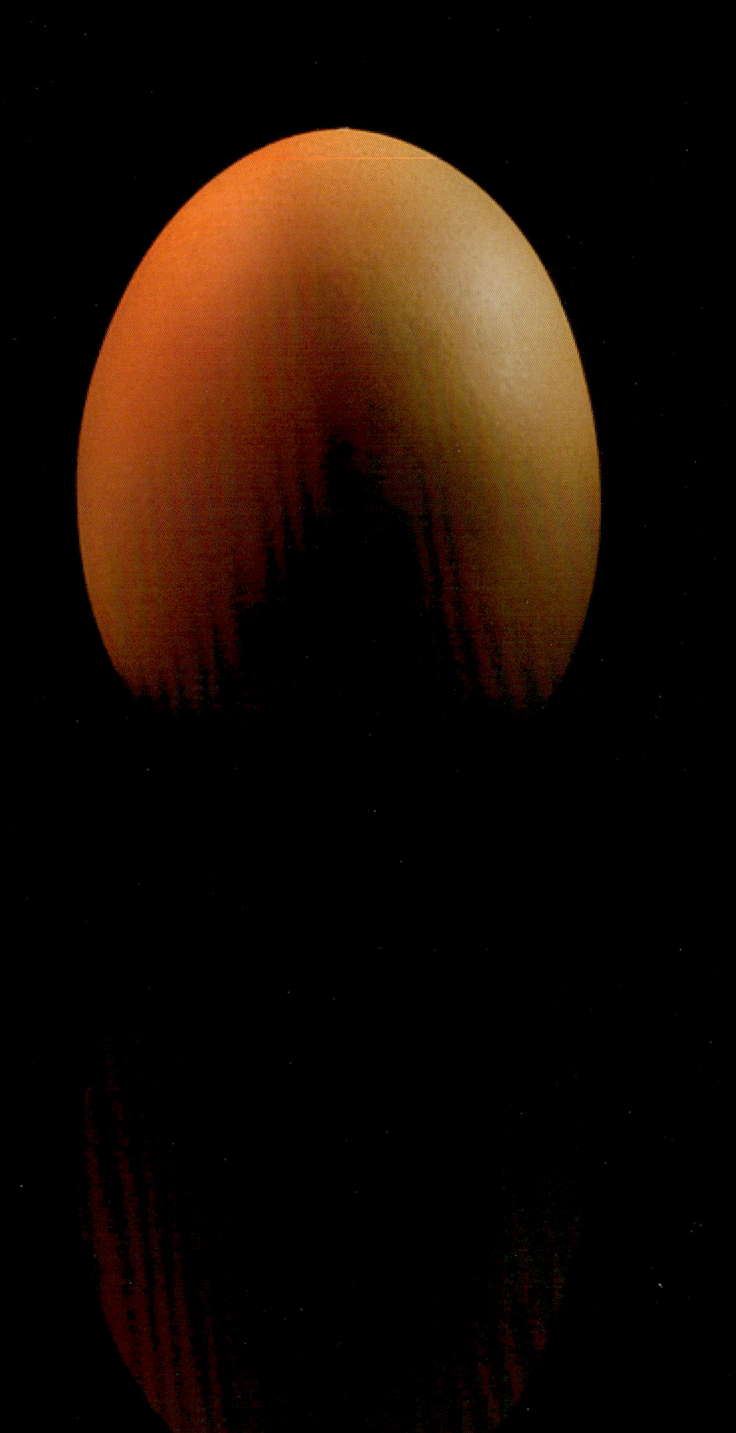

EGGS

When I crack open an egg from my friends at Path Valley Farms, I know I'm going to be greeted by a cheery yolk that's more orange than the stereotypical yellow. The clementine-colored cores are so full of flavor; they're almost buttery. They remind me of an after school snack my mother used to make: raw yolk whipped with sugar. It was so simple, but it tasted like a rare extravagance. That's when my passion for eggs first began. As a chef I love them, because they are tools of transformation: changing textures, boosting richness, and adding protein. I cannot stress enough the importance of sourcing great eggs, preferably cage free and organic. You'll know you've gotten the right dozen when you crack the first one open.

1

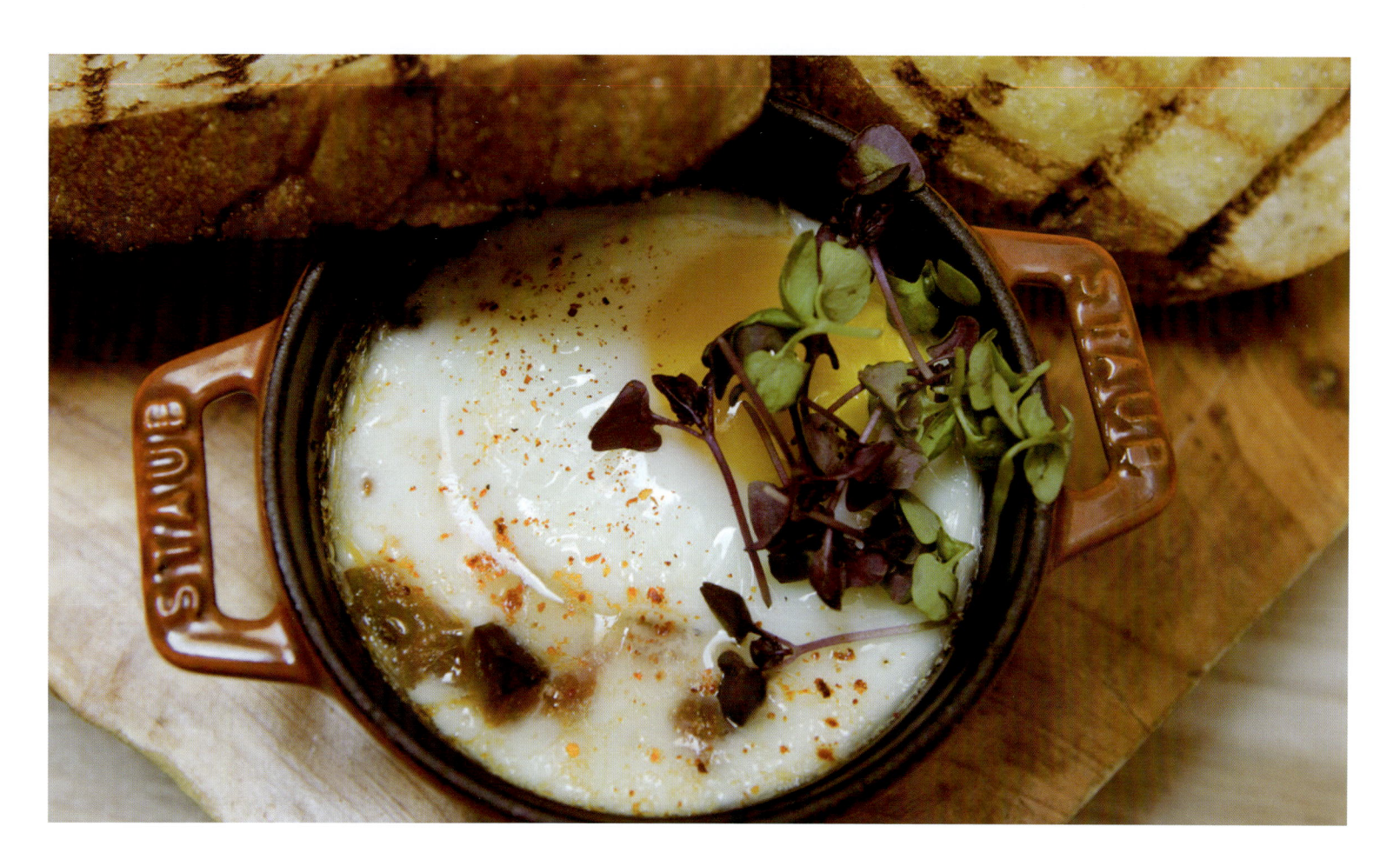

SERVES
8

Eggs Cocotte with Vegetable Ratatouille

My ratatouille features the usual suspects— eggplant, red and yellow bell peppers, onions, tomatoes, and zucchini. Though it's is generally eaten at lunch or dinner, I like starting my day with it. Topping off the thick stew with a sunnyside-up egg, I serve it in a small cast-iron cocotte. I recommend popping the yolk with a slice of grilled country bread and mixing it in to add a silky sensibility to the vegetable medley.

INGREDIENTS

1. One 28-ounce (800 gram) can whole peeled San Marzano tomatoes
2. 1 cup (200 grams) extra virgin olive oil, divided, plus more for brushing and drizzling
3. 1 medium Italian eggplant, diced small
4. Kosher salt and freshly ground black pepper
5. 1 medium zucchini, diced small
6. 4 cloves garlic, finely chopped
7. 1 large yellow onion, diced small
8. 1 red bell pepper, diced small
9. 1 yellow bell pepper, diced small
10. 2 sprigs fresh thyme
11. 1 dried bay leaf
12. 1 1/2 teaspoon (3 grams) Espelette pepper
13. 8 large eggs (400 grams)
14. 8 large slices country bread
    Microgreens for garnish

DIRECTIONS

Using an immersion blender or food processor fitted with the stainless-steel blade, blend the tomatoes and their juices into a puree. Set aside.

In a medium sauté pan over high heat, warm 1/4 cup (50 grams) of the olive oil until slightly smoking. Sauté the eggplant, 1/2 teaspoon (2 grams) salt, and 1/4 teaspoon (1 grams) black pepper until softened and golden brown,

4 to 5 minutes. Remove the eggplant from the pan and place it in a colander set over a sheet pan to let the excess oil drip off. Add another 1/4 cup (50 grams) of the olive oil to the sauté pan and return it to the heat. Add the zucchini and cook until slightly browned, about 2 minutes. Remove the zucchini from the pan and place in the colander

In a medium pot over medium heat, combine the remaining 1/2 cup (50 grams) olive oil, the garlic, and onion. Let them cook, stirring constantly, until translucent but not browned, about 10 minutes. Add the red and yellow bell peppers. Let them cook, stirring constantly, until they have softened, about 10 minutes. Add the thyme, bay leaf, pureed tomatoes, 1 teaspoon (5 grams) salt, and the Espelette pepper. Turn the heat down to low and simmer, stirring occasionally, until the liquid has reduced by half, about 20 minutes. Add the Eggs Cocotte with Vegetable Ratatouille21 eggplant and zucchini and cook until the mixture looks like a thick stew, about 25 minutes. Season to taste with salt and black pepper.

Preheat the oven to 350°F (175°C)

Take 8 small cocottes (approximately 4 inches/10 cm wide and 2 inches/5 cm high) and fill each one with the ratatouille. Remove and discard the bay leaf. Crack an egg in the center of the vegetables. Place the cocottes on a sheet pan and bake for approximately 25 minutes, until the whites are cooked but the yolks are still runny.

Remove from oven and let sit for 5 minutes. Meanwhile, brush one side of each piece of bread with olive oil. Toast in a toaster or under the broiler until golden brown. Garnish each cocotte with microgreens and drizzle with olive oil. Serve each with a slice of toasted country bread

Smoked Salmon Benedict

We are well known at Et Voila! for our brunch, where our smoked salmon Benedict is a star. If you don't feel like coming in to see us, don't worry—it's relatively effortless to make at home. Hollandaise sauce seems imposing to those who haven't made it before, but it simply requires precision and focus. Make sure the clarified butter you're using is warm, or it will give your hollandaise an unpleasantly mayonnaise-like consistency. Any high-quality cold-smoked salmon will do the trick; I'm a big fan of Ivy City Smokehouse's NOVA Style Smoked Salmon myself.

SERVES 4

DIRECTIONS

To make the eggs, fill a medium bowl with ice and cold water. Fill a large pot halfway with water, add the vinegar, and bring to a boil over high heat. Gently crack the eggs one at a time into the water, taking care not to break the yolks. Reduce the heat to a gentle simmer and cook the eggs for 3 ½ to 4 minutes, until the whites are set. Remove them from the water with a slotted spoon and place them in the ice water. Set aside.

To make the hollandaise sauce, in a medium stainless steel bowl, whisk together the egg yolks, lemon juice, and wine until the mixture is thickened and doubled in volume.

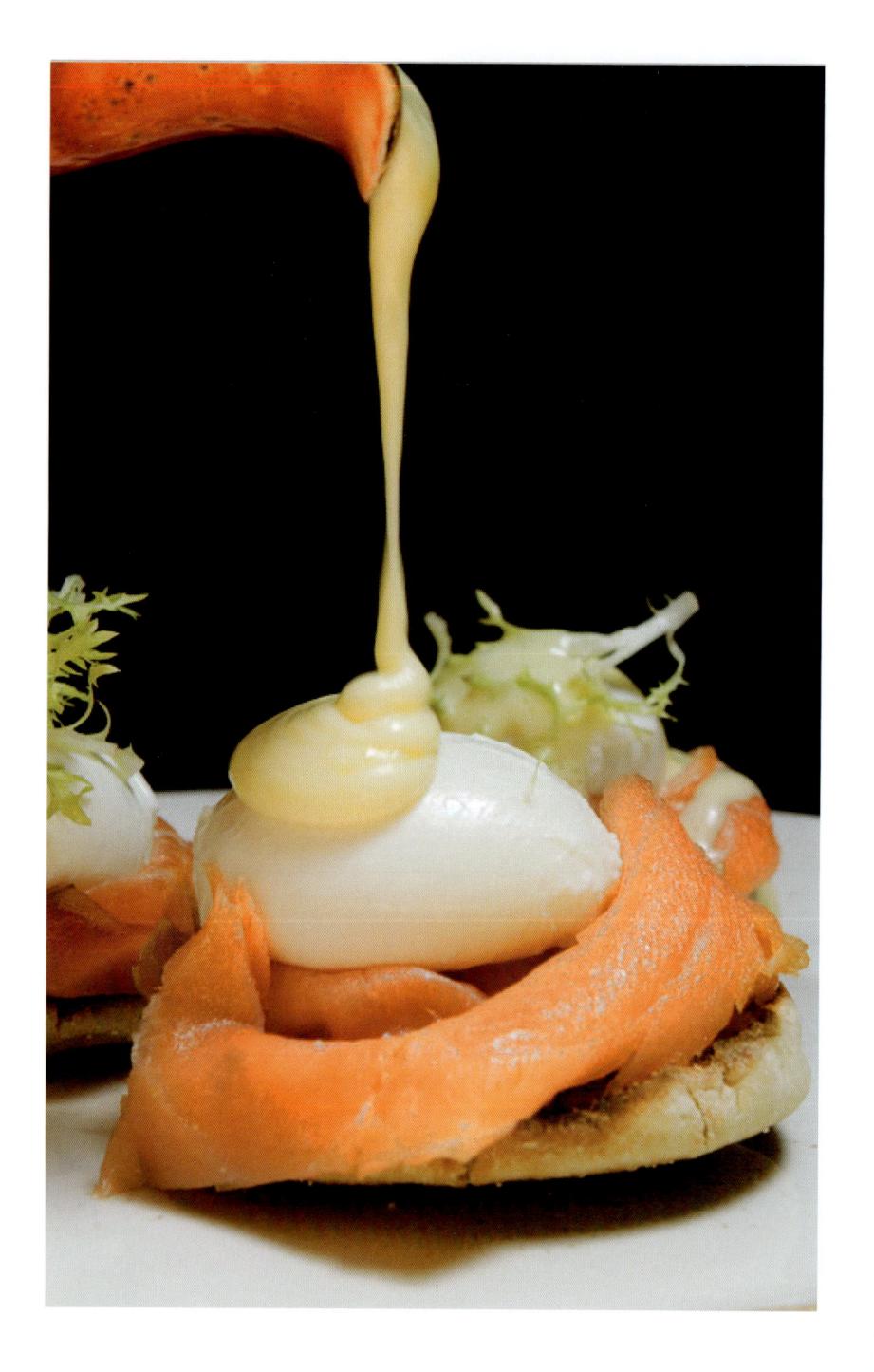

INGREDIENTS

1. One 28-ounce (800 gram) can whole peeled San Marzano tomatoes
2. 1 cup (200 grams) extra virgin olive oil, divided, plus more for brushing and drizzling
3. 1 medium Italian eggplant, diced small
4. Kosher salt and freshly ground black pepper
5. 1 medium zucchini, diced small
6. 4 cloves garlic, finely chopped
7. 1 large yellow onion, diced small
8. 1 red bell pepper, diced small
9. 1 yellow bell pepper, diced small
10. 2 sprigs fresh thyme
11. 1 dried bay leaf
12. 1 1/2 teaspoon (3 grams) Espelette pepper
13. 8 large eggs (400 grams)
14. 8 large slices country bread
    Microgreens for garnish

Fill a large pot with just enough water so the bottom of the stainless-steel bowl does not touch the water when placed over it. Over medium heat, bring the water to a gentle simmer.

Place the stainless-steel bowl over the water, balancing it on the rim of the pot. Continue to whisk rapidly until the mixture has thickened enough that when you pull out the whisk, the mixture drips off in long ribbons. Do not let the eggs get too hot or they will scramble.

Remove the bowl from the pot and slowly whisk in the clarified butter. The sauce will thicken and double in volume. Whisk in the salt and Espelette pepper. Cover with plastic wrap and set aside in a warm spot until ready to use.

To warm up the eggs, place a large pot filled halfway with water over medium-high heat and bring to a boil. Once boiling, turn off the heat. Use a slotted spoon to gently transfer the eggs to the water to warm for 5 minutes. Toast the English muffins, cut sides up. To assemble, lay a slice of the smoked salmon on top of each toasted English muffin half. Remove a poached egg from the hot water with a slotted spoon, drain it briefly, and place on the salmon. Spoon hollandaise sauce over the eggs. Garnish with chopped parsley

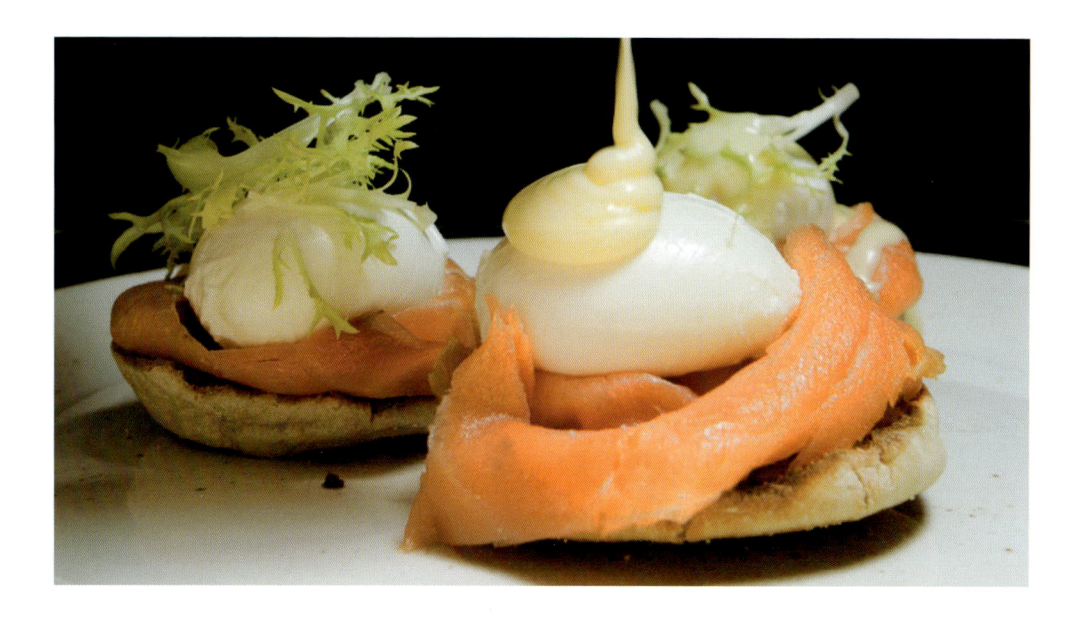

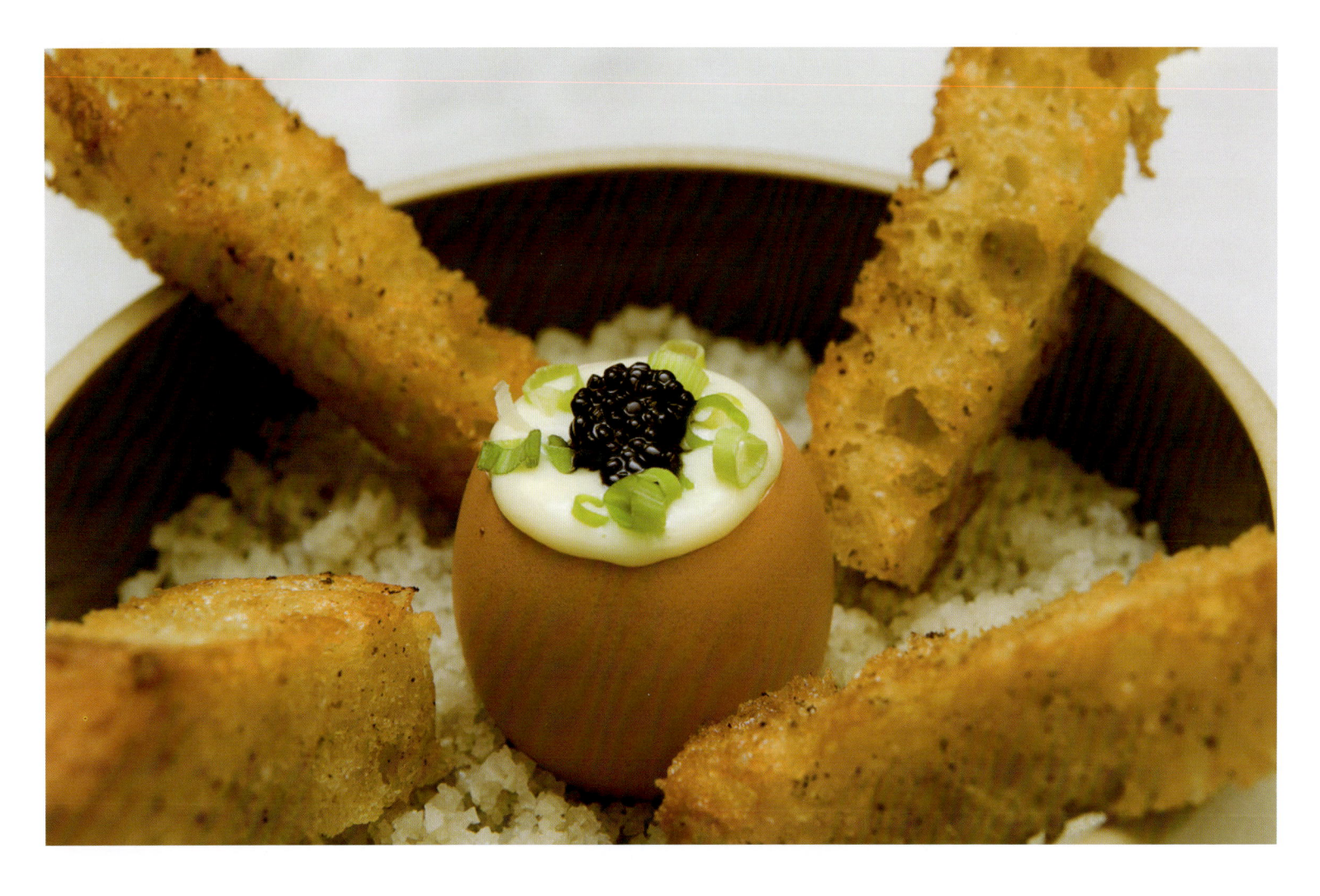

Eggs à la Coque

with Potato Puree, Smoked Eel, and Caviar

(Step By Step)

INGREDIENTS

1. 1 pound (450 grams) fingerling potatoes, peeled
2. 1 teaspoon (5 grams) kosher salt
3. 1 1/4 cups (300 grams) heavy cream
4. 4 slices white Pullman bread (store-bought, or page 215)
5. 8 tablespoons (1 stick/125 grams) unsalted butter
6. 8 large eggs (400 grams)
7. 4 1/4 ounces (120 grams) smoked eel fillet, diced small
8. 1 green onion (white and green parts), thinly sliced
9. 1 ounce (30 grams) caviar

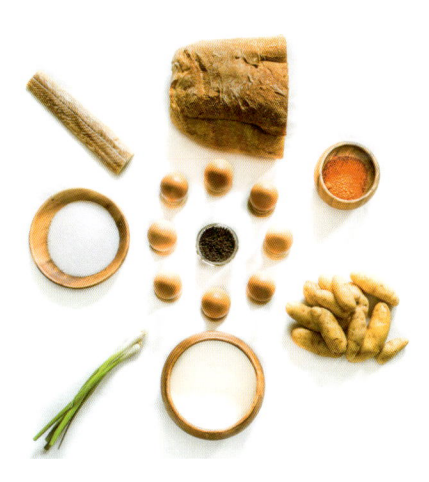

DIRECTIONS

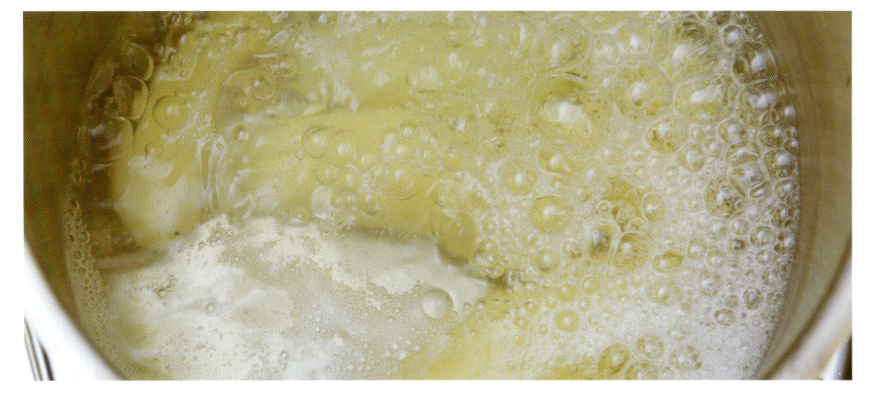

1. In a medium pot over high heat, place the potatoes, salt, and enough water to cover. Bring to a boil and cook until potatoes are softened but there's still some resistance when you poke them with a fork, about 20 minutes. Set a strainer in the sink and pour in the potatoes to drain. Return them to the pot.

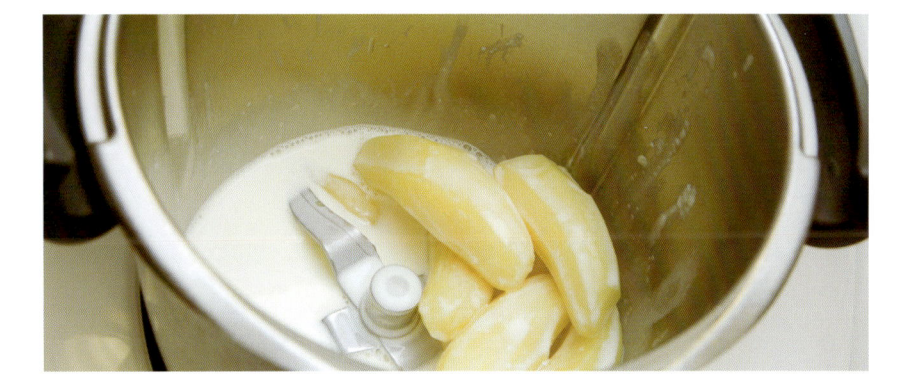

2. Turn the heat down to medium-low, add the cream, and continue cooking the potatoes until a fork passes through them with no resistance, 15 to 20 minutes. Remove from the heat and let cool. Pour the potatoes and cream into a blender and process until smooth and creamy. Set aside.

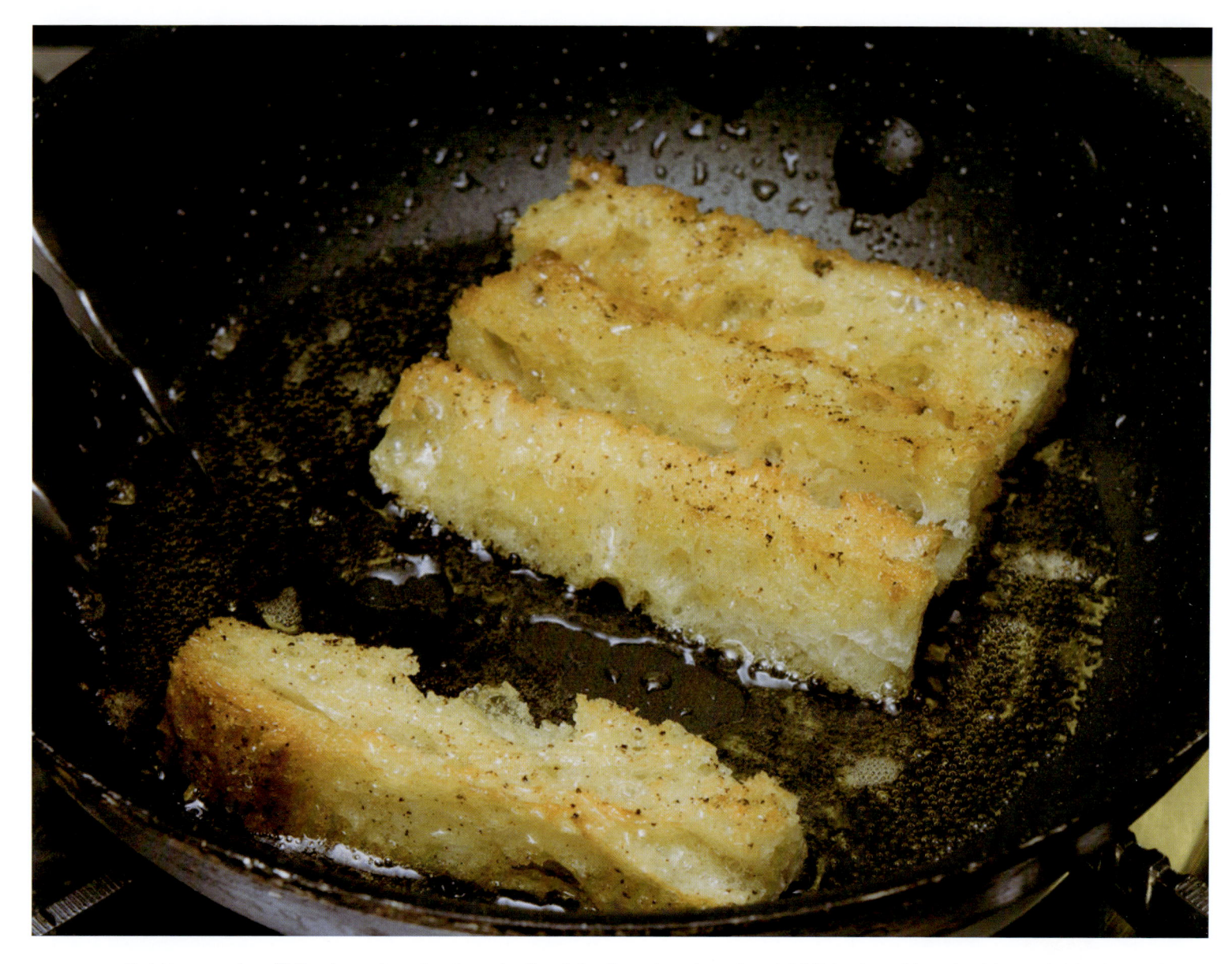

3. Cut the crusts off the bread and cut each slice into 2 rectangles about 1 1/2 inches (4 cm) wide and 4 inches (10 cm) long. Cover a plate with a paper towel. In a medium sauté pan, melt the butter, then add the bread. Cook until the bottoms are golden brown, then flip them over and brown the other side. Set aside on the plate

4.

Using the egg topper, cut off the tops of the eggshells; discard the tops. One at a time, carefully pour out the eggs and separate the yolks from the whites. Place the yolks back into the shells. Store the whites for another use.

5.

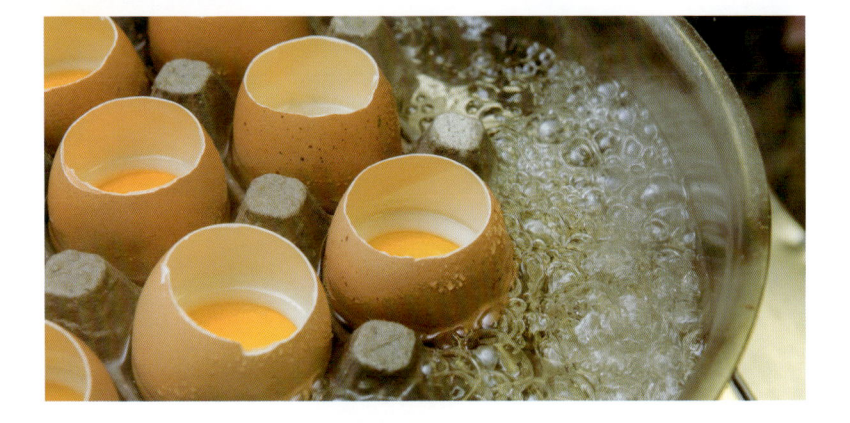

In a medium brazier pot, place a cardboard egg carton with the top cut off and place the eggshells in it. Fill the pot with water until the cardboard is just covered. Over high heat, without the lid, bring the water to a boil and poach the yolks until just firm, 3 to 3 1/2 minutes.

6.

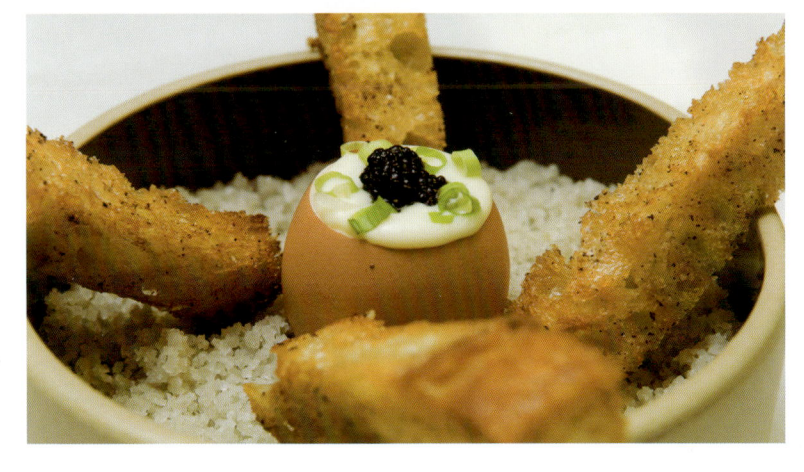

Drain off any water that managed to get into the eggshell and then place each eggshell in an egg cup. Fill each eggshell with 1 tablespoon (15 grams) of the eel, a sprinkle of green onion, potato puree almost up to the rim, and 1/2 teaspoon (3.75 grams) caviar. Serve immediately with the toasted bread on the side

PAGE 26

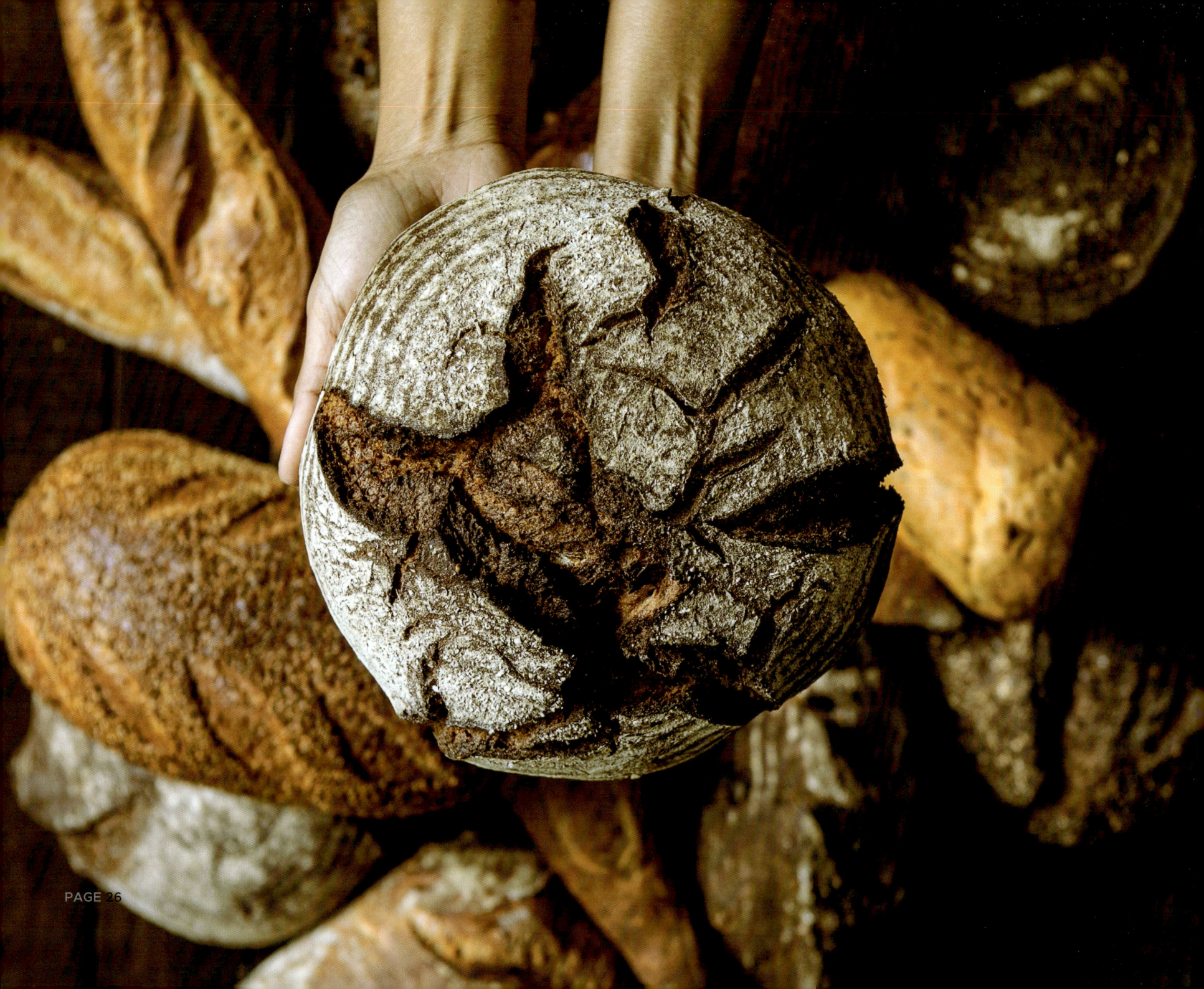

BREAD

I'm very passionate about bread. When I go out to eat, I first judge the restaurant by its bread basket. Though I've never been a baker, I became familiar with the work when I was an apprentice to a pastry chef. Later, when I worked for famed Belgian chef Roland DeBuyst, I was in charge of baking small rolls, focaccia, and brioche. I still love to bake, though I mostly do it for my family and myself. These recipes are reminders of the days when I had more time to roll up my sleeves, get dusted in flour, and work the dough

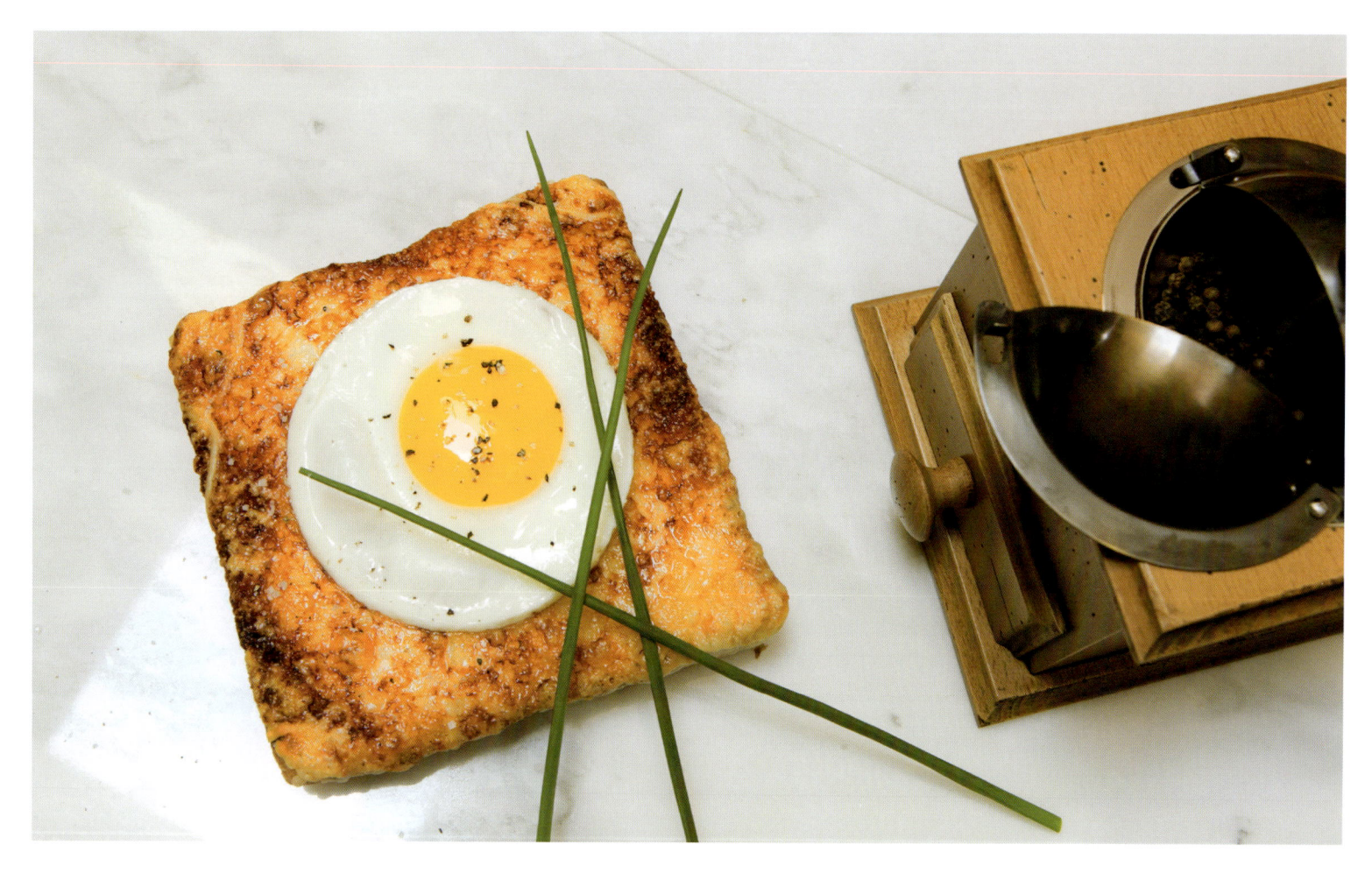

Croque Monsieur

The foundation of any great croque monsieur is great bread. Ideally, you would source pain de mie, the crustless French bread with just a touch of sweetness. If that's not available, get a good Pullman loaf from a local baker. The other keys to a memorable croque are smooth béchamel sauce, good Gruyère cheese (or a nice Comté if you're in a pinch), and quality ham, such as those from producers like Madrange, Leoncini, or Levoni, which can be purchased from good import stores or online

INGREDIENTS

1. 2 1/4 cups (500 grams) whole milk
2. 1 1/4 teaspoons (4 grams) flaky sea salt
3. 3/4 teaspoon (2 grams) freshly grated nutmeg
4. 1 teaspoon (3 grams) Espelette pepper
5. 14 tablespoons (1 3/4 sticks/210 grams) unsalted butter, divided
6. 1/4 cup + 2 tablespoons (50 grams) all-purpose flour
7. 8 slices white bread (about 1/2 inch/1 cm thick)
8. 1 tablespoon + 1 teaspoon (20 grams) Dijon mustard
9. 4 slices deli ham
10. 2 cups (226 grams) grated Swiss or Gruyère cheese
11. 1/4 cup (10 grams) chopped fresh chives

DIRECTIONS

To make the béchamel sauce, place the milk, salt, nutmeg, and Espelette pepper in a medium pot over medium heat. Bring to a boil, turn off the heat, and set aside.

In a separate medium saucepan over medium heat, melt 6 tablespoons (90 grams) of the butter until it's bubbling slightly. Slowly add the flour while whisking constantly, until a thick paste has formed. Turn down the heat to low and, whisking constantly, cook until the flour very lightly browned, 10 to 15 minutes. Add the milk while whisking constantly until smooth and cook until the sauce has thickened, 8 to 10 minutes. Remove the mixture from the heat and pass it through a fine-mesh strainer into a medium bowl. Set aside.

Using a spatula, brush 4 pieces of the bread with the Dijon mustard and 1 tablespoon (18 grams) of the béchamel sauce. Lay a piece of ham on each slice and sprinkle each with 1/4 cup (28 grams) of the cheese. Top each with another slice of bread to form sandwiches. Preheat the oven to 360°F (180°C).

In a medium sauté pan over medium heat, melt 2 tablespoons (30 grams) of the butter until it's bubbling. One at a time, place a sandwich in the pan and griddle it until the bottom is golden brown, 2 to 3 minutes. Set aside on a cooling rack while cooking the others. Wipe out the pan before adding 2 tablespoons (30 grams) of the butter to the pan and let it melt until it's bubbling before adding another sandwich.

Spread the remaining béchamel on top of the sandwiches and sprinkle each sandwich with another 1/4 cup (28 grams) of the cheese. Place the sandwiches on a parchment paper–lined baking sheet and bake until the cheese on top is melted, slightly crispy, and golden, 10 to 15 minutes. Serve immediatel

5

MAKES 10 4 OPEN-FACED SANDWICHES

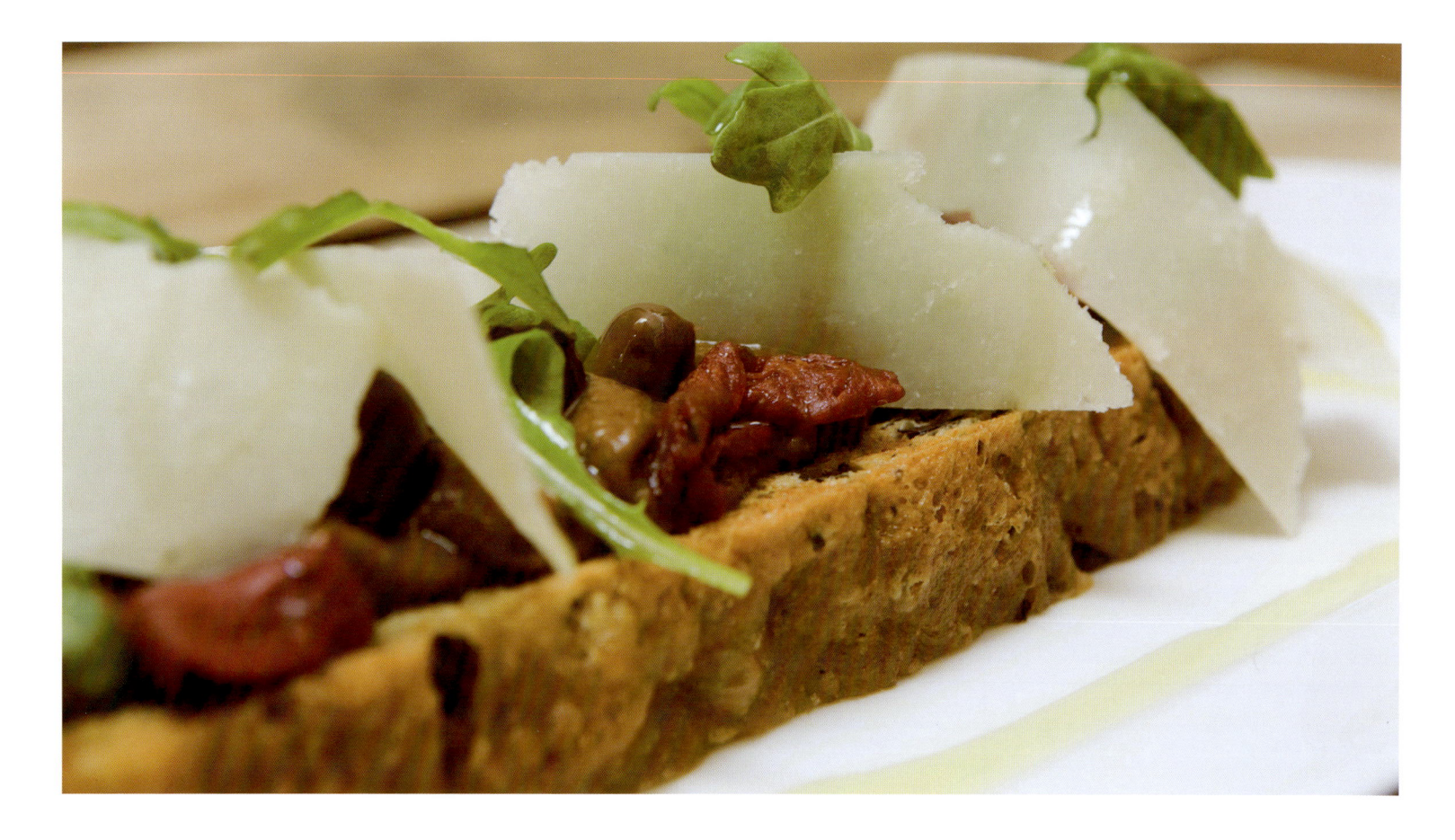

Grilled Focaccia

with Smoked Eggplant Caviar, Sun-Dried Tomatoes, and Parmesan

Focaccia is an excellent starting point for beginner bakers. It's a straightforward process and the dough is very forgiving, so untrained hands can still produce memorable bread. The soft yet sturdy consistency makes it the perfect base for lighter sandwiches, like this open-faced vegetarian option that has been a longtime favorite of my guests at Et Voila!. You can also use the smoked eggplant caviar to garnish roasted lamb loin, slather on crostini, or as a base for a cold soup. You'll need high-gluten flour. King Arthur makes the best; it's available online and in many fine grocery stores. Ibérico de Bellota is easy to find at specialty food stores—my favorite is by Cinco Jotas—but prosciutto works as well.

INGREDIENTS

Focaccia

1. 1/4 cup + 3 tablespoons (60 grams) active dry yeast
2. 8 1/4 cups (1 kilogram) high-gluten flour
3. 2 1/2 teaspoons (12 grams) kosher salt
4. Pinch of Espelette pepper
5. 1/4 cup + 1 tablespoon (60 grams) extra virgin olive oil,
6. plus more for the pan and brushing
7. 3 cloves garlic, finely diced
8. 3 sprigs fresh rosemary, roughly chopped
9. 1 teaspoon (6 grams) flaky sea salt

Eggplant caviar

1. 5 medium Italian eggplants
2. 3 sprigs fresh thyme, roughly chopped
3. 1/4 cup (60 grams) extra virgin olive oil, divided
4. 2 1/2 teaspoons (15 grams) flaky sea salt
5. 3 medium shallots, finely diced
6. 4 cloves garlic, finely diced
7. 1/2 cup (60 grams) grated Grana Padano cheese
8. Pinch of Espelette pepper

To assemble

1. 1/2 cup + 2 tablespoons (150 grams) sherry vinegar

DIRECTIONS

To make the focaccia

warm 3 cups (660 grams) water to approximately 75°F (25°C) and place it in a medium bowl with the yeast. Whisk gently until the yeast is completely dissolved. Set aside.

In the bowl of a stand mixer fitted with the dough hook attachment, mix the flour, kosher salt, and Espelette pepper on medium speed until thoroughly combined. Slowly pour in the water and olive oil and mix until the dough is starting to pull away from the sides of the bowl and bunch around the hook. Remove the bowl from the mixer, form the dough into a ball, and place it back into the bowl. Cover the bowl with a damp kitchen towel and set it in a warm place until the dough has doubled in size, about 1 hour.

Generously grease with olive oil a 13 by 9-inch (33 by 23 cm) baking pan. Place the dough in the pan and using your fingers, press the dough evenly across it. Cover again with the kitchen towel and set it in a warm place until the dough has again doubled in size, about 1 hour.

Preheat the oven to 360°F (180°C).

Brush the top of the dough with olive oil and sprinkle on the garlic, rosemary, and sea salt. Bake the focaccia on the middle rack until a toothpick inserted into its center comes out dry, 30 to 35 minutes. Remove the focaccia from oven but do not turn off the oven. Let the focaccia cool in the pan on a cooling rack for 10 minutes before removing the bread from the pan. Set the bread aside on the rack to cool completely.

To make the eggplant caviar,

while the bread is cooling, cut the eggplants in half lengthwise and place them cut side up on a sheet pan covered with parchment paper. Top each eggplant half with thyme, drizzle with 1 tablespoon (15 milliliters) of the olive oil, and sprinkle with 1/4 teaspoon (1 gram) of the sea salt. Bake until the tops are dark brown and

... (continued on next page)

2. 2 tablespoons (30 grams) extra virgin olive oil
3. 5 ounces (150 grams) baby arugula
4. 1 1/2 teaspoons (8.4 grams) balsamic dressing (storebought, or page 201)
5. 10 slices Ibérico de Bellota ham or prosciutto
6. 1 cup (100 grams) shaved Parmigiano-Reggiano
7. cheese
8. 20 petals tomato confit (page 212)
9. Flaky sea salt for garnish

completely soft, about 40 minutes. Using a spoon, scoop out all the softened flesh of the eggplants and discard the skins.

In a medium stew pot over medium heat, place the remaining 3 tablespoons (45 milliliters) olive oil, the shallots, garlic, and eggplant flesh. Cook, stirring occasionally and making sure it does not stick to the bottom of the pan, until all the water from the eggplants has cooked off and the mixture has dried, about 30 minutes. Transfer to a food processor fitted with the stainless-steel blade and process until pureed. Place the eggplant puree in a medium bowl, add the cheese and Espelette pepper, and mix thoroughly with a wooden spoon. Set aside.

Place the sherry vinegar in small saucepan over medium-high heat and let it reduce by one half and has become syrupy, about 10 minutes. Remove from the heat and set aside.

To make the sandwiches,

preheat the broiler and move the rack to the top position.

Slice the focaccia into 10 pieces. Place them on a sheet pan and drizzle with olive oil. Toast under the broiler until golden brown and crispy, about 3 minutes.

In a medium bowl, toss the arugula with the balsamic dressing.

Spread eggplant caviar on the toasted focaccia and top each with a slice of ham. Divide the arugula on top of the ham, followed by Parmigiano and 2 petals of tomato confit. Finish with a drizzle of the reduced sherry vinegar and a sprinkle of sea salt.

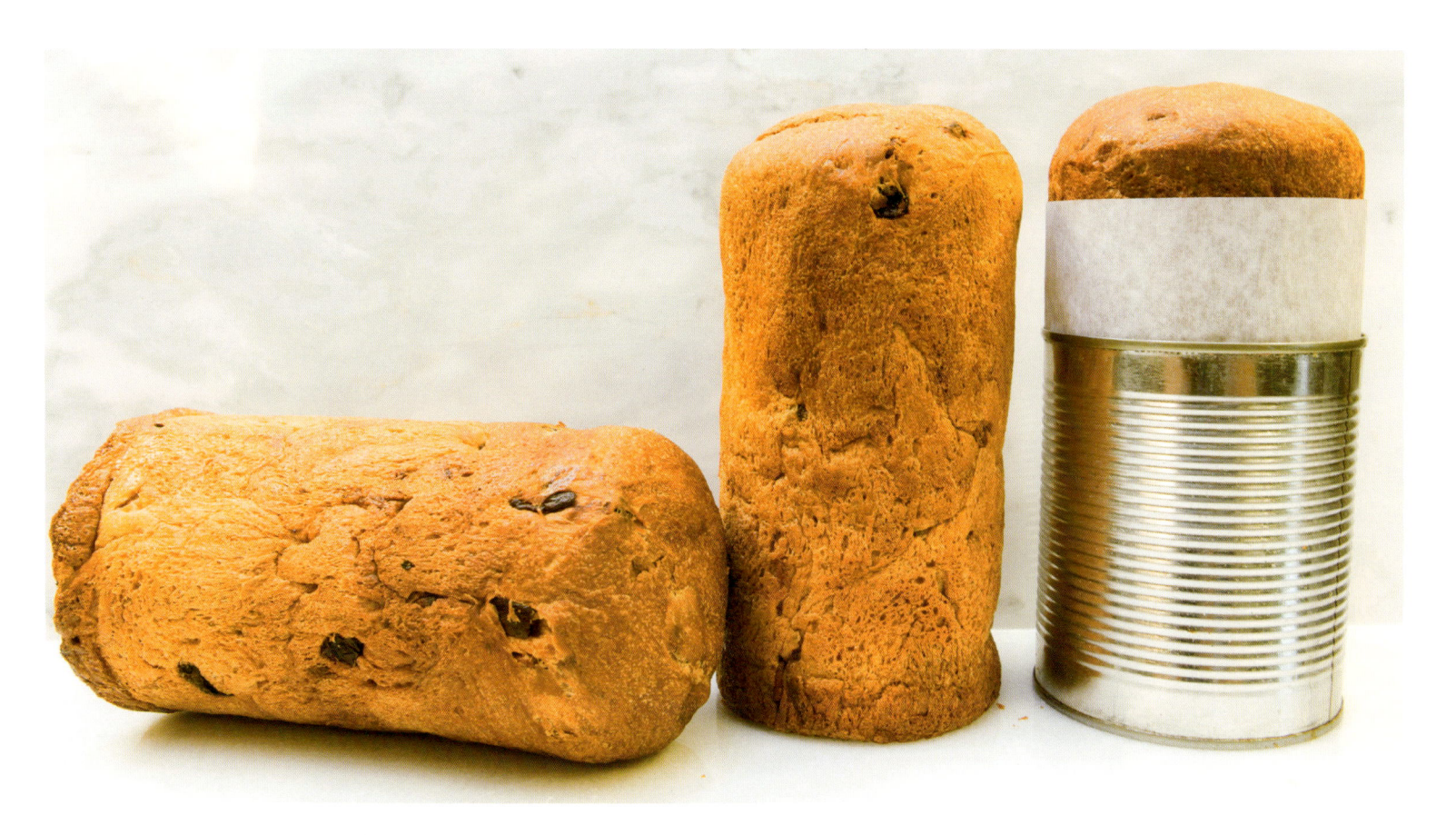

Pear And Pecan Brioche
(Step By Step)

Light and airy, dotted with bits of dried pears and pecans and sweetened with honey, this brioche hits all the right notes. After a slice spends a moment in the toaster, it becomes gilded with a golden crust, creating just the right amount of crunch. That makes this bread the perfect accompaniment to our Laphroaig whiskey–marinated foie gras torchon at Et Voila!. It's also a good starting point for novice bakers, because it's a straightforward recipe that's almost foolproof. I bake our loaves in 28-ounce (800 gram) cans with the top lids removed (make sure they don't have a plastic lining); I'm sure you have a few in your pantry at home. You'll need high-gluten flour. King Arthur makes the best; it's available online and in many fine grocery stores.

MAKES 2 LOAVES

INGREDIENTS

Makes 2 loaves

1. 3 tablespoons (50 grams) raisins
2. 1 tablespoon + 2 teaspoons (25 grams) dark rum
3. 4 cups (500 grams) high-gluten flour
4. 2 teaspoons (6 grams) kosher salt
5. 1/2 cup + 2 tablespoons (150 grams) whole milk
6. 5 tablespoons (100 grams) honey
7. 1 tablespoon + 2 teaspoons (15 grams) instant yeast
8. 4 large eggs (200 grams)
9. 1/2 pound (2 sticks/250 grams) unsalted butter, cubed, at room temperature
10.
11. 3/4 cup (100 grams) diced dried

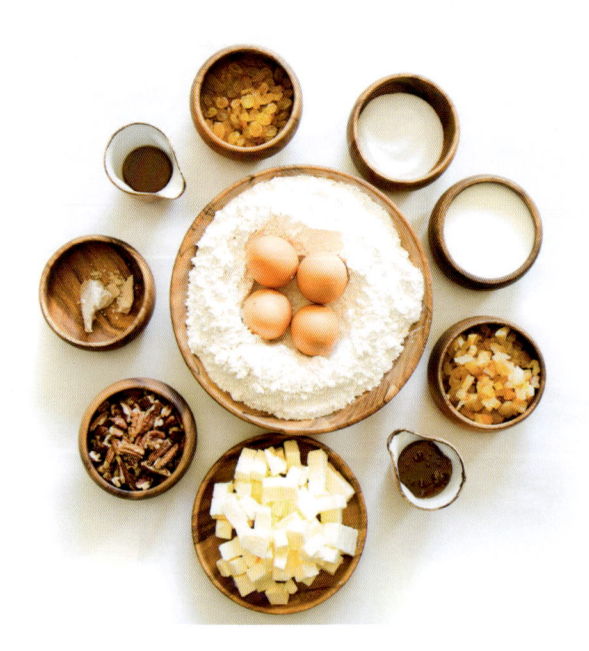

DIRECTIONS

In a small bowl, mix together the raisins and rum. Set aside for 1 hour or until the raisins have absorbed the rum.

In the bowl of a stand mixer fitted with the dough hook attachment, blend the flour and salt on medium speed until fully combined, approximately 1 minute. Set aside.

In a small saucepan over low heat, warm the milk and honey and whisk gently until the honey is completely dissolved. Remove from the heat, add the yeast, and whisk until it is completely dissolved. Add the milk mixture to the flour mixture and mix on medium speed until fully incorporated. Add the eggs and mix on medium speed until they are fully incorporated.

Reduce the speed to low and add the butter, mixing until fully incorporated. Increase the speed to medium and mix until the dough forms a ball, begins to come off the side of the bowl, and feels elastic.

With a small strainer, drain the raisins. Add the raisins and pecans to the dough and mix on low speed until they are fully incorporated, about 5 minutes. Remove the bowl from the mixer and the dough hook from the dough. Cover the bowl with a damp kitchen towel and place it in a warm place until the dough has doubled in size, about 1 hour.

While the dough is rising, spray nonstick cooking spray on the inside of two clean 28-ounce (800 gram) cans with the tops taken off. Cut a round pieces of parchment paper to cover the bottoms. Cut another piece of parchment paper that when rolled up is twice the length of the can; insert it into the can.

Divide the dough into two equally sized balls and put one in each can. Place the cans in a warm place until the dough has once again doubled in size, about 1 hour.

Preheat the oven to 300°F (150°C). Place the cans on the middle rack of the oven and bake for 70 minutes, until the loaves are a brownish gold and a long skewer inserted into their centers comes out clean. Remove the cans from the oven, ease the loaves out of the cans and let them cool on a cooling rack. To enjoy peak texture and flavor, use this bread within 24 hours.

PAGE 35

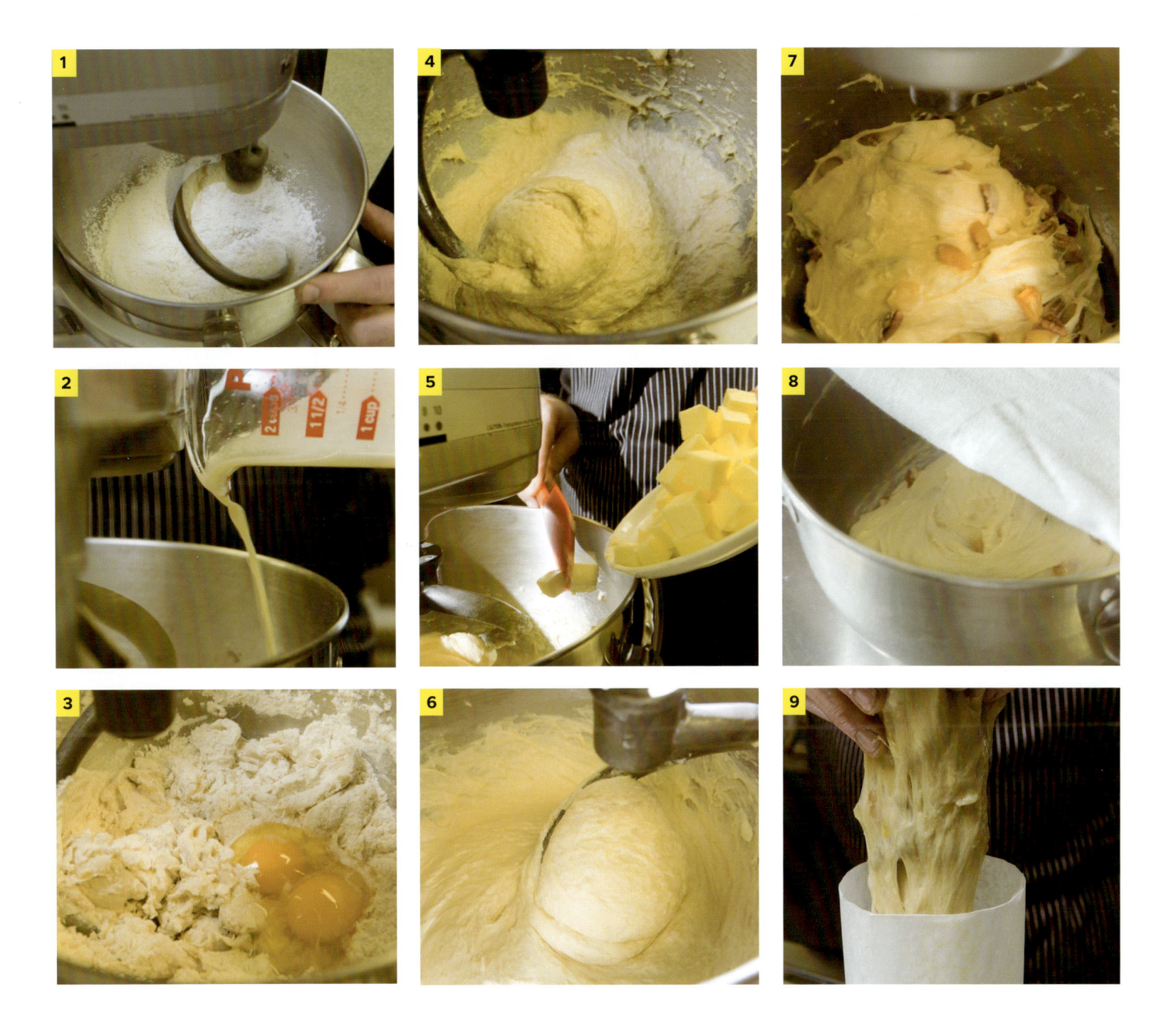

PAGE 36

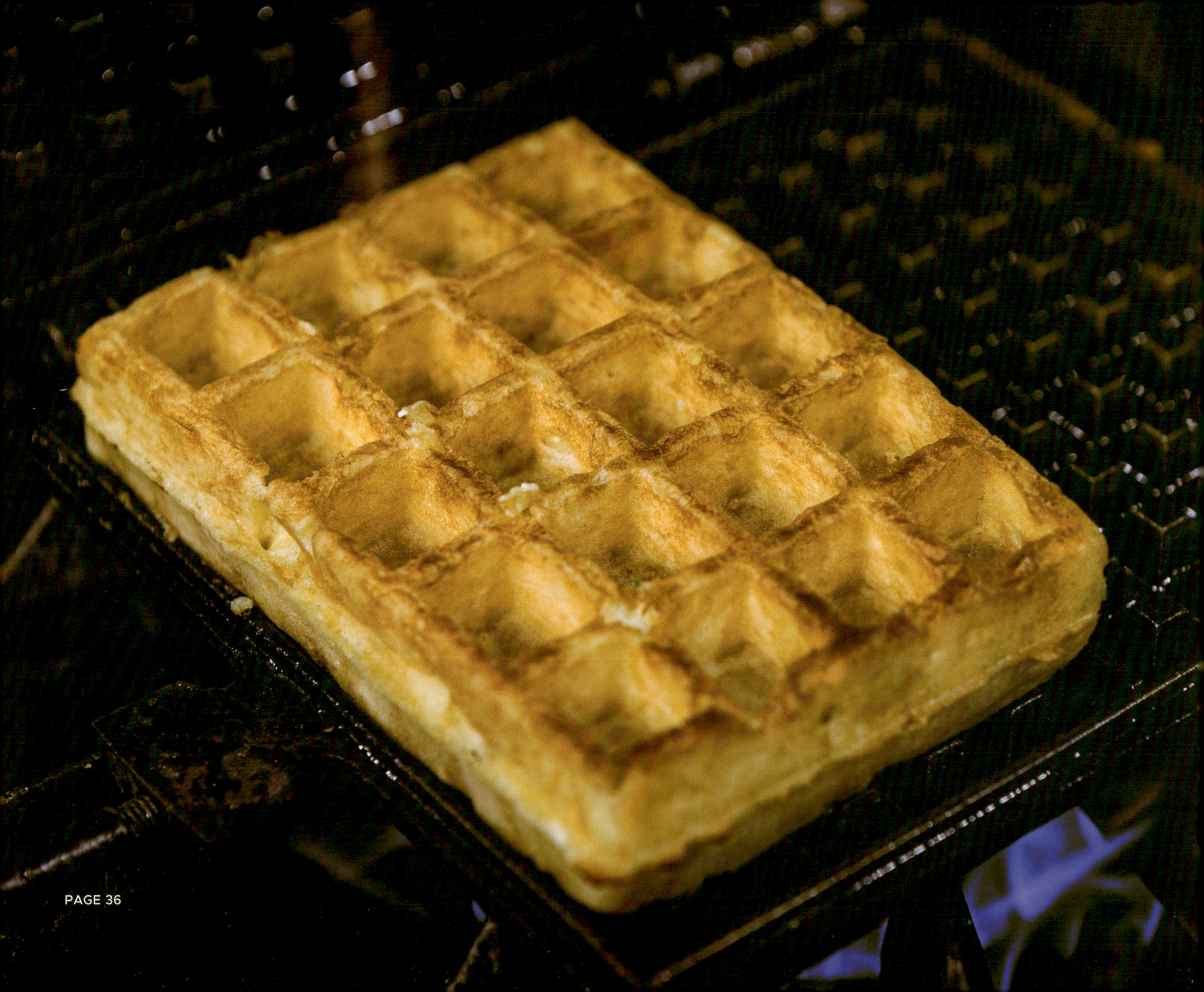

WAFFLES

We take our waffles seriously in Belgium. There are two distinct types, and we love bickering over which is superior. Made with yeasted dough, the Brussels waffle is fluffy and airy on the inside, with a crispy exterior. These golden, honeycombed rounds are traditionally topped with some combination of confectioners' sugar, whipped cream, fruits, chocolate sauce, and/or Nutella. On the other hand, classic Liège waffles are forged from butter-rich brioche-like dough and dotted with clusters of Belgian pearl sugar, which caramelize when the waffle is cooked in a sizzling hot iron. This adds a rich sweetness and an unforgettable crunch. Depending on my mood, I'm happy with either one— especially if I'm enjoying it back home

SERVES
4

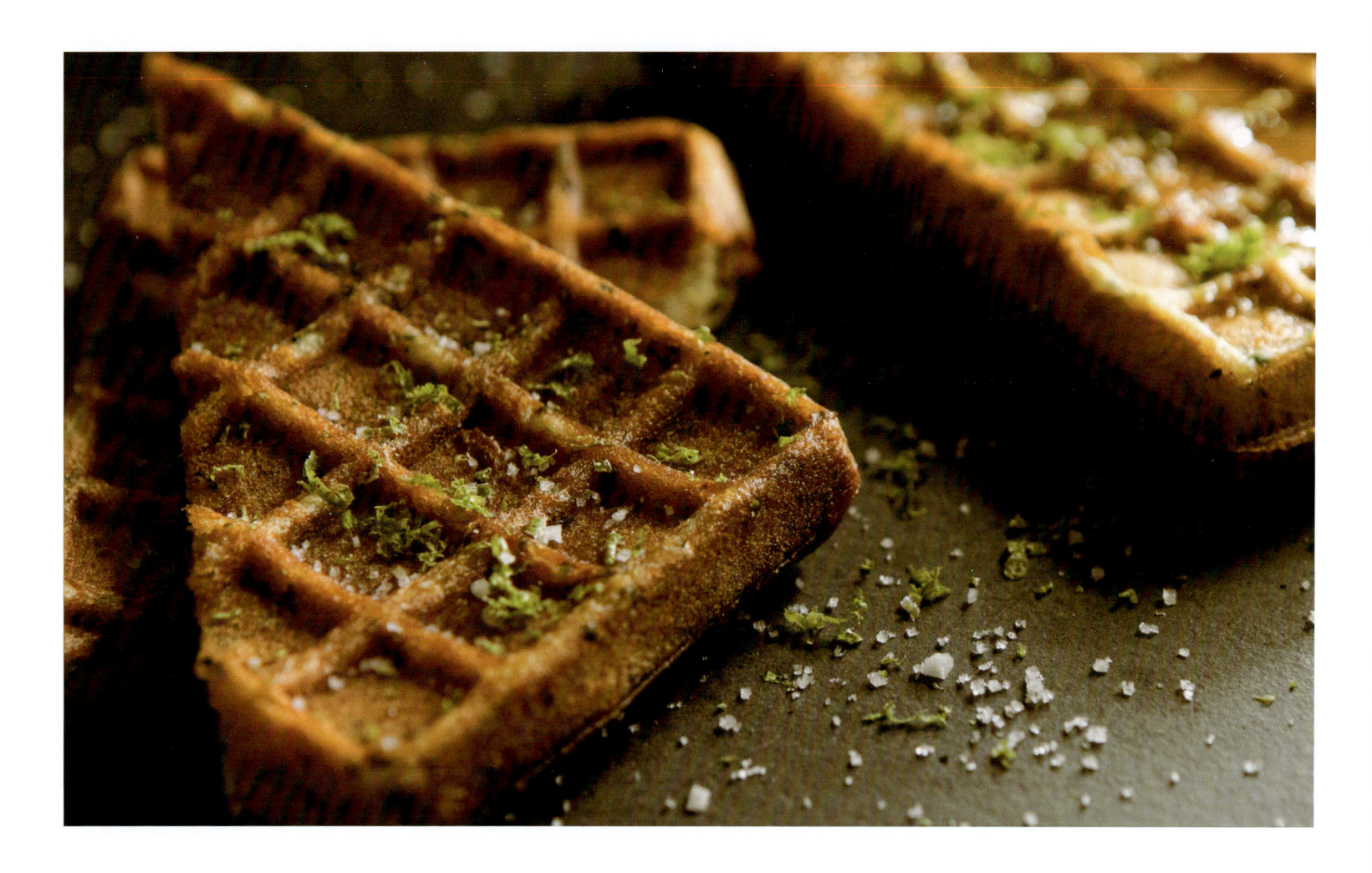

Cod Waffles

Obviously, we're known for our waffles in Belgium. I was looking to transform the sweet breakfast version into a more savory, brunch-ier option, so I decided to stuff them with cod. When I want to take them to the next level, I top them with whipped crème fraîche laced with horseradish and sprinkle on salmon roe. They were always a big hit when I served them at events at the Belgian Embassy, and I know they'll be a smashing success at your next brunch.

INGREDIENTS

1. 1 1/2 teaspoons (3.6 grams) flaky sea salt
2. 1 pound (450 grams) fresh cod fillets
3. 1/2 cup (125 milliliters) heavy cream
4. 1 cup (250 milliliters) fish stock (store-bought, or page
5. 206), divided
6. 5 garlic cloves, finely diced
7. 1 dried bay leaf
8. 1 sprig fresh thyme
9. Pinch of Espelette pepper
10. 6 large egg whites (180 grams)
11. 1 1/4 cups + 2 tablespoons (200 grams) all-purpose
12. flour
13. 1 1/4 teaspoons (5 grams) baking powder
14. 2 large egg yolks (40 grams)
15. 1/2 cup (125 grams) whole milk
16. 4 tablespoons (1/2 stick/60 grams) unsalted butter, melted
17. 1/4 cup (50 grams) extra virgin olive oil
18. Grated zest of 2 lemons

DIRECTIONS

Sprinkle the salt on the cod fillets and place them in a large saucepan. Add the cream, fish stock, garlic, bay leaf, thyme, and Espelette pepper. Cook over medium heat until the fish has cooked through, about 15 minutes. Take out the fish and set aside. Strain out the herbs and garlic and set the liquid aside.

Using an immersion blender, whip the egg whites until firm peaks appear. Set aside.

In the bowl of a stand mixer fitted with the paddle attachment, mix together the cod, the reserved cooking liquid, flour, baking powder, egg yolks, and milk on low speed until well combined, 3 to 5 minutes.

Preheat a waffle iron and coat both plates with nonstick spray.

Remove the bowl from the stand mixer and use a spatula to mix in the melted butter, olive oil, and lemon zest. Gently fold in the egg whites.

Scoop about 3/4 cup (180 milliliters) of the batter onto the center of the waffle iron and close. Cook until golden brown on both sides, about 6 minutes. Keep the waffles warm in the oven at 300°F (150°C) until you are ready to serve them

8

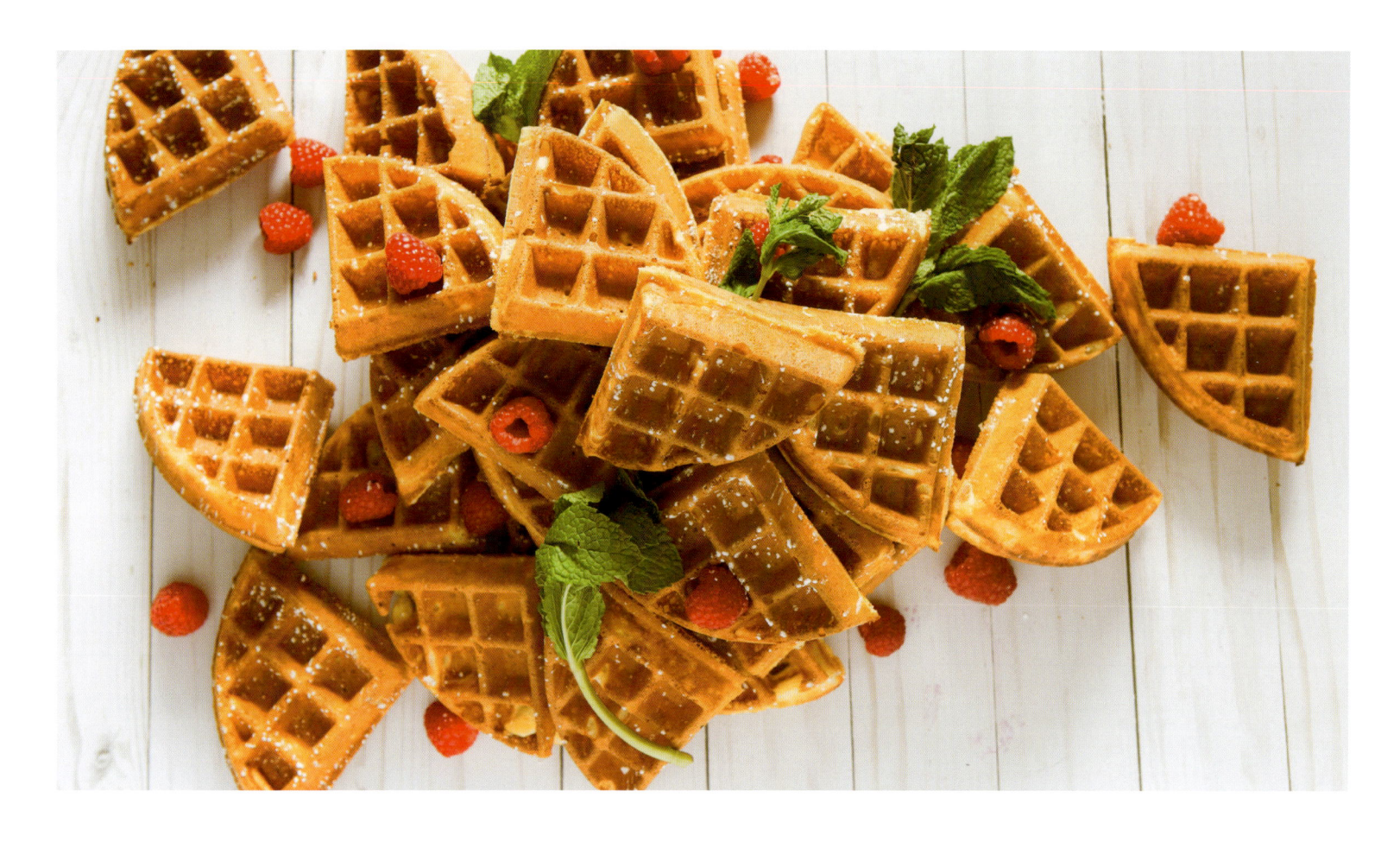

PREPARATION
30 MIN

SERVES
10

Classic Brussels Waffles

The simplest foods can be the most difficult to execute well. That's the case with these iconic waffles made with only milk, yeast, flour, granulated sugar, and eggs, so make sure you use only the finest ingredients. Make the whole batch at once, keeping them warm in the oven at 300°F (150°C) until you're ready to serve them all. You can eat them plain or dress them up. Just make sure to enjoy them quickly, so they don't deflate. A waffle iron is required. A reliable brand is Cuisinart—no need to get anything fancier than their classic model, which is widely available online and in good cookware stores. Top the waffles with chocolate sauce, maple syrup, fresh fruit, whipped cream, or whatever your heart desires.

INGREDIENTS

1. 1 quart (1 liter) whole milk
2. 1/4 cup + 1 teaspoon (40 grams) fresh yeast or 5 teaspoons (14 grams) active dry yeast
3. 14 tablespoons (1 3/4 sticks/210 grams) unsalted butter
4. 7 large eggs, separated (140 grams yolks, 210 grams whites)
5. 5 cups (650 grams) pastry flour
6. Confectioners' sugar for sprinkling

DIRECTIONS

In a large saucepan over low heat, warm the milk to about 90°F (30°C), being careful to not bring it to a boil. Turn off the heat, add the yeast and stir with a wooden spoon until it is dissolved completely. Set aside.

In a small saucepan, melt the butter; set it aside.

In the bowl of a stand mixer fitted with the whisk attachment, whip the egg whites on high speed until firm peaks form. Set aside

In a large mixing bowl, using a whisk, mix the flour and egg yolks until thoroughly combined. Add the melted butter and mix until thoroughly combined. Add the milk mixture and mix until thoroughly combined. Using a spatula, gently fold in the whipped white eggs. Let the waffle batter sit at room temperature for 25 minutes, until it has risen slightly and is a little bubbly.

Preheat the oven to 250°F (120°C). Preheat a waffle iron and coat both plates with nonstick spray. When the waffle iron is hot, ladle 1 cup (240 milliliters) of the batter on the center, close the waffle iron, and cook until the waffle is gold and crispy, about 3 to 4 minutes. As they are finished, place the waffles on a cooling rack over a sheet pan and keep them warm in the oven.

Sprinkle the finished waffles with confectioners' sugar.

Potato Waffles

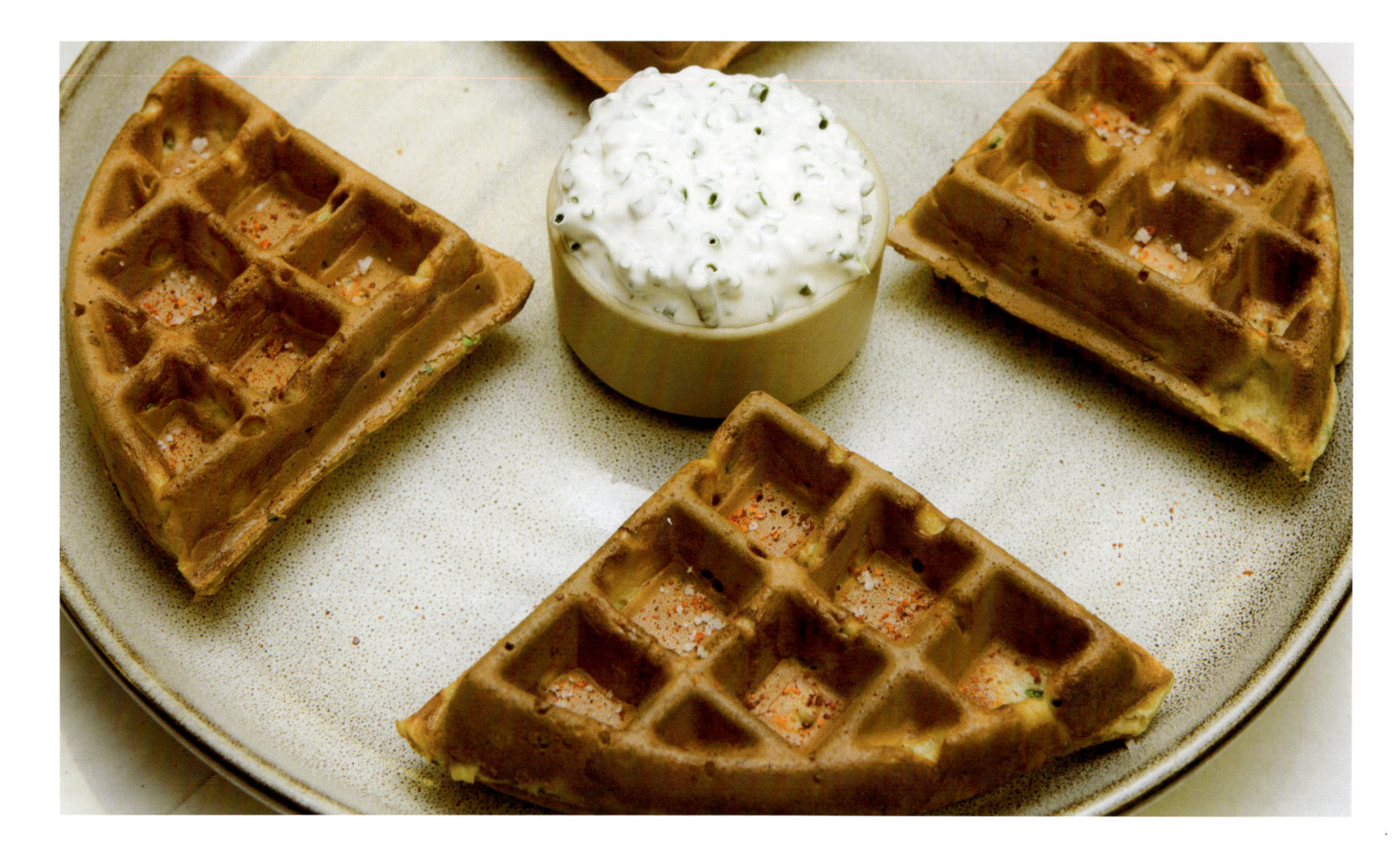

(Step By Step)

Made with russet potatoes, these feathery waffles with crispy edges are pepped with garlic, chive, and horseradish. Consider them the Belgian answer to the French crêpe vonnassienne. They're a great complement to seafood, so I often top them off with ribbons of gravlax or a lump crab salad. Or you can serve them instead of hash browns as a side dish to fill out a classic breakfast plate with eggs and your choice of meat.

9

SERVES
8

INGREDIENTS

1. 1 tablespoon + 1 teaspoon (18 grams) kosher salt,
2. divided
3. 2 large russet potatoes (about 6.5 ounces/200 grams
4. each), peeled
5. 3/4 cup (100 grams) all-purpose flour
6. 1/2 cup + 2 tablespoons (150 grams) heavy cream
7. 1 large egg (50 grams)
8. 2 large egg yolks (40 grams)
9. 1 small clove garlic, finely diced
10. 2 tablespoons + 2 teaspoons (40 grams) shredded
11. fresh horseradish
12. Scant 1/2 teaspoon (2.5 grams) baking soda
13. 2 tablespoons (20 grams) chopped shallots
14. 2 tablespoons (20 grams) chopped fresh chives

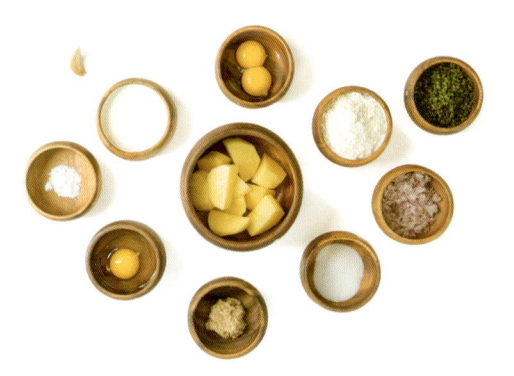

DIRECTIONS

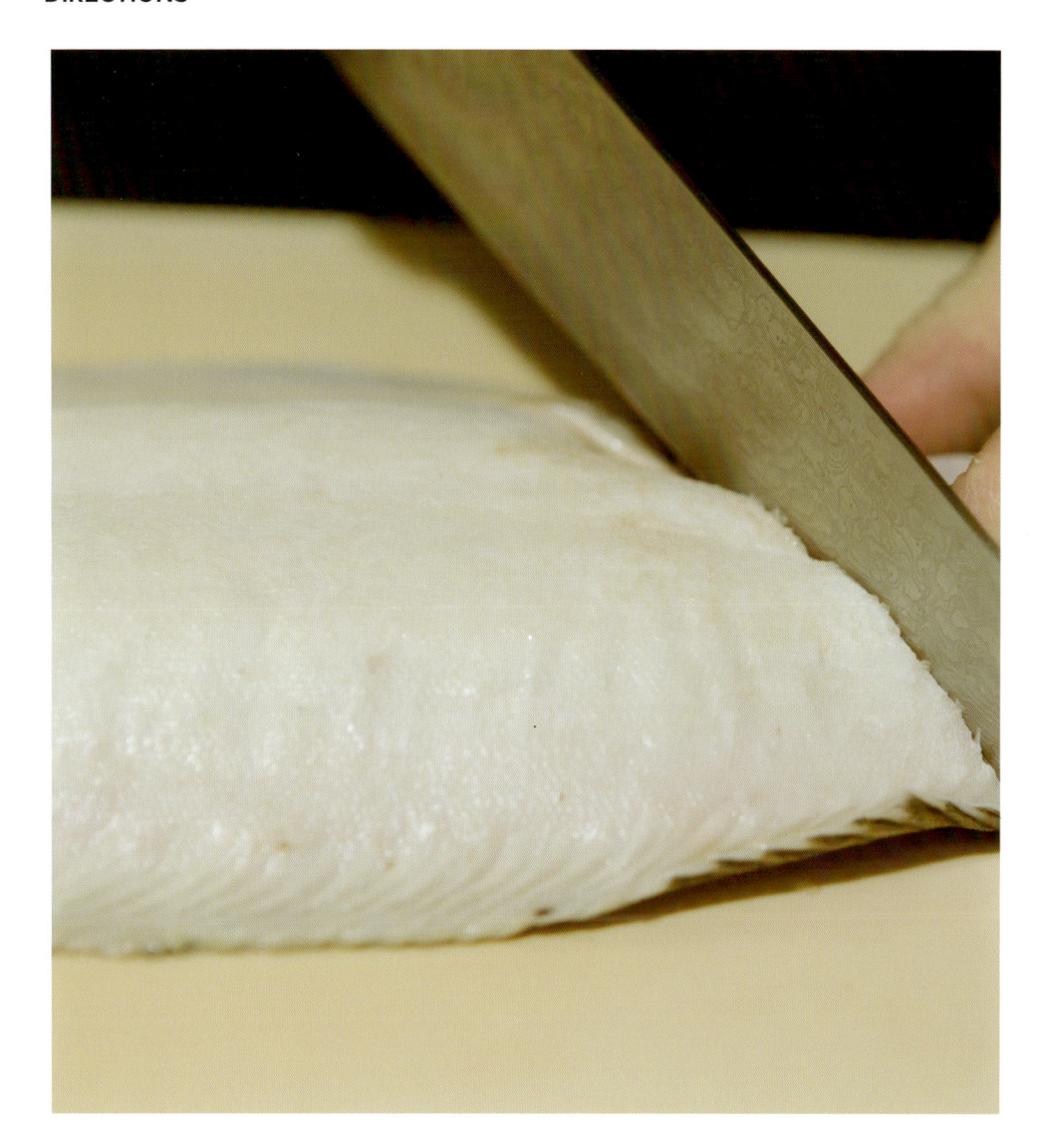

1. Fill a large pot halfway with water, add 1 1/2 teaspoons (4 grams) of the salt, and bring to a boil over high heat. Add the potatoes and cook until a knife passes through them without resistance, about 1 hour. Drain them in a strainer in the sink and let them cool for about 10 minutes

PAGE 43

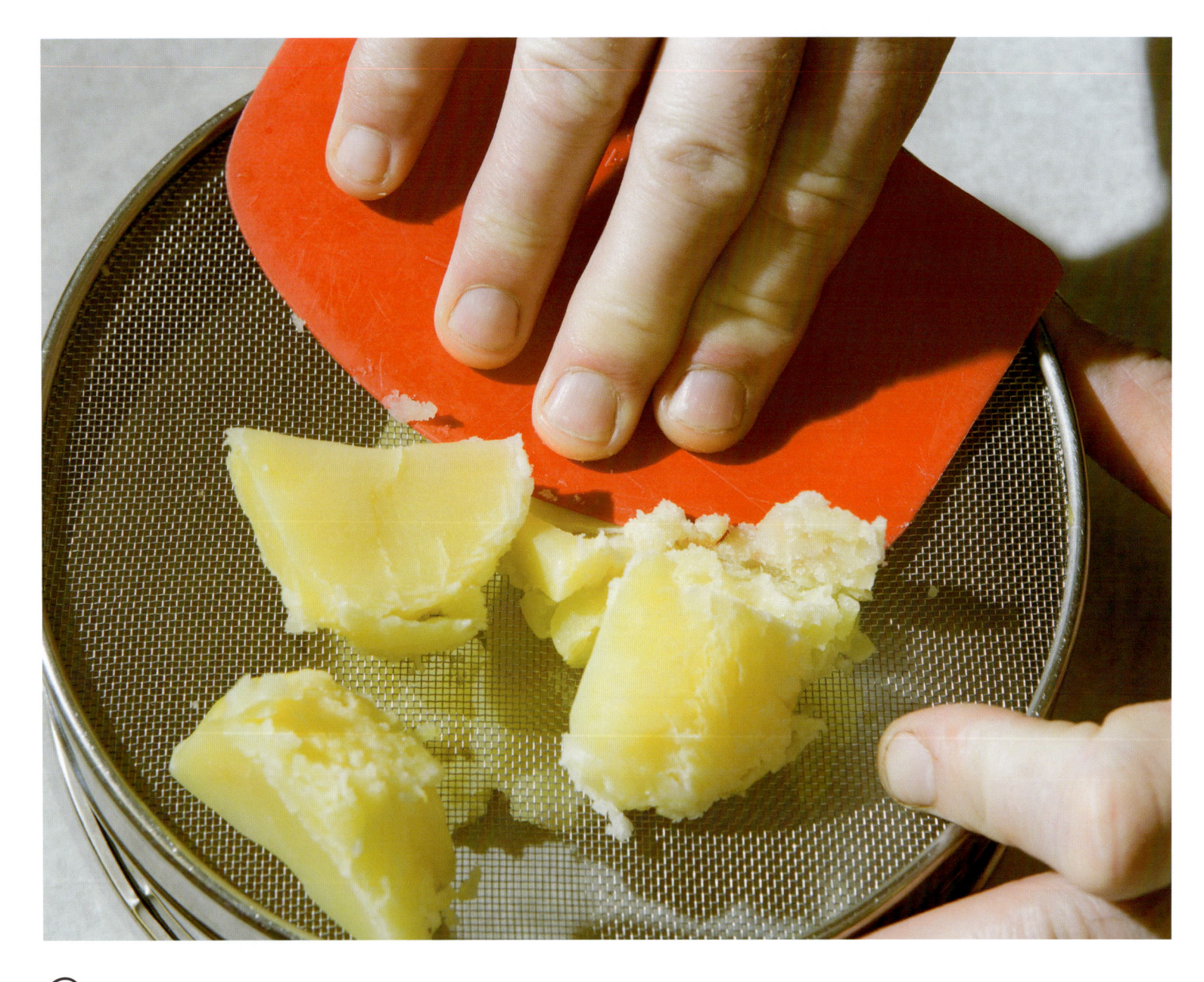

2. Mash the potatoes in the bowl of a stand mixer, or pass them through a sieve into the bowl.

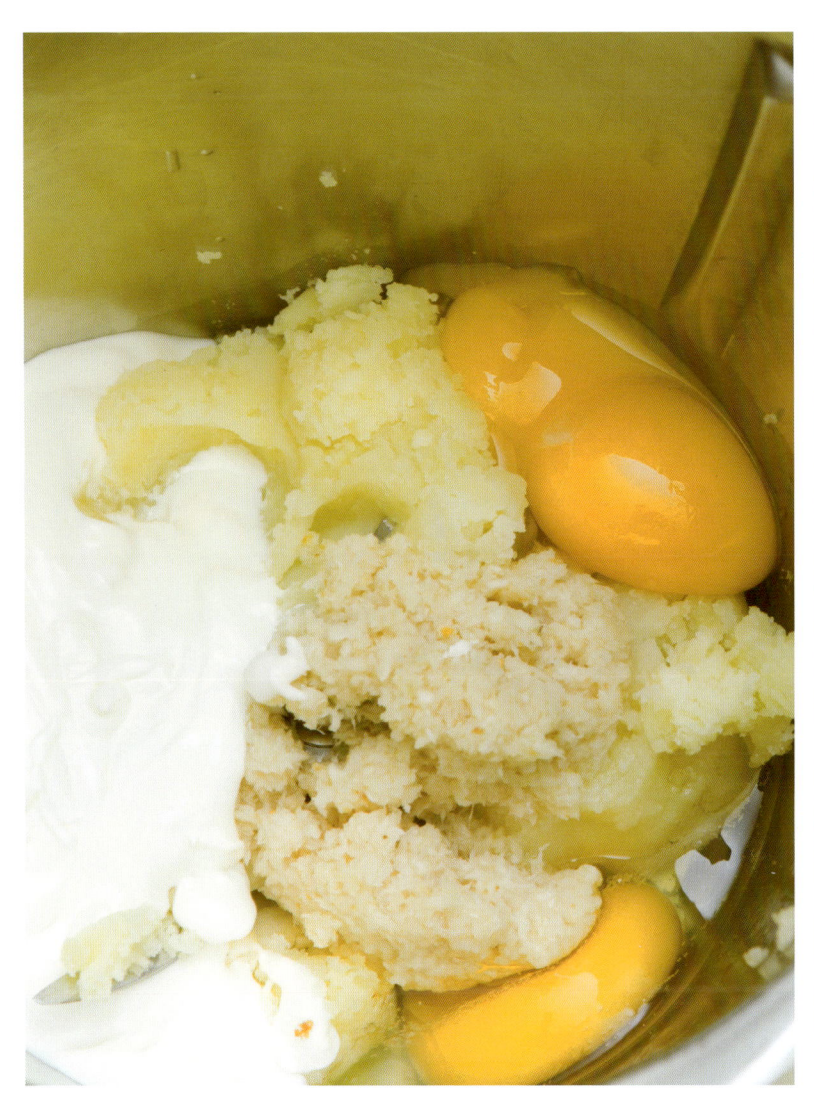

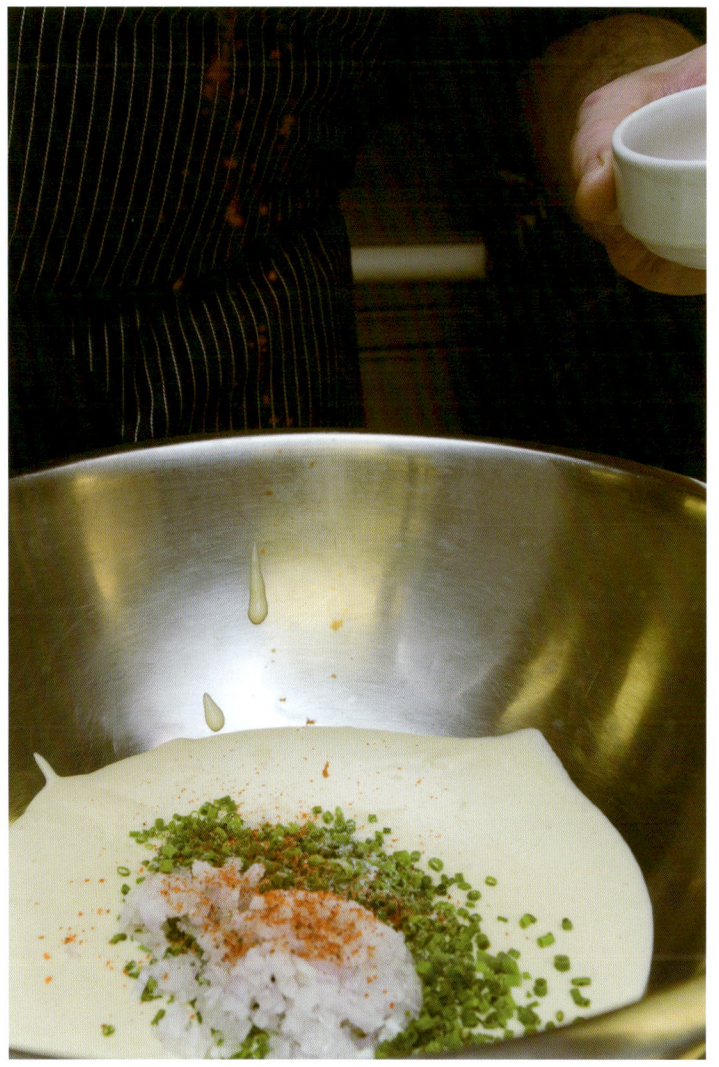

3. Fit the paddle attachment onto the mixer, and on medium speed mix the potatoes with the flour, cream, egg, egg yolks, garlic, horseradish, baking soda, shallots, and chives until fully combined, 3 to 4 minutes

4. Preheat the oven to 300°F (150°C). Preheat the waffle iron and coat both plates with nonstick spray. Scoop 1 cup (240 milliliters) of the batter onto the waffle iron and cook until both sides are golden brown, about 3 to 4 minutes. As they are finished, place the waffles on a cooling rack over a sheet pan and keep them warm in the oven.

PAGE 46

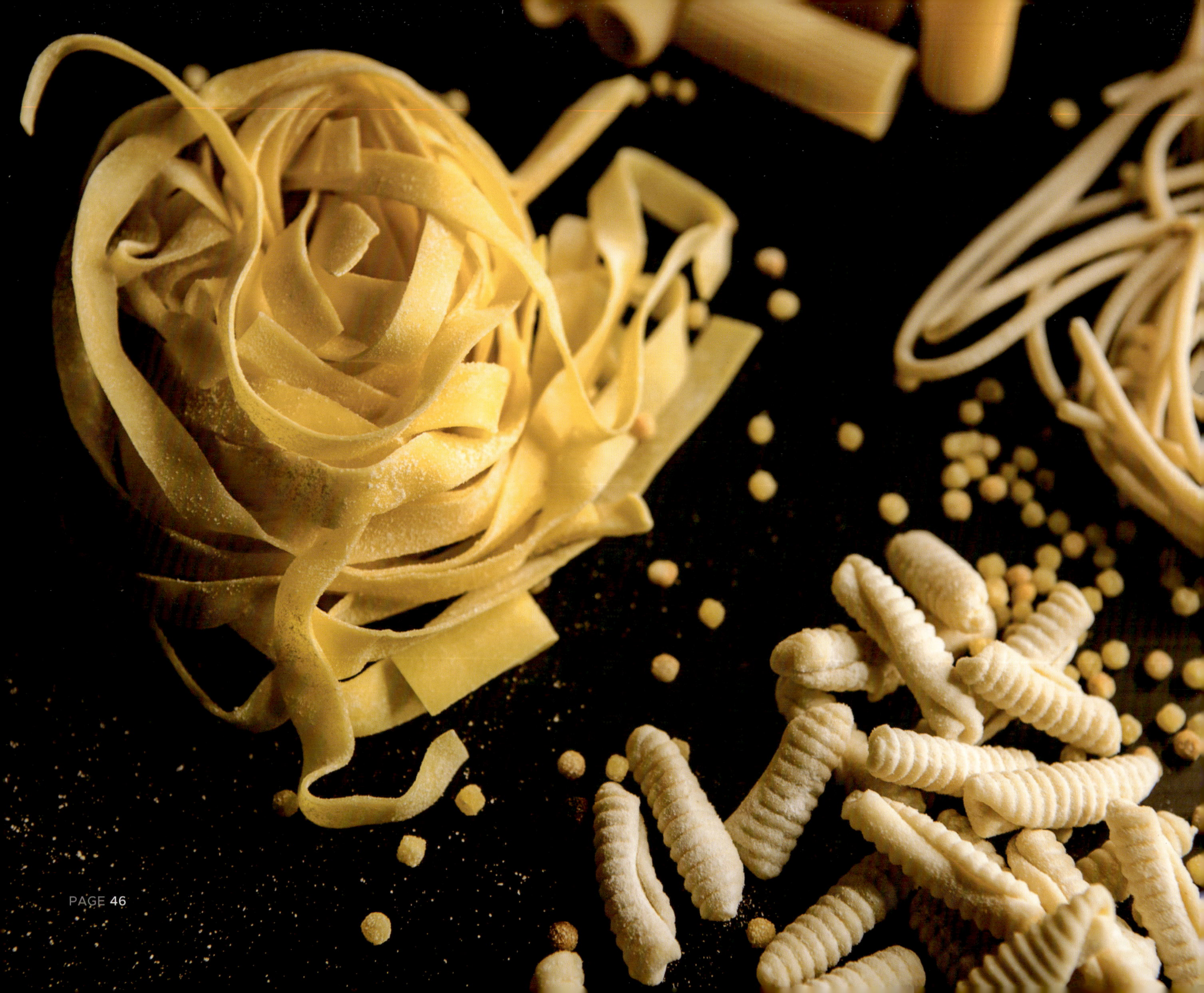

PASTA

Seeking to pass along one of her most beloved traditions, my mother taught me how to make pasta when I first began working in the kitchen of my father's traiteur. It was a precise, painstaking process. I remember cracking dozens of eggs at a time, carefully weighing the semolina flour, and working the dough with my hands. I learned to get a feel for a good dough with just the right amount of moisture and perfect pliability. I still love making it as a way of honoring my roots. It's a way to take myself back to my earliest forays into cooking, when it was just my mother and me working side by side at the counter

SERVES 8

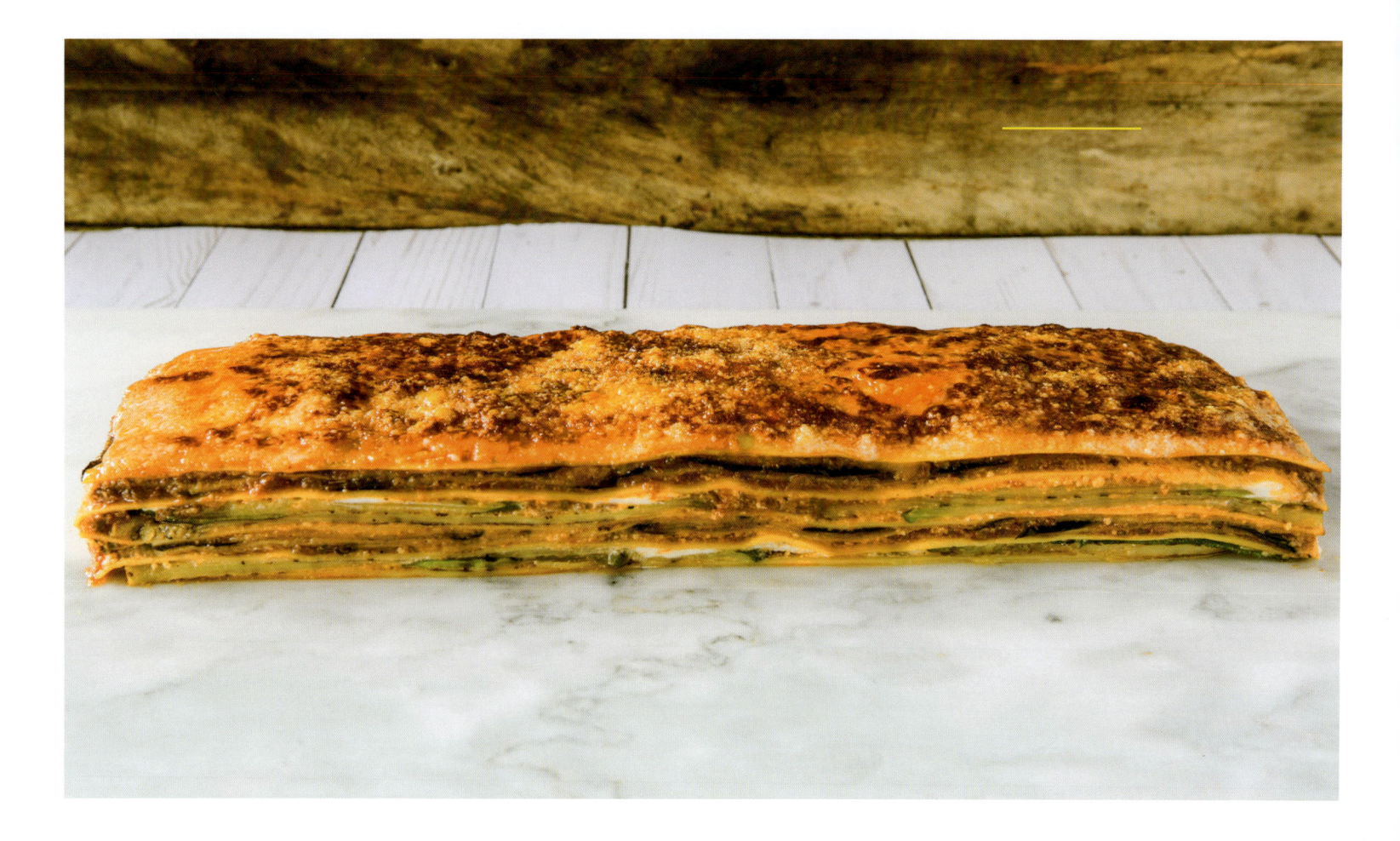

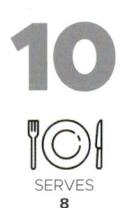

Vegetable Lasagna

Perfect for vegetarians but hearty enough to satisfy a hungry carnivore, this lasagna has been a favorite at Et Voila! for years. It's layered with crispy fried eggplant, seared zucchini strips, fresh basil, creamy goat cheese, Grana Padano for a hit of salty umami, and a slow-cooked tomato sauce rich with onions. The finishing touch is a drizzle of marjoram-infused olive oil. If you can't find one online or at a specialty food store, you can make it by warming 2 cups (400 grams) high-quality extra virgin olive oil to 175°F (80°C) and adding a bunch of whole fresh marjoram sprigs. Remove from the heat and infuse the oil for 1 hour before straining out the herbs. It will last for 3 months stored at room temperature in a tightly closed container.

INGREDIENTS

1. Tomato sauce
2. 1/4 cup (50 grams) extra virgin olive oil
3. 1 large yellow onion, diced
4. 8 garlic cloves, chopped
5. Two 28-ounce (800 grams) cans whole peeled San
6. Marzano tomatoes
7. 2 1/2 teaspoons (12 grams) kosher salt
8. 1 teaspoon (12 grams) granulated sugar
9. 1 tablespoon (10 grams) chopped fresh oregano
10. 2 dried bay leaves
11. 1 sprig fresh thyme
12. Tomato concassé
13. 5 pounds (2.25 kilograms) Roma tomatoes
14. 1/4 cup (50 grams) extra virgin olive oil
15. 1/2 cup + 2 tablespoons (100 grams) chopped shallots
16. 1/4 cup + 1 tablespoon (50 grams) chopped garlic
17. 1 dried bay leaf
18. 1 sprig fresh thyme
19. 1 teaspoon (5 grams) kosher salt
20. 1 1/4 teaspoons (5 grams) granulated sugar
21. 2 teaspoons (5 grams) Espelette pepper

DIRECTIONS

To make the tomato sauce, in a large saucepan heat the olive oil over medium heat until shimmering. Add the onions and garlic. Cook, stirring occasionally, until softened but not browned, 5 to 10 minutes. Add the tomatoes and their juices, the salt, sugar, oregano, bay leaves, and thyme. Simmer while stirring occasionally until the sauce has reduced slightly and thickened, about 1 1/2 hours. Remove from heat and take out the bay leaves and thyme sprigs. Let cool completely and then blend in a blender until smooth (work in batches if necessary). Set aside 2 1/2 cup (450 grams) of the tomato sauce. Store the remainder in an airtight container for other uses; it will last for a week in the refrigerator and six months or more in the freezer.

To make the tomato concassé, fill a large bowl with ice and cold water. Cut out the core of the tomatoes and slice an X into the skin at the other end of the tomatoes. Fill a large pot with water and bring to a boil over high heat. Boil the tomatoes for 10 seconds; using a mesh skimmer, immediately place them into the ice water. Once cooled, place them in a strainer and peel them. Vegetable Lasagna 55 Cut the tomatoes lengthwise and then remove the seeds and centers. Dice the tomatoes and set aside. In a large saucepan, heat the olive oil over medium heat until shimmering. Add the shallots and garlic. Cook, stirring occasionally, until softened but not browned, 5 to 10 minutes. Turn down the heat to low and add the tomatoes, bay leaf, thyme, salt, sugar, and Espelette pepper. Cook until all the moisture has evaporated, stirring occasionally, about 2 hours. Place the concassé in a strainer set in the sink; remove the bay leaf.

To assemble, cut the eggplant lengthwise into slices approximately 1/4 inch (6 mm) thick. Cover two sheet pans with paper towels and place the eggplant slices on them. Sprinkle each slice with 1/4 teaspoon (1 gram) salt, then cover the eggplant with more paper towels. (The towels are to soak up the moisture the eggplant will release.). Set aside until water beads on top of the eggplant, 30 to 45 minutes. Dab off the water with the paper towels.

Place the flour on a plate and dredge the eggplant in the flour on both sides. Tap off any excess flour. Set aside on a plate. Cover a sheet pan or large plate with paper towels. Place the vegetable oil in a large frying pan and warm over medium-high heat. When the oil reaches 300°F (150°C), fry the eggplant slices..

... *(continued on next page)*

TO ASSEMBLE

1. 4 large Italian eggplants
2. Kosher salt
3. 2 1/2 cups (300 grams) all-purpose flour
4. 2 cups + 2 tablespoons (425 grams) vegetable oil
5. 5 large green zucchinis
6. 2 tablespoons (27 grams) extra virgin olive oil
7. 1/2 pound (220 grams) fresh goat cheese, crumbled
8. 2 1/2 cups (450 grams) tomato concassé (above)
9. 1 pound (450 grams) lasagna noodles (store-bought, or
10. page 216, about 1/2 batch)
11. 3 cups (300 grams) grated Grana Padano cheese
12. 10 fresh leaves basil
13. Marjoram-infused olive oil for drizzling (see headnote)

... in batches, making sure not to overcrowd the pan, until golden brown on both sides, about 4 minutes. Place the fried eggplant slices on the sheet pan or plate to remove the excess oil. Set aside.

Cut the zucchini lengthwise into slices approximately 1/4 inch (6 mm) thick. Lightly season with salt. In large cast-iron skillet over high heat, heat the olive oil until it starts to smoke slightly. Working in batches and making sure not to overcrowd the pan, sear both sides of the zucchini slices until light brown, about 2 minutes a side. Set aside.

To prepare the lasagna noodles, fill a large pot with water and season with 1 teaspoon (3 grams) salt. Bring to a boil over high heat. Meanwhile, fill a large bowl with cold water. Place the noodles in the boiling water and cook until al dente, about 7 minutes (or according to manufacturer's instructions if using store-bought noodles). Using a mesh skimmer, remove the noodles and place them into the cold water until chilled, about 10 minutes. Remove the noodles from the water and lay them out on a kitchen towel to dry, about 5 minutes

Preheat the oven to 350°F (175°C).

In a 13 by 9-inch (33 by 23 cm) metal baking pan, put 1/2 cup (120 milliliters) of the tomato sauce and spread it to cover the entire bottom of the pan. Next, layer lasagna noodles in the pan (cut any edges so it fits perfectly), then evenly spread with 2 tablespoons (30 milliliters) of the tomato concassé. Next, lay the eggplant slices side by side to form an even layer. Sprinkle with about one-seventh of the Grana Padano and about one-sixth of the goat cheese. Cover with a layer of the lasagna sheets, then add of tomato sauce, tomato concassé, Grana Padano and goat cheese. Top with a layer of the grilled zucchini. Repeat the layering process, alternating levels with eggplant and zucchini (there should be three levels of each). After the last layer of zucchini, top with lasagna noodles, then cover 56 with any remaining tomato sauce, the fresh basil leaves, and Grana Padano. Store any remaining tomato concassé in an airtight container for other uses; it will last for a week in the refrigerator and six months or more in the freezer.

Bake until bubbling at the edges and the cheese on top is light golden brown, about 25 minutes. Turn on the broiler, move a rack as close as possible, and broil the lasagna until the cheese on top is golden brown and crispy, 4 to 5 minutes. Remove from the broiler and let rest 15 minutes before serving. Before serving, drizzle with marjoram-infused oil.

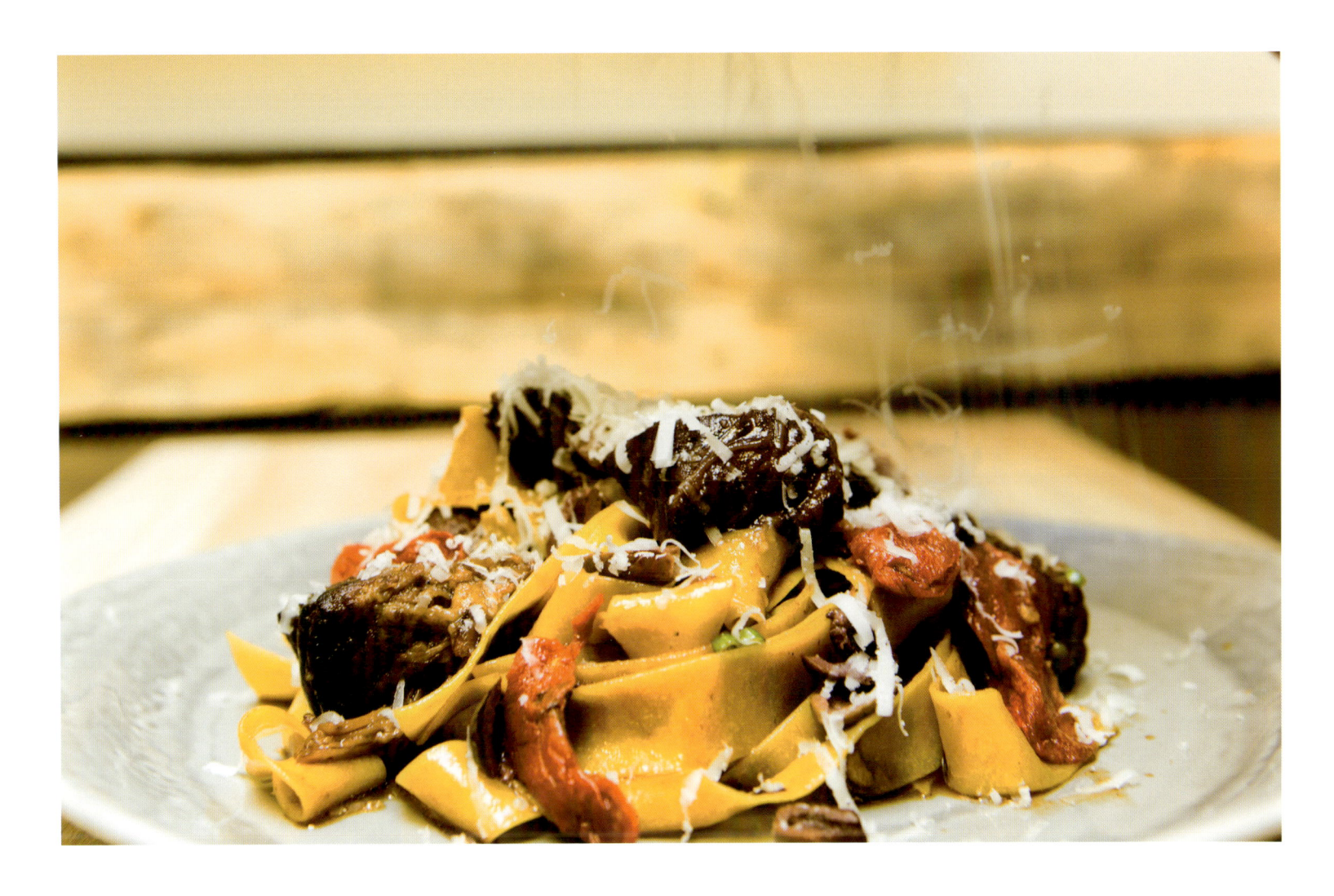

Pappardelle with Pork Shoulder and Olives

The idea for this dish came from a pulled pork sandwich. I love the interplay between the smoky, savory, and salty tones, which are offset by a little sweetness. Hearty and heartwarming, this pasta is perfect for a Sunday dinner during the winter months.

SERVES 10

INGREDIENTS

1. 3 1/2 pounds (1.5 kilograms) boneless pork shoulder Kosher salt
2. 1 cup (200 grams) extra virgin olive oil, divided, plus
3. more for garnishing
4. 20 slices (about 1 pound/450 grams) applewoodsmoked bacon, cut into 2-inch (5 cm) pieces
5. 1 stalk lemongrass, cut in half lengthwise and crushed
6. with the back of a knife
7. 2 large carrots, diced large
8. 2 stalks celery, diced large
9. 1 1/3 ounces (40 grams) peeled and finely diced fresh ginger
10. 2 medium yellow onions
11. 4 cloves garlic, peeled and smashed
12. 4 sprigs fresh thyme
13. 4 dried bay leaves
14. 1 quart (1 liter) dry red wine
15. One 28-ounce (850 grams) can whole peeled San Marzano tomatoes
16. 2 quarts (2 liters) chicken stock (store-bought, or page 208)
17. 2 quarts (2 liters) veal stock (store-bought, or page 207)
18. 2 1/2 teaspoons (6 grams) cayenne pepper
19. Leaves from 1 bunch fresh marjoram, roughly chopped
20. 1/2 cup (100 grams) Taggiasca or kalamata olives, pitted
21. 2 1/4 pounds (1 kilogram) fresh pappardelle (storebought, or page 216, 1 batch)
22. 40 petals tomato confit (page 212)
23. 2 cups (200 grams) freshly grated Pecorino Romano cheese

Cut the pork shoulder into three large pieces and season all sides with salt. In a large sauté pan over high heat, warm 1/2 cup (100 grams) of the olive oil until shimmering hot. Sear the meat on all sides until dark brown all over. Set aside.

Preheat the oven to 350°F (175°C).

In a very large stew pot over medium-high heat, place the remaining 1/2 cup (100 grams) olive oil, the bacon, lemongrass, carrots, celery, ginger, onions, and garlic. Cook until everything is softened and lightly browned, 8 to 10 minutes. Add the thyme, bay leaves, and red wine and cook until the liquid is reduced by half, about 10 minutes. Add the seared pork, tomatoes, chicken stock, veal stock, and cayenne pepper and bring to a boil. Remove from heat and cover the pot with aluminum foil. Place in the oven to cook until the meat is so well cooked it breaks apart when you press a finger into it, about 2 hours.

Remove the pork from the sauce and set aside. Pass the remaining vegetables and bacon through a fine mesh strainer so the liquid goes back into the pot. Place the pot over medium-high heat and bring to a boil. Skim the fat from the surface of the liquid and then turn down the heat to low. Pull the pork apart into shreds and return to the sauce. Add marjoram and olives and mix until fully combined. Keep warm over low heat.

Bring a large pot filled with salted water to boil over medium-high heat. Cook pappardelle until al dente, about 7 minutes (or according to manufacturer's instructions if using store-bought noodles). Drain the pasta in a strainer set in the sink, then toss with 1 tablespoon (15 milliliters) olive oil.

To serve, place the pasta in a large bowl and ladle the sauce over it. Gently toss the sauce with the pasta. Top with tomato confit, sprinkle with the pecorino, and drizzle with olive oil

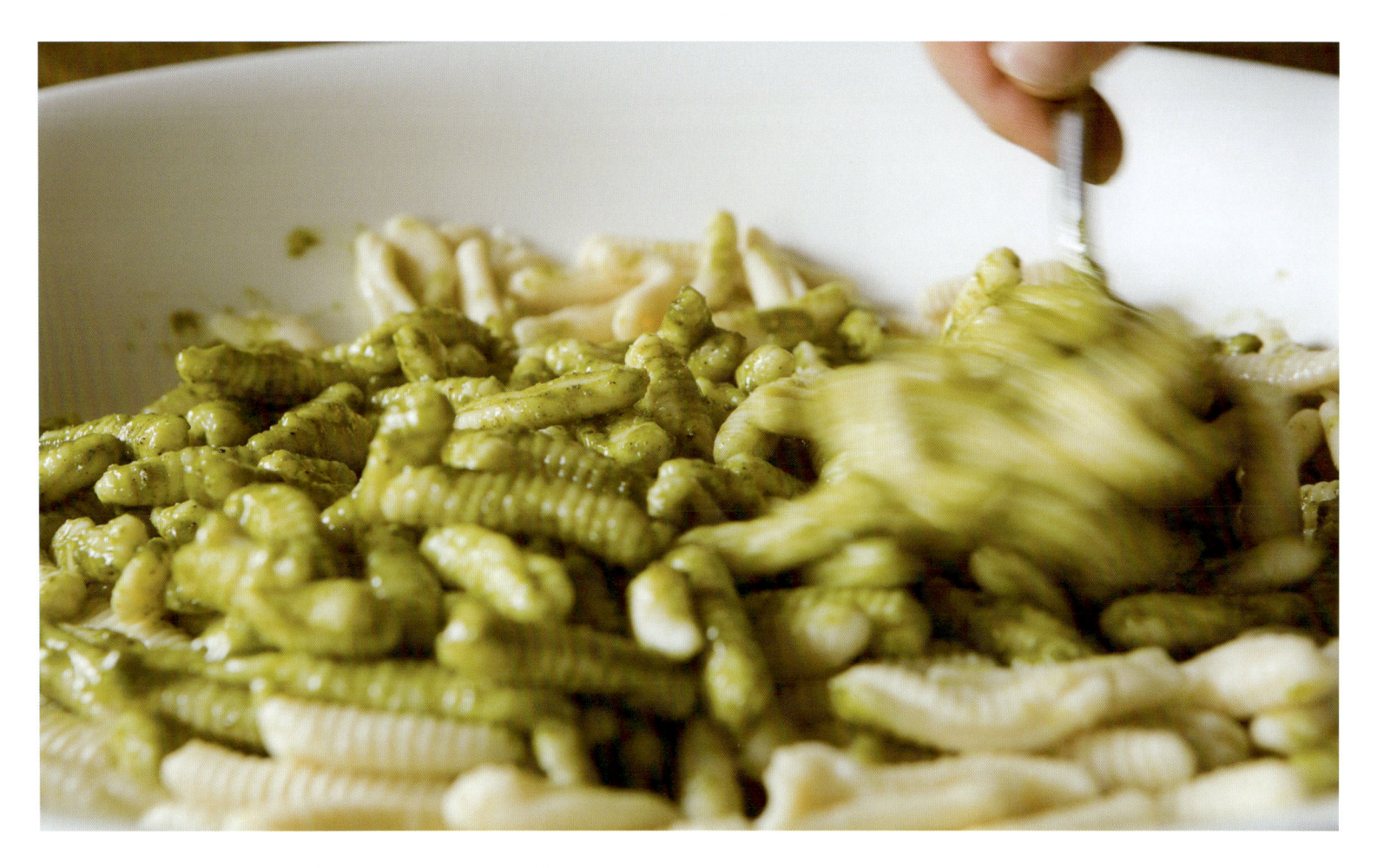

Ricotta Cavatelli

(Step By Step)

12

SERVES 10

Because the valley running up their centers is great for trapping liquids, cavatelli are the perfect foil for stews and sauces. Sometimes I'll toss them with a lobster mushroom broth and garnish them with sautéed sunchokes deglazed with chicken stock; other times I'll employ nothing more than pomodoro and plenty of Parmigiano. I make them with ricotta cheese—I prefer buffalo ricotta, which you can purchase at any respectable grocery or Italian deli—which adds an intense milky flavor to the pasta. You will need a cavatelli maker, which is readily available at kitchenware stores and online. Fantes brand machines are a good bet.

INGREDIENTS

1. 4 cups (500 grams) 00 flour
2. 1 1/2 cups (375 grams) ricotta cheese
3. 2 large egg yolks (40 grams)
4. 2 tablespoons + 2 teaspoons (40 grams) whole milk
5. 2 teaspoons (9 grams) kosher salt
6. Semolina flour for rolling and shaping
7. Extra virgin olive oil for garnish

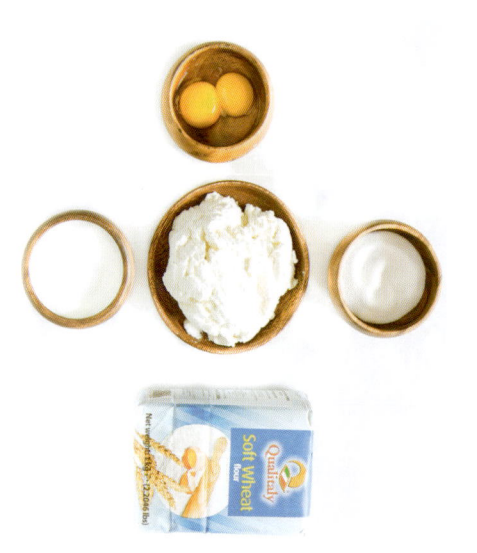

DIRECTIONS

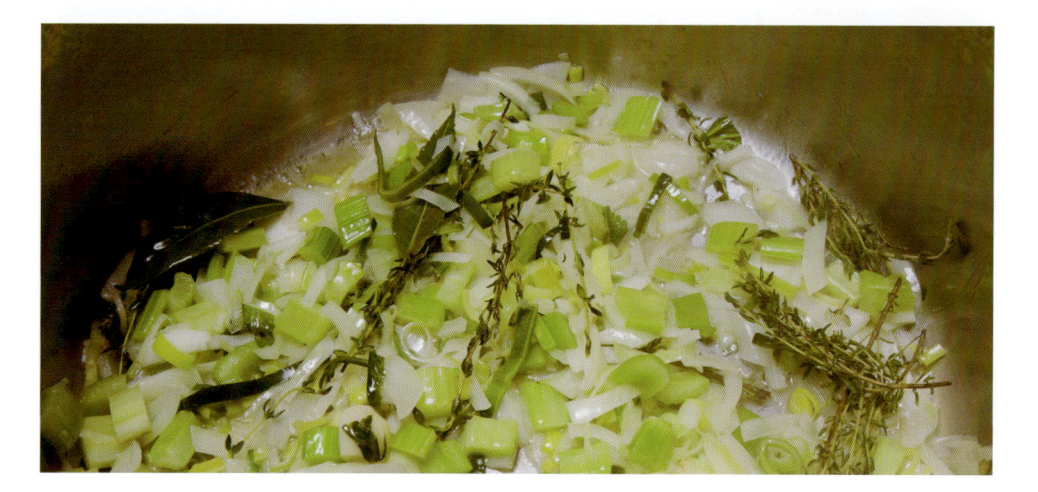

In the bowl of a stand mixer fitted with the dough hook attachment, mix the 00 flour and ricotta until fully combined.

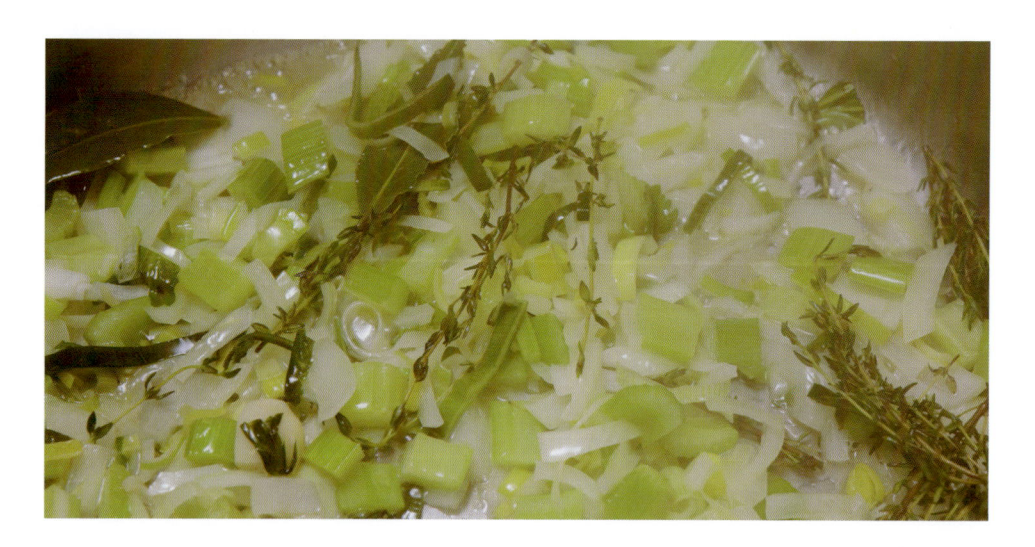

Add the egg yolks, milk, and salt and mix until the dough becomes a ball, approximately 10 minutes

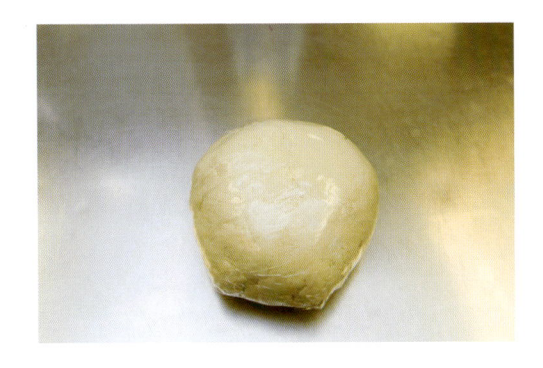

Wrap the dough in plastic wrap and let it chill in the refrigerator for 24 hours

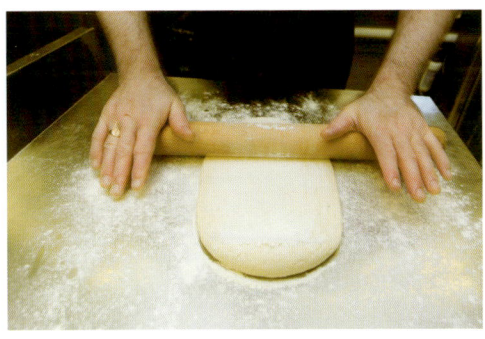

The next day, divide the dough into two balls of equal size. On a surface well floured with semolina flour, with a well floured rolling pin, roll out the dough into a 1/2-inch-thick (1 cm) rounded square.

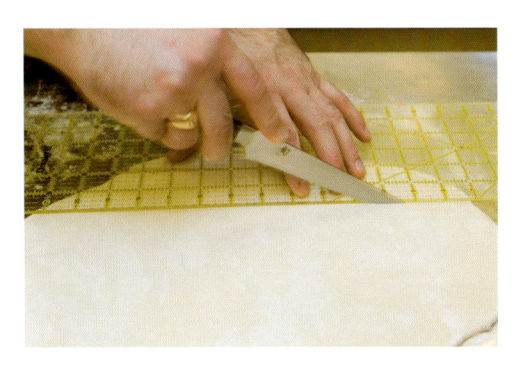

Using a sharp knife, cut the dough into 1- inch-wide (2.5 cm) strips

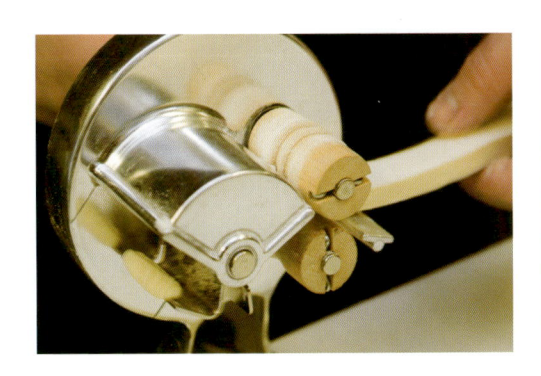

One by one, pass the strips through the cavatelli maker to create the cavatelli. Place them on a sheet pan dusted with semolina flour, cover them with plastic wrap, and refrigerate until use, up to 5 days. The cavatelli may also be frozen for 2 months for longer. Do not thaw them before cooking

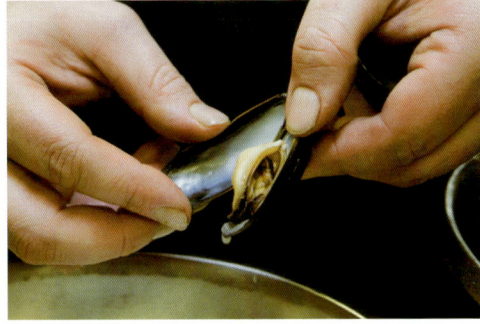

To cook the cavatelli, fill a large pot half-full with well-salted water and bring it to a boil over high heat. Place the cavatelli in the boiling water and wait for them to float to the surface and stay there for 30 seconds.

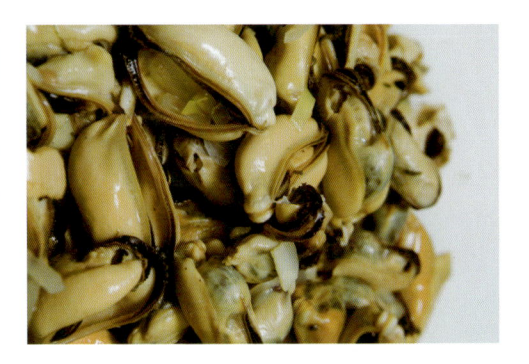

Remove them with a slotted spoon and place in a strainer in the sink. Toss them with a little olive oil and serve them with your sauce of choice.

PAGE 55

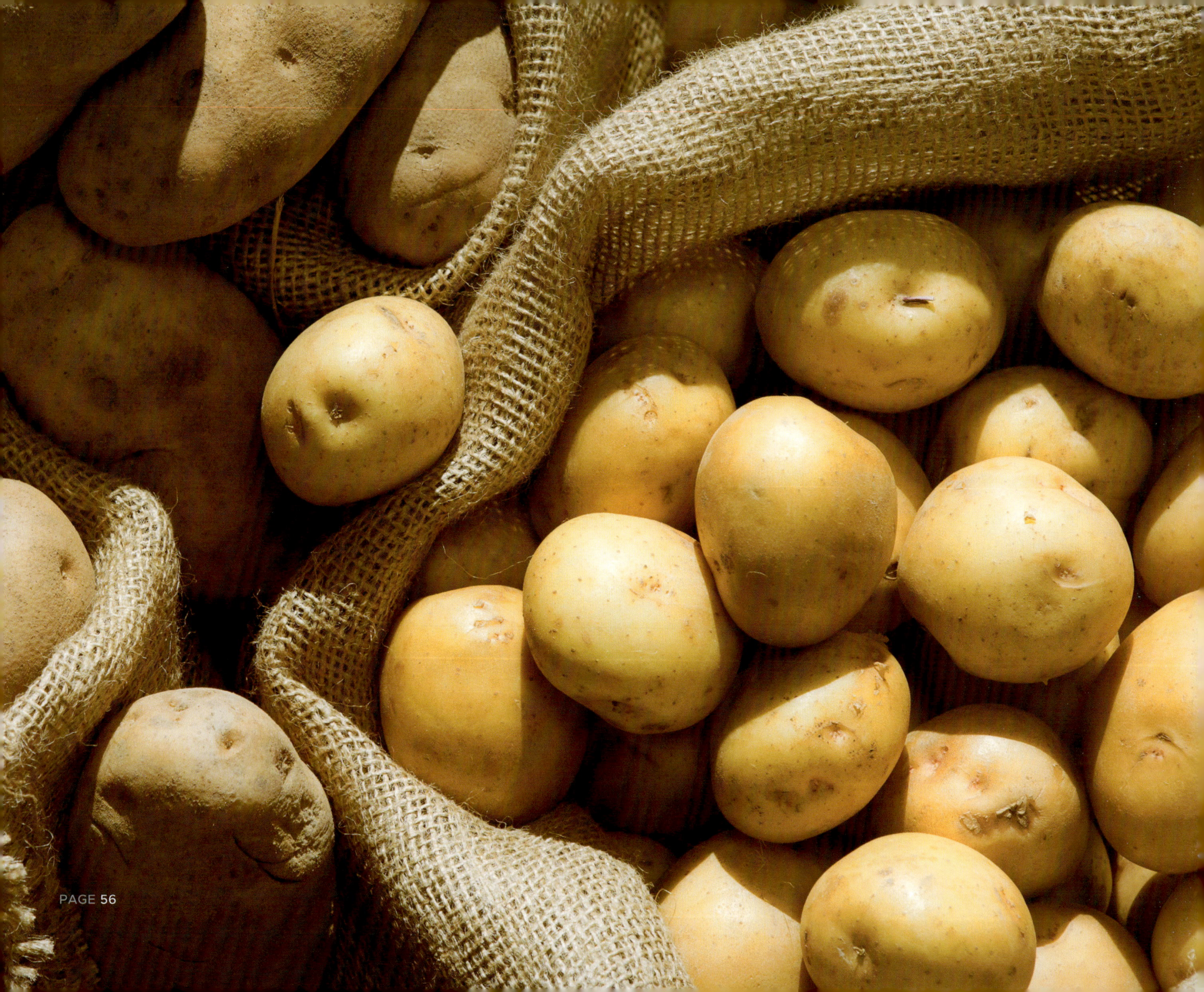

POTATOES

Potatoes are a huge part of the traditional Belgian diet, often appearing at breakfast, lunch, and dinner —and sometimes in between. We have different varieties back home, so it took me several years of R&D to determine which American varieties work best for my recipes. Yukon golds are ideal for purees; nothing beats fingerlings for pommes Lyonnaise; and a good gratin should be built with russets. No matter what kind I'm using, I always cut a few in half to check that their flesh is white and clean. If the potato has a granulated quality, has started to go soft anywhere, or has begun to sprout, you should throw it out or, better yet, compost it

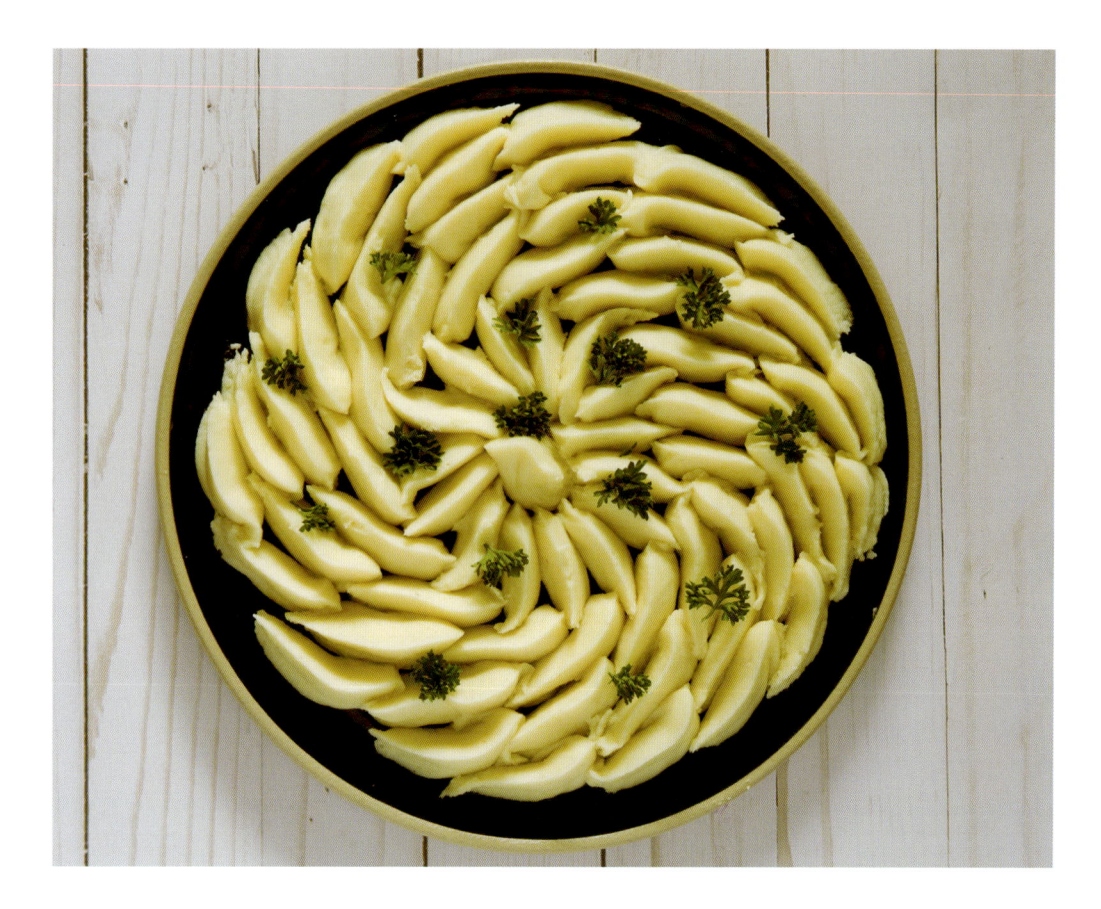

Mashed Potatoes

SERVES 10

This recipe could not be simpler. You add an avalanche of warm dairy—heavy cream, whole milk, and butter—to a mound of boiled potatoes and vigorously whip them. I prefer using a KitchenAid fitted with the whisk attachment, but you're welcome to do it by hand. A pinch of nutmeg adds a dusky nuttiness. Yukon golds are the perfect foundation this recipe, producing fluffy, velvety drifts of potatoes. In my mind, mashed potatoes go well with anything, but they're an especially welcome complement to Endive Gratin (page 87), Flemish Beef Stew (Carbonnade à la Flamande) (page 122) or Pork Chops with Blackwell Sauce (page 130)

INGREDIENTS

1. 6 pounds (3 kilograms) Yukon gold potatoes, washed and peeled
2. Kosher salt
3. 1 1/4 cups (300 grams) whole milk
4. 1 1/4 cups (300 grams) heavy cream
5. 12 tablespoons (1 1/2 sticks/180 grams) unsalted butter
6. 1/4 teaspoon (0.5 gram) freshly grated nutmeg

DIRECTIONS

Place potatoes in a large pot, cover with cold water, and stir in 1 tablespoon (8 grams) salt. Place over high heat and cook until a knife inserted into the potatoes meets no resistance, about 1 hour. Drain the potatoes completely in a colander set in the sink.

In a medium saucepan over medium-high heat, place the milk, cream, butter, and nutmeg and bring to a boil, whisking occasionally. Remove from heat.

In a large bowl, mash the potatoes thoroughly. Add the milk mixture and whip together with wooden spoon until fully incorporated and there are no lumps. Serve immediately.

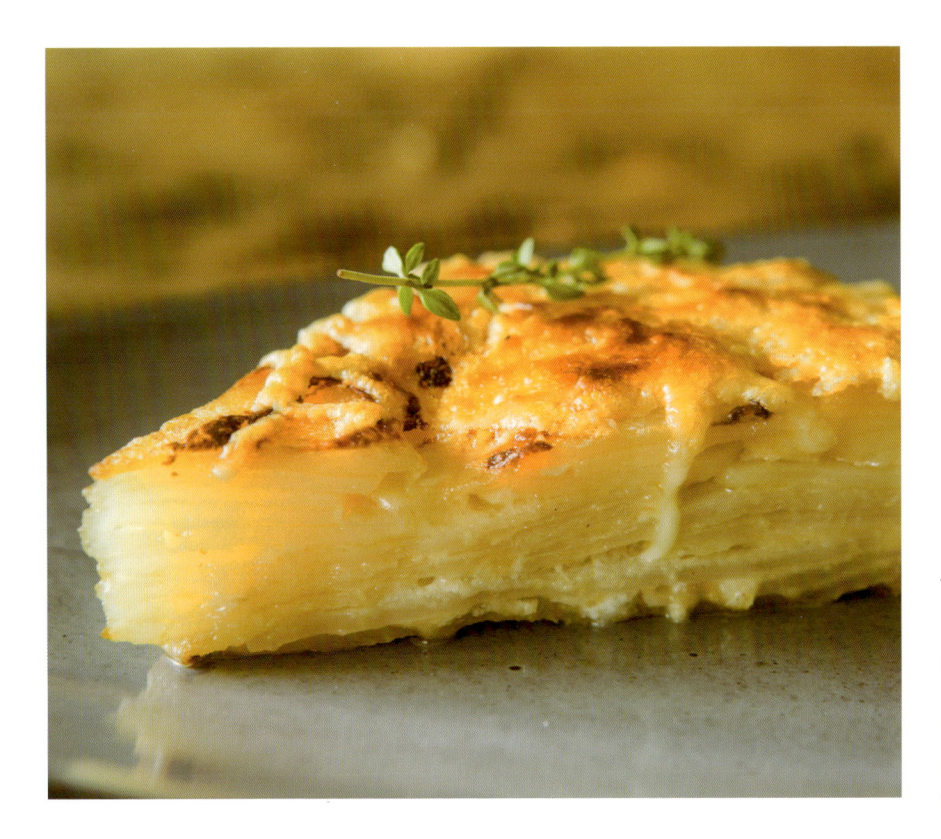

Potato and Kohlrabi Gratin

I discovered turnip-like kohlrabi while working at the German Embassy. They possess a nice spicy note and just a touch of acidity. Plus, they are texturally complementary to russet potatoes, which is why I combine them in this gratin, containing a mixture of the two vegetables on each layer. When you're choosing kohlrabi at your farmers' market or at the grocery story, make sure they're firm all over. Soft spots will indicate interior rot. Bigger isn't better. Chose kohlrabi with smaller bulbs—about 3 inches (8 cm) in diameter—as they will be more tender and flavorful

INGREDIENTS

1. 8 tablespoons (1 stick/125 grams) unsalted butter, divided
2. 1 3/4 cups (400 grams) heavy cream
3. 2 cloves garlic, finely diced
4. 2 sprigs fresh thyme
5. 2 1/2 teaspoons (12 grams) kosher salt
6. 1/4 teaspoon (1 gram) freshly ground black pepper
7. 1/4 teaspoon (0.5 gram) ground nutmeg
8. 2 large russet potatoes, washed and peeled
9. 10 small kohlrabi, washed and peeled
10. 1 1/2 cups (200 grams) shredded Gruyère cheese

DIRECTIONS

Preheat the oven to 325°F (165°C). Butter a 13 by 9- inch (33 by 23 cm) metal baking pan with 1 tablespoon (14 grams) of the butter. In a large saucepan over medium heat, bring the cream, garlic, the remaining butter, the thyme, salt, pepper, and nutmeg to a boil. Remove from the heat.

Using a mandoline, thinly slice the potatoes and kohlrabi. Add to the cream mixture and toss to coat thoroughly. Evenly layer the potatoes and kohlrabi in the prepared pan. Pour the remaining liquid over them. Bake until the vegetables are tender and the top is browned, about 1 hour.

Remove the gratin from the oven. Turn on the broiler. Spread the Gruyère on top of the gratin, and broil until the cheese is completely melted and crispy, 4 to 5 minutes. Remove from the broiler and let sit for about 15 minutes before serving

14

SERVES
4

Belgian Frites
(Step By Step)

Belgium is the home to the world's best frying potato variety, bintje. Boasting high moisture contrasted with low starch, they have a creamy consistency that holds up under the high heat. They're the only potato you'll find being used at any respectable frikot (fry stand) dishing out paper cones full of salt-speckled frites served with a side of mayonnaise or sauce américaine.

15

SERVES
8-10

INGREDIENTS

1. Canola oil as needed
2. 6 pounds (3 kilograms) russet potatoes, peeled and washed with cold water
3. Kosher salt

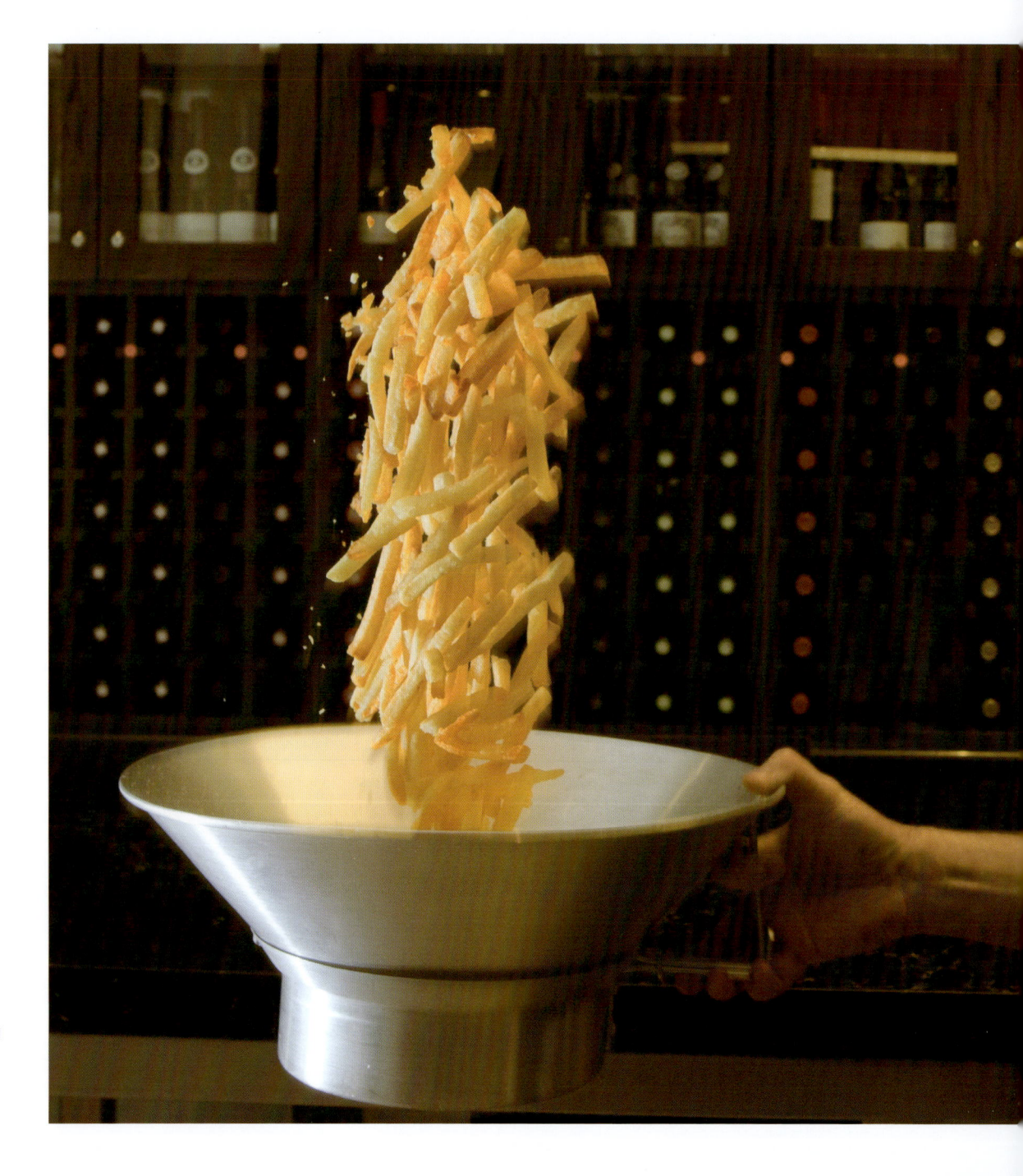

DIRECTIONS

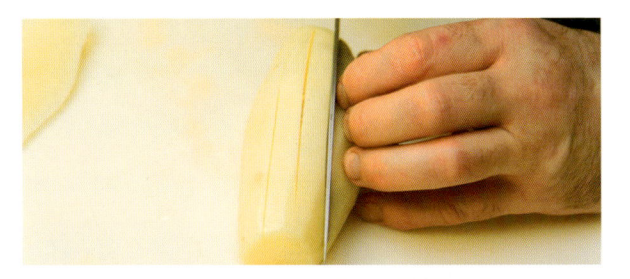

1. Following the manufacturer's instructions, fill a deep-fryer with oil and heat it to 300°F (150°C). Cut the potatoes lengthwise into 1/2-inch-square (1 cm) rods

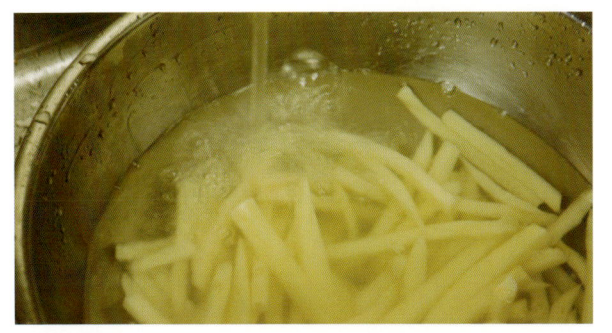

2. Rinse the potatoes again with cold water, and then place them on a sheet pan lined with kitchen towels. With another towel, pat them dry, making sure you get off as much moisture as you can. Transfer them to a sheet pan covered with parchment paper.

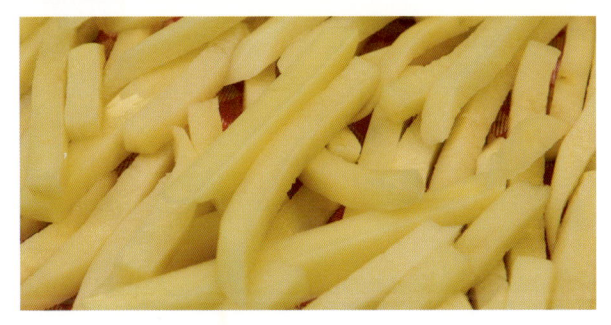

3. Place the potatoes in the fryer, making sure not to overcrowd it, frying in batches if necessary. Let the potatoes cook until they are soft—remove one with a slotted spoon and press it between your fingers to check—but not yet turning golden, about 5 minutes. Remove them from the oil using a slotted spoon and place them on the sheet pan covered with parchment paper. Let the fries cool for 3 hours or up to overnight, leaving them uncovered. Leave the oil in the fryer.

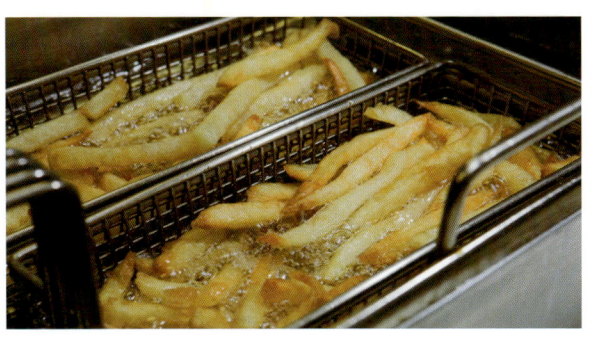

4. Using the same oil, heat the deep-fryer to 350°F (175°C). Put the fries back into the oil and fry until they're golden brown, about 5 to 6 minutes per batch.
Remove from the oil with a slotted spoon, shake to remove excess oil, and place in a large bowl. Add salt to taste and toss until they are evenly seasoned. Serve immediately with your choice of condiments.

PAGE 62

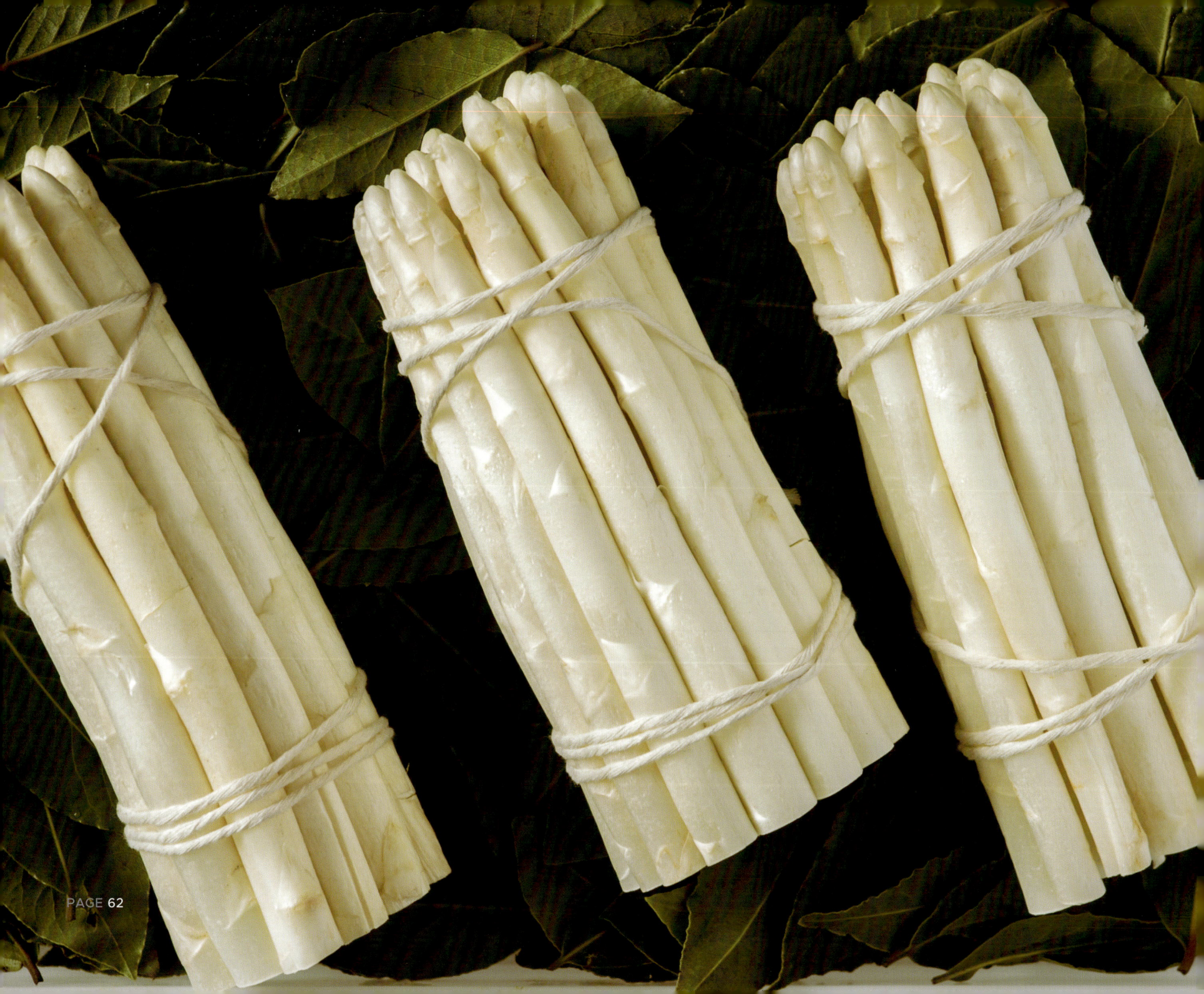

ASPARAGUS

There are two main types of asparagus: green and white. Both are in season from mid-April through early July in a good year, but that's where their similarities end. I find the white variety slightly sweeter, a tiny bit thicker, and more tender than its green siblings, though I'm fond of both. The ivory stalks can be difficult to find in the States. Locally grown options can sometimes be purchased at the farmers' market, while imported varieties from France, Holland, and Peru are often available at good grocery stores.

16

SERVES 4

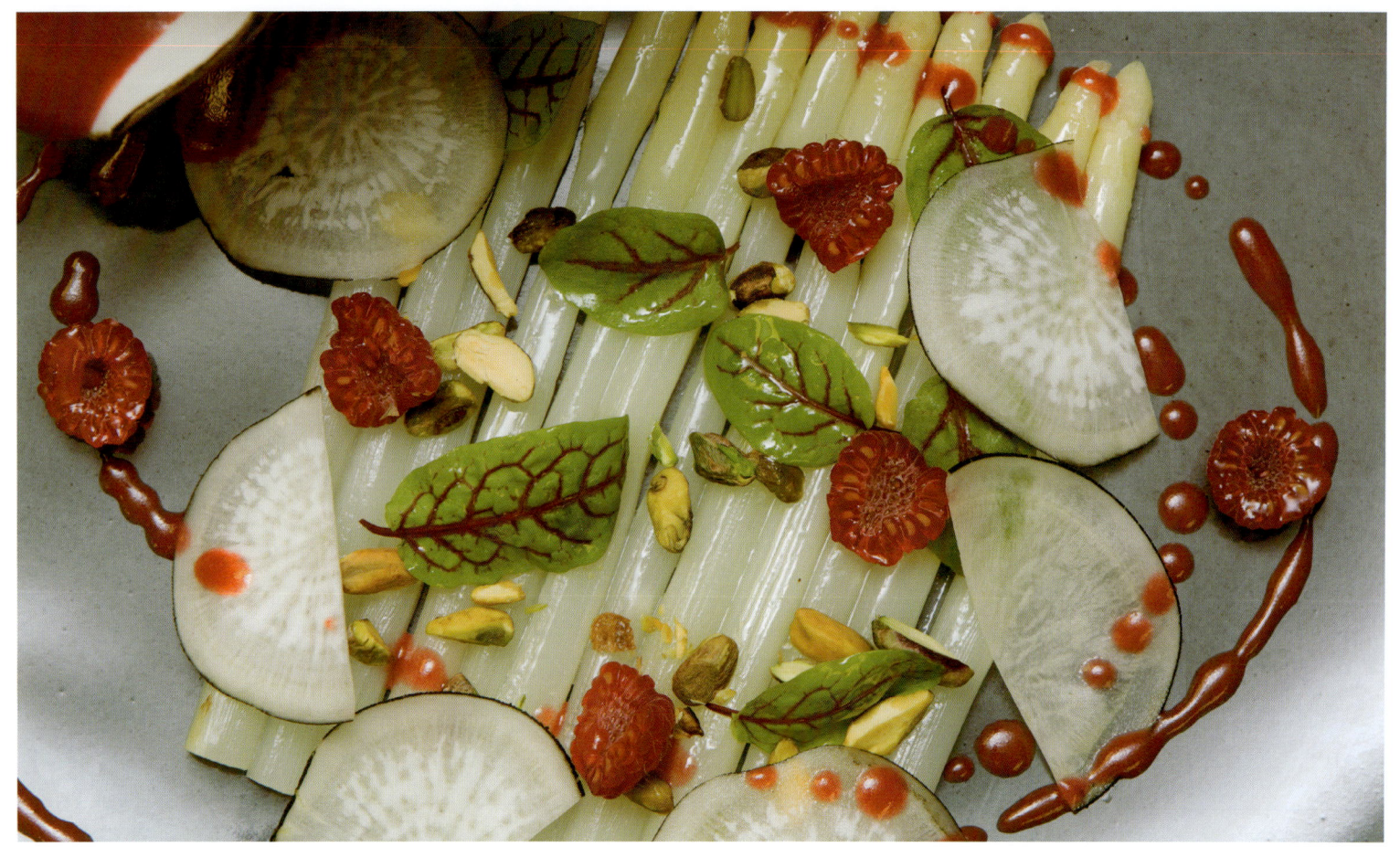

White Asparagus

with Raspberry-Hibiscus Dressing

Lemon vinaigrette is a classic pairing with white asparagus, but I wanted to push past tradition. So I created a punchy dressing with hibiscus vinegar, mashed raspberries, and a touch of Dijon mustard. Perky and peppy, it really dances on the palate, while playing well with the other components on the plate: pistachios, paper thin slices of radish, and red vein sorrel. Serve this as an appetizer at a springtime dinner party and your guests will be wowed from the get go. You can purchase hibiscus vinegar at Et Voila!'s market; raspberry vinegar also works well and is available from Williams Sonoma and other retailers

INGREDIENTS

1. Kosher salt
2. 2 bunches (about 2 pounds/1 kilogram) large white asparagus, stems peeled
3. 1 tablespoon (15 grams) freshly squeezed lemon juice
4. 1/2 cup + 2 tablespoons (125 grams) extra virgin olive oil, divided
5. 1 medium radish, washed, thinly sliced, soaked in cold water, and dried on paper towels
6. 3/4 cup (100 grams) fresh raspberries
7. 1/4 cup (55 grams) hibiscus vinegar
8. 2 teaspoons (10 grams) Dijon mustard
9. 2 tablespoons (15 grams) finely chopped unsalted
10. pistachios (Sicilian, if available)
11. 1 bunch red vein sorrel, washed and dried

DIRECTIONS

Place a large pot of well-salted water over high heat and bring to a boil. Add the asparagus and cook for 8 minutes, until tender. Remove the pot from the heat and let the asparagus cool in the water. When they've cooled, remove them from the pot and lay them on a sheet pan covered with a kitchen towel to help to remove the excess water.

In a medium bowl, whisk together the lemon juice, a pinch of salt, and 1 tablespoon (15 milliliters) of the olive oil. Add the sliced radish and stir to combine. Set aside.

In a separate medium bowl, whisk together the raspberries, hibiscus vinegar, mustard, and 2 1/2 teaspoons (12 grams) kosher salt. With an immersion blender, mix until fully incorporated. Gradually add the olive, whisking or mixing constantly until smooth and creamy. Set aside.

When ready to serve, divide the asparagus between four plates. Drizzle 1 tablespoon (15 milliliters) of the hibiscus dressing on each, then evenly sprinkle with chopped pistachios. Drain the radishes, pat them dry, and place 3 or 4 slices on each plate. Garnish with red vein sorrel.

Store remaining hibiscus dressing in a bottle and refrigerate for up to three months. Bring it to room temperature before using.

17

SERVES 4

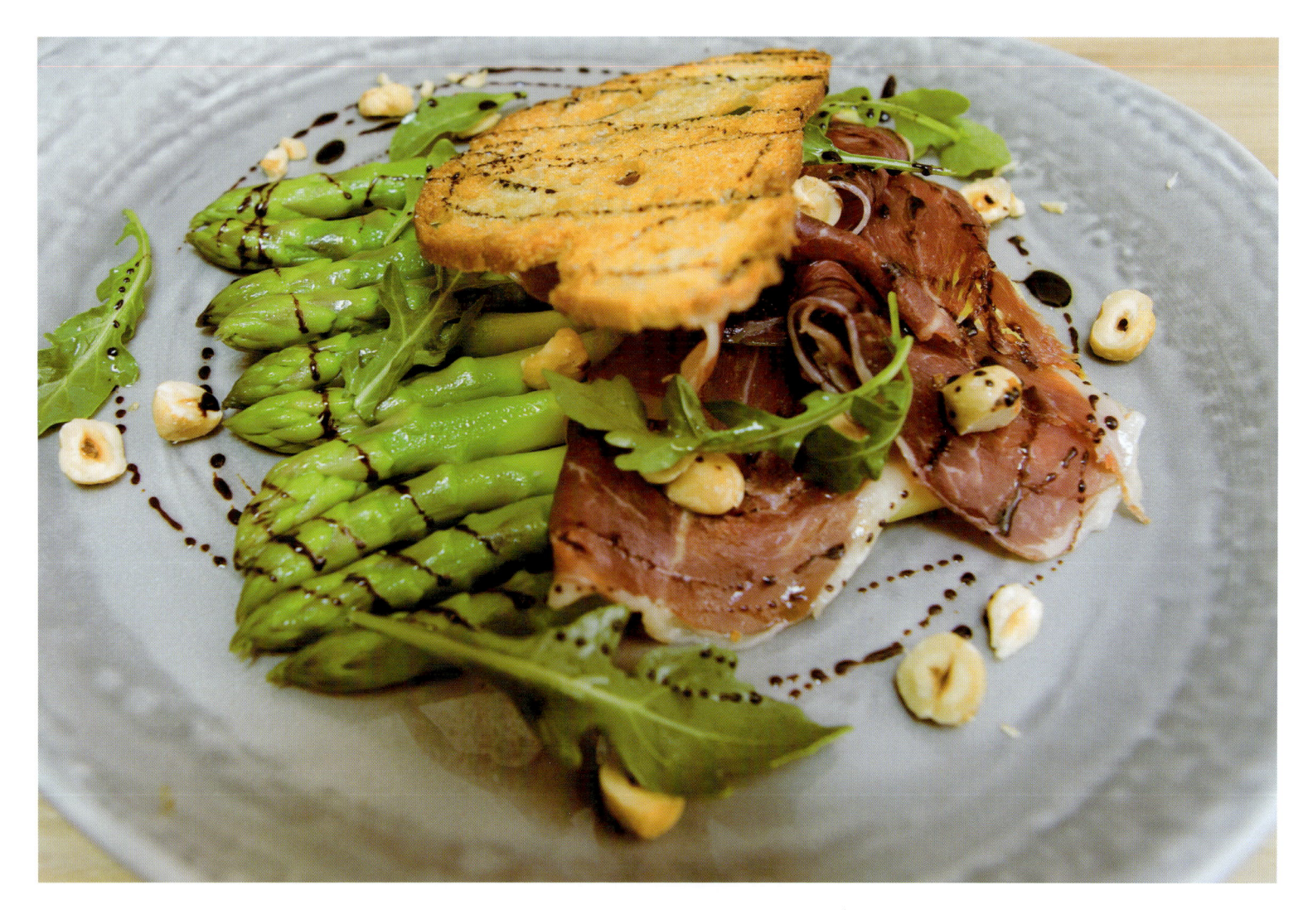

Green Asparagus
with Hazelnuts and Prosciutto

We've all enjoyed prosciutto-wrapped melon. This springy starter plays with similar flavors, but switches in green stalks of asparagus for the usual half-moons of cantaloupe. I dress up my preparation with a zigzag of sherry vinegar reduction, crushed Piedmont hazelnuts, thin ribbons of ham, and crisped-up slices of French baguette. It's a simple preparation that's simply delicious

INGREDIENTS

1. 1 baguette
2. Kosher salt
3. 2 large bunches (about 2 pounds/1 kilogram) green
4. asparagus, stems peeled
5. 3 tablespoons (42 grams) extra virgin olive oil, divided, plus more for brushing
6. 7 tablespoons (100 grams) sherry vinegar (preferably
7. 10-year-old Jerez)
8. 1 clove garlic, peeled
9. 3 cups (100 grams) lightly packed baby arugula
10. 1 teaspoon (5 grams) hazelnut oil, plus more for garnishing
11. 8 to 12 slices Ibérico de Bellota ham or prosciutto
12. 1/4 cup (30 grams) finely chopped skin-off roasted
13. hazelnuts (preferably from Piedmont

DIRECTIONS

Cut the baguette into 3 equal parts and place in the freezer until half frozen, about 1 hour.

Fill a large bowl with cold water and ice. Set aside.

Place a large stew pot filled with well-salted water over high heat and bring to a boil. Add the asparagus and cook until tender but al dente, about 5 minutes. With a large slotted spoon, remove the asparagus from the boiling water and put them in the ice bath. Let sit until chilled, about 10 minutes, then remove with the spoon and set aside on a sheet pan covered with a kitchen towel.

Preheat the oven to 300°F (150°C).

Line a sheet pan with parchment paper, then brush the parchment with a light coating of olive oil. Remove the bread from the freezer and use a serrated knife to cut 4 slices on the diagonal, each about 1/8 inch (3 mm) thick and 6 inches (15 cm) long. (Save the remaining baguette in the freezer for another project.) Place the bread slices in a single layer on the prepared pan, then lightly brush each slice with 1 1/2 teaspoons (8 milliliters) of the olive oil. Toast the bread in the oven until brown and crisp, about 8 minutes. Set aside.

Meanwhile, place the sherry vinegar in a small saucepan and bring to a simmer over medium heat. Cook the vinegar until reduced by half, about 8 minutes. Pour into a small bowl and set aside.

In a large sauté pan over medium heat, heat 1 tablespoon (15 milliliters) of the olive oil until shimmering. Add the garlic and cook until fragrant, 30 to 60 seconds. Add the asparagus and season with a pinch of salt. Cook for 3 to 4 minutes, until al dente. Remove the asparagus from the pan and place on a paper towel–lined plate to remove the excess oil

In a small bowl, combine the arugula, hazelnut oil, and a pinch of salt. Toss together until well combined.

To serve, divide the asparagus between 4 plates. Top the asparagus with 2 or 3 slices of the ham each, then drizzle with the sherry reduction and sprinkle with hazelnuts. Place a mound of dressed arugula on top. Finish with a slice of the crispy bread and drizzle with hazelnut oil

18

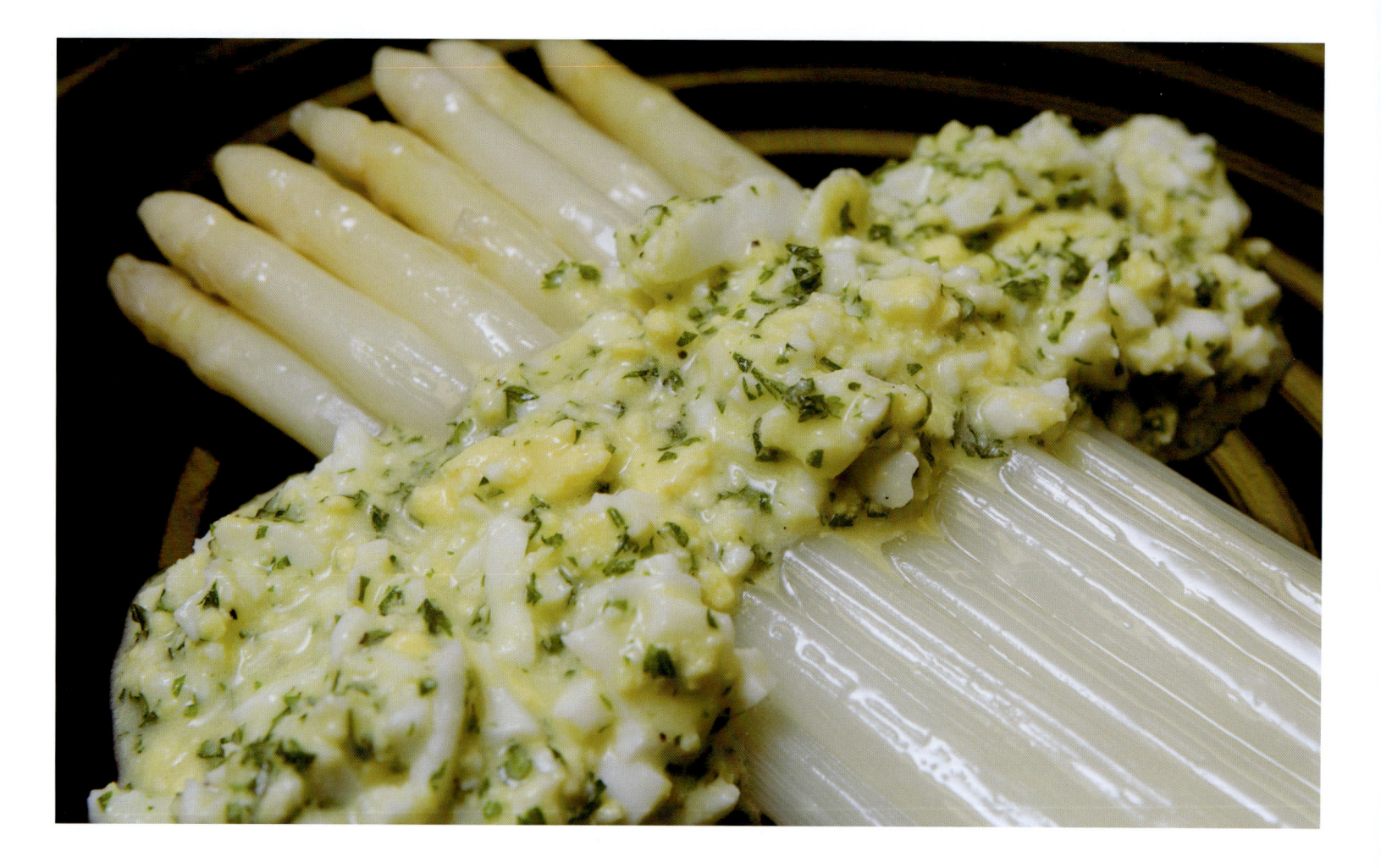

SERVES
4

White Asparagus à la Flamande

(Step By Step)

Back home in Belgium, we call white asparagus wit goud (white gold), because it's so sought after and people always pay a premium for it. When it's in season, I make this classic dish every single day. It's a very straightforward: after being boiled, the ivory stalks are topped with mashed hard-boiled eggs and seasoned melted butter. Given the simplicity, it's a fun dish to make alongside young cooks in your family who want to work on their kitchen skills

INGREDIENTS

1. Kosher salt
2. 2 bunches (about 2 pounds/1 kilogram) large white asparagus, stems peeled
3. 4 large eggs in the shell (200 grams)
4. 8 tablespoons (1 stick/125 grams) unsalted butter, divided
5. 1/4 teaspoon (1 gram) freshly ground nutmeg
6. 1/4 teaspoon (1 gram) freshly ground black pepper
7. 6 sprigs curly parsley, finely chopped

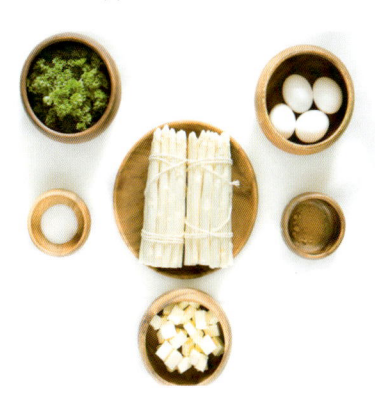

DIRECTIONS

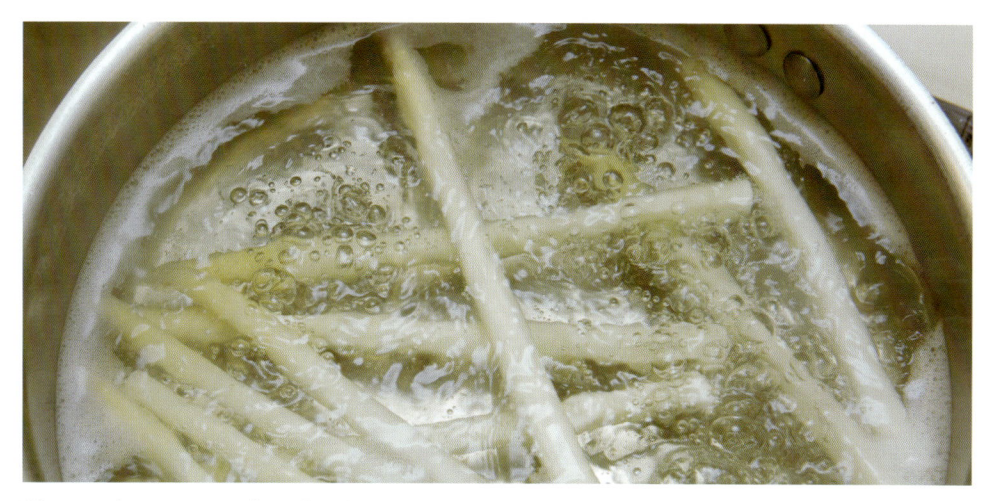

Place a large pot of well-salted water over high heat and bring to a boil. Add the asparagus and cook for 8 minutes, until tender. Remove the pot from the heat and let the asparagus cool in the water.

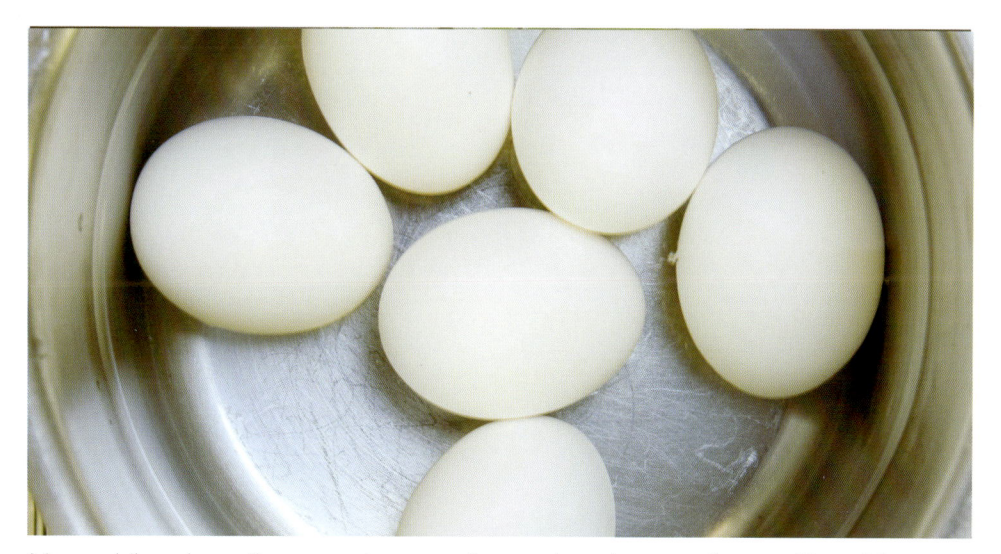

Meanwhile, place the eggs in a medium pot and cover them with cold water. Place the pot over high heat and bring to a boil. Cook the eggs for 8 minutes. Remove the eggs from the pot and rinse them under cold water until cool.

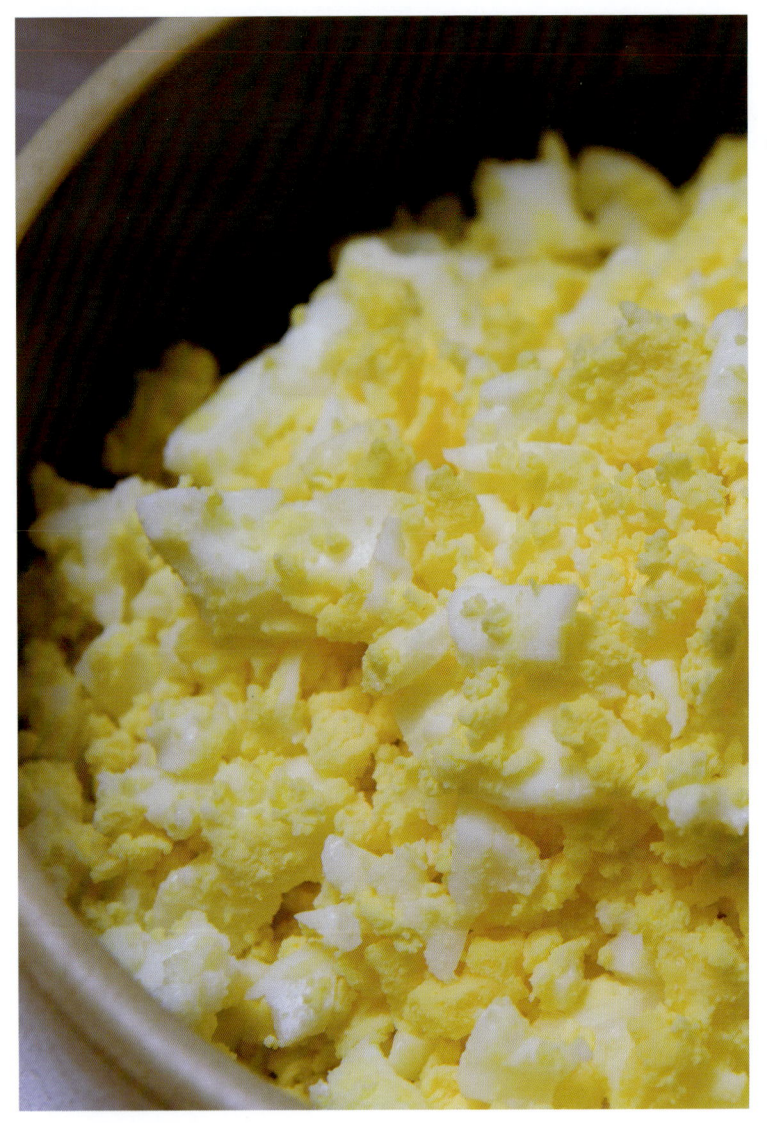

Remove the eggshells and rinse the eggs. In a medium bowl, use a fork to smash 1 egg at a time to create a crumbled consistency. Set aside

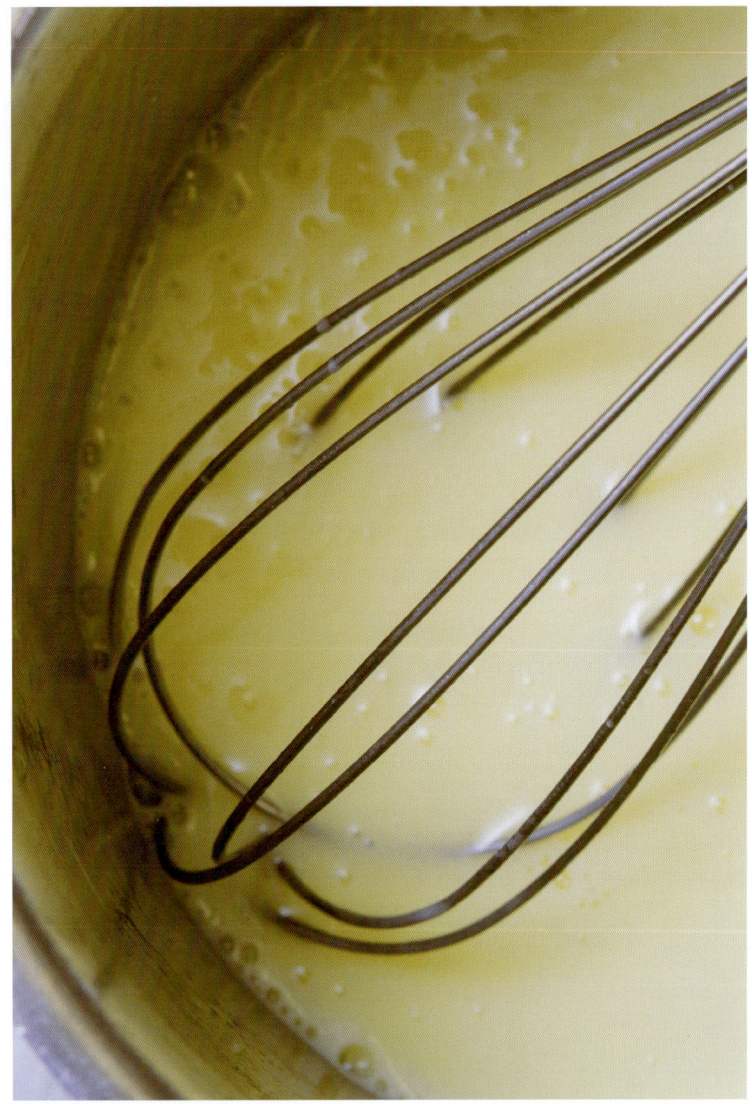

In a large saucepan over medium heat, bring 3/4 cup (180 milliliters) of the asparagus water to a simmer. Whisk in 4 tablespoons (60 grams) of the butter until fully melted and then whisk in the remaining 4 tablespoons until fully melted. Whisk in 1 teaspoon (8 grams) salt, the nutmeg, black pepper, and parsley.

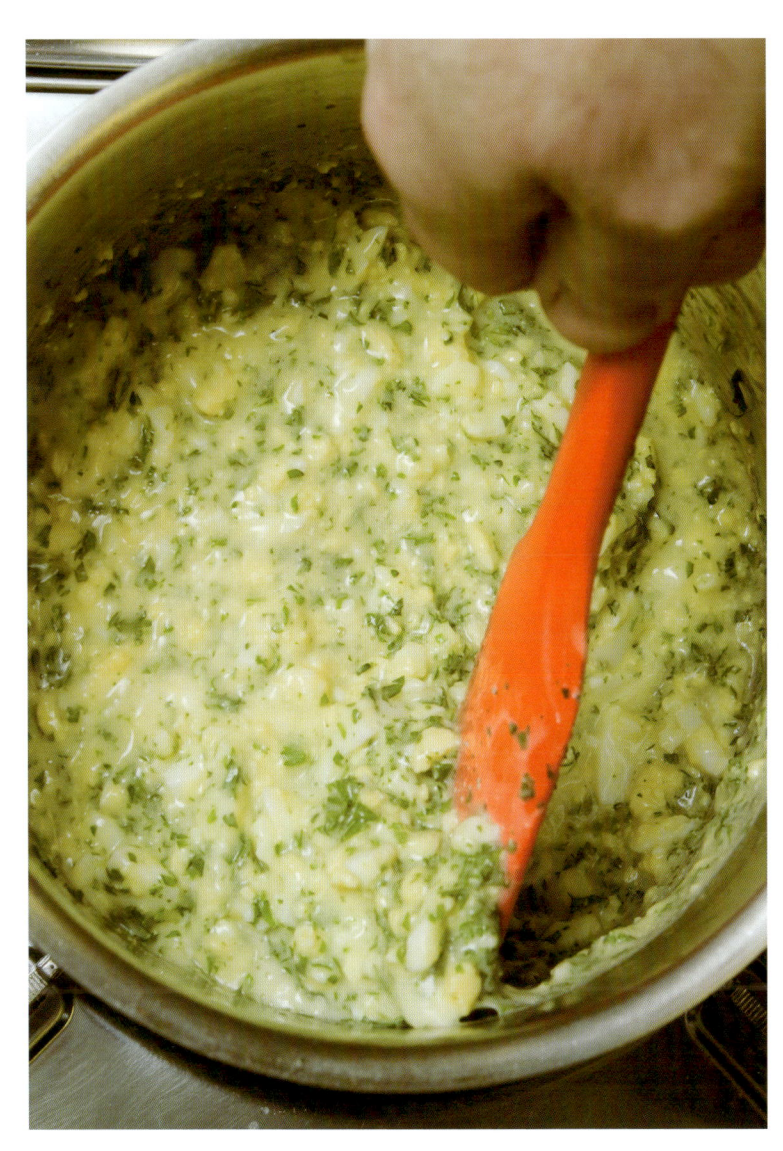

Add the smashed eggs and gently mix with a wooden spoon until just combined.

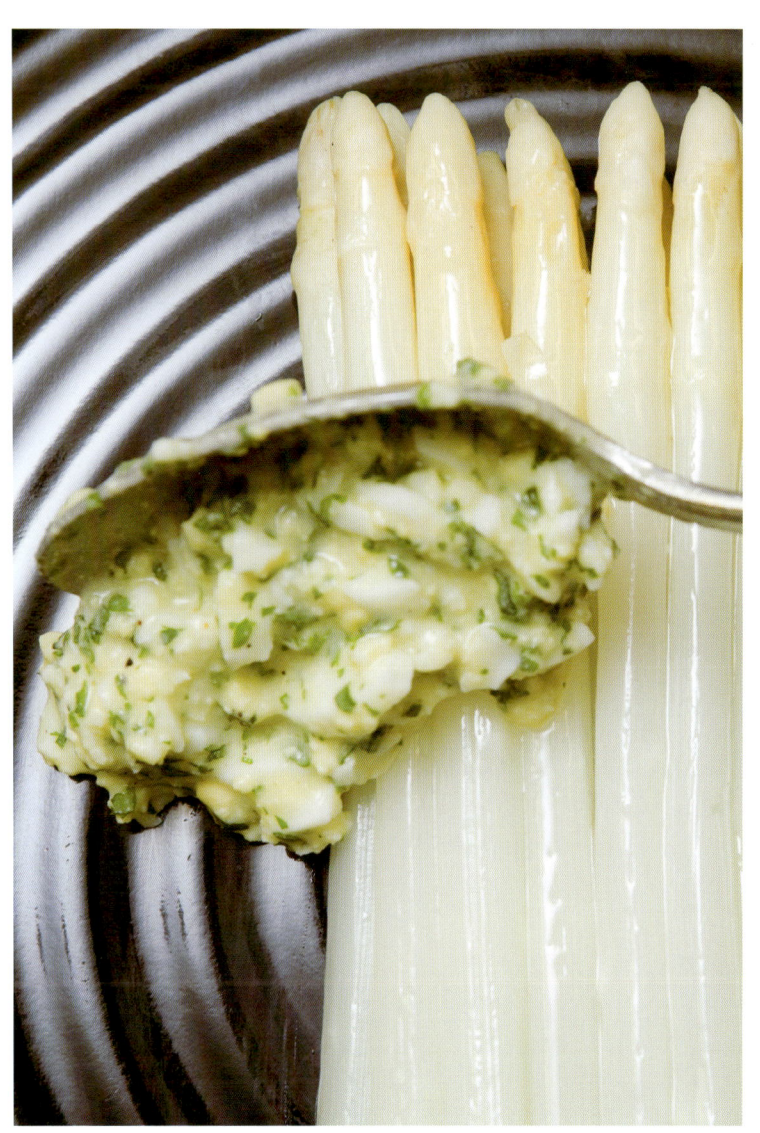

Remove the asparagus from the water, drain them briefly on a clean kitchen towel, and divide them evenly between four plates. Cover them with the egg sauce and serve immediately

PAGE 72

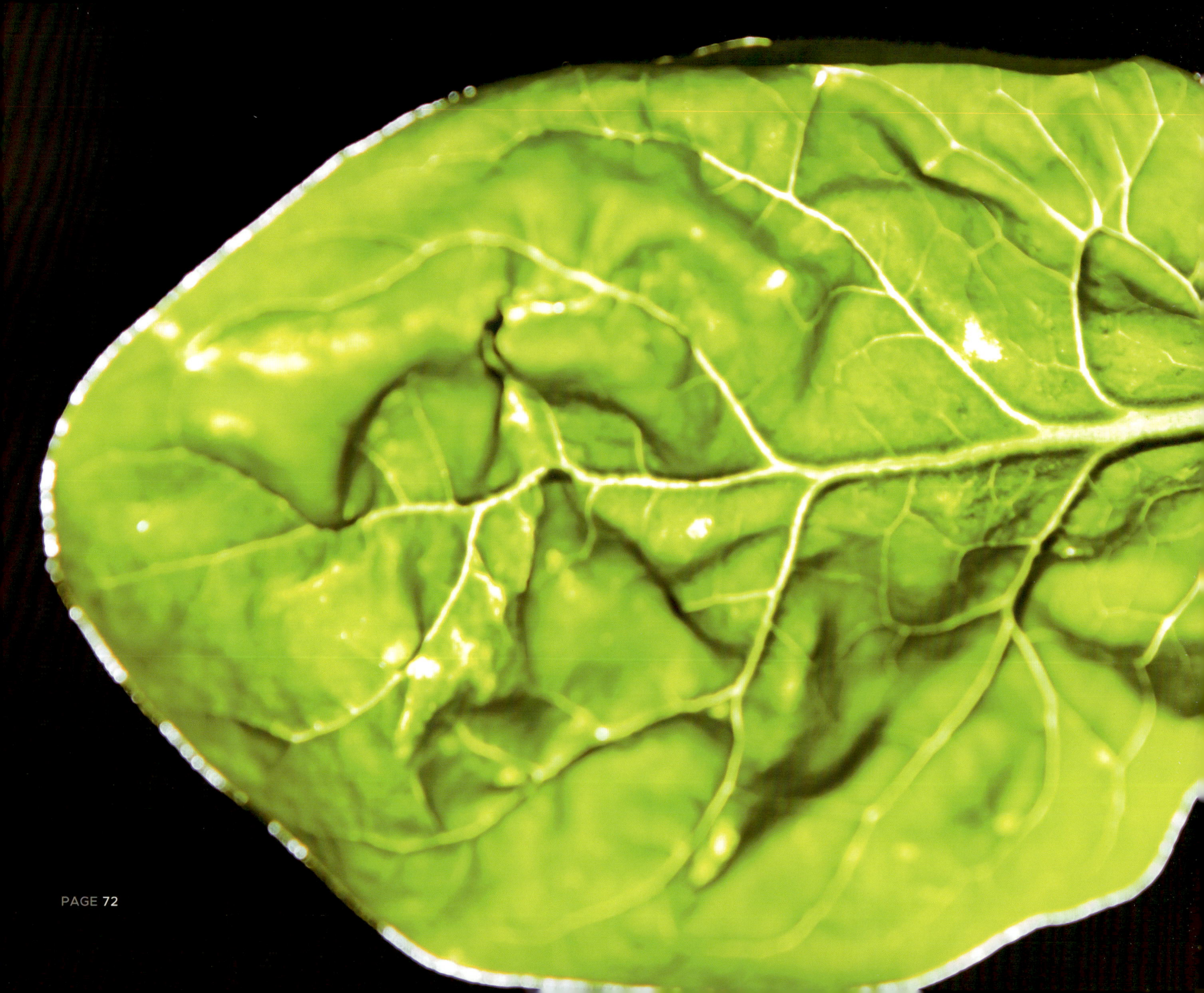

BABY SPINACH

When I was a young cook, I cleaned a lot of spinach. A lot. It was a painstaking process, because the spine had to be removed from the leaves, which were then washed three or four times. If the chef I was working for ever tasted the slightest hint of grit, he would insist I throw everything out and bring him a fresh batch. Now it's my job to inspect the spinach my team has prepped—and I'm just as particular as my mentors. You have to respect the products you're handling, making sure they are represented as well as they can be in your cooking. Spinach is a humble ingredient, but it can shine brightly if you handle it the right way

19

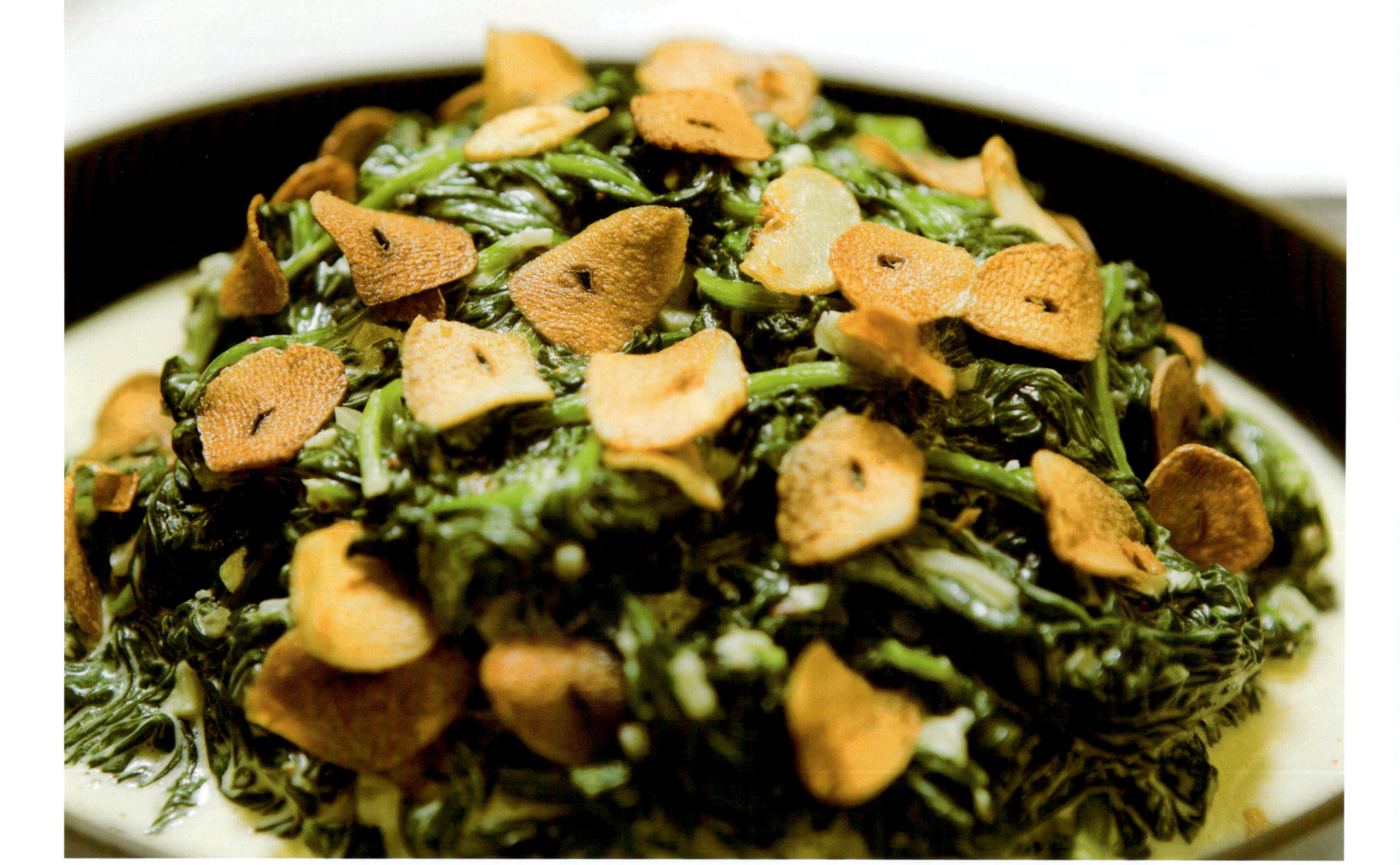

SERVES
6

Creamy and Garlicky Baby Spinach

The timeless steakhouse side gets a lift from a scattering of crispy fried garlic chips. I love this dish because the leftovers are so versatile. The day after, use it to smother roast chicken or sautéed fish. Add some ricotta and stuff it into cannelloni. Or toss it with your favorite pasta

INGREDIENTS

1. 8 cloves garlic, peeled, divided
2. 4 cups (1 liter) whole milk, divided
3. 8 tablespoons (1 stick/125 grams) unsalted butter
4. 2 pounds (900 grams) fresh baby spinach, washed well
5. 1 tablespoon (9 grams) kosher salt, divided
6. 1/2 teaspoon (2 grams) Espelette pepper
7. 2 1/4 cups (500 grams) heavy cream
8. Canola oil for frying

DIRECTIONS

The day before you wish to serve the dish, use a mandoline to cut 6 of the cloves lengthwise into very thin slices. Place them in a small bowl and cover with 2 cups (500 milliliters) of the milk. Refrigerate for 6 hours.

Remove the garlic from the milk and rinse it with cold water. Discard the milk and clean out the bowl. Place the garlic slices back in the bowl and cover with the remaining milk. Refrigerate for 6 more hours.

Remove the garlic from the milk and rinse with it cold water. Discard the milk. Place the garlic on sheet pan covered with a kitchen towel, cover with plastic wrap, and chill in your refrigerator until ready to use the next day.

Finely chop the remaining 2 garlic cloves. In a large stew pot over medium heat, melt the butter. Add the garlic and cook the garlic until fragrant, 30 to 60 seconds, then stir in the spinach. Season with 1 teaspoon (8 grams) of the salt and the Espelette pepper. Continue cooking, stirring frequently, until the spinach is cooked down, about 3 minutes. Drain the cooked spinach and set aside.

Meanwhile, place the cream in a small saucepan over medium heat. Simmer the cream until reduced by half, 15 to 20 minutes. Set aside.

Following the manufacturer's instructions, fill a deep fryer with oil and heat it to 350°F (175°C). Using a slotted spoon and working in batches if necessary, gently place the garlic slices in the oil and cook until golden brown, about 1 to 2 minutes, keeping a close eye on them so they don't burn. Remove them from the fryer and place on a paper towel–lined plate. Sprinkle with the remaining 1/2 teaspoon (2 grams) salt.

In a food processor, place the reduced cream and cooked spinach and process until the spinach is completely combined with the cream, about 5 minutes. Pour the mixture into a serving bowl. If necessary, warm the spinach in the microwave on medium for about 2 1/2 minutes, until hot. Garnish with the fried garlic chips and serve.

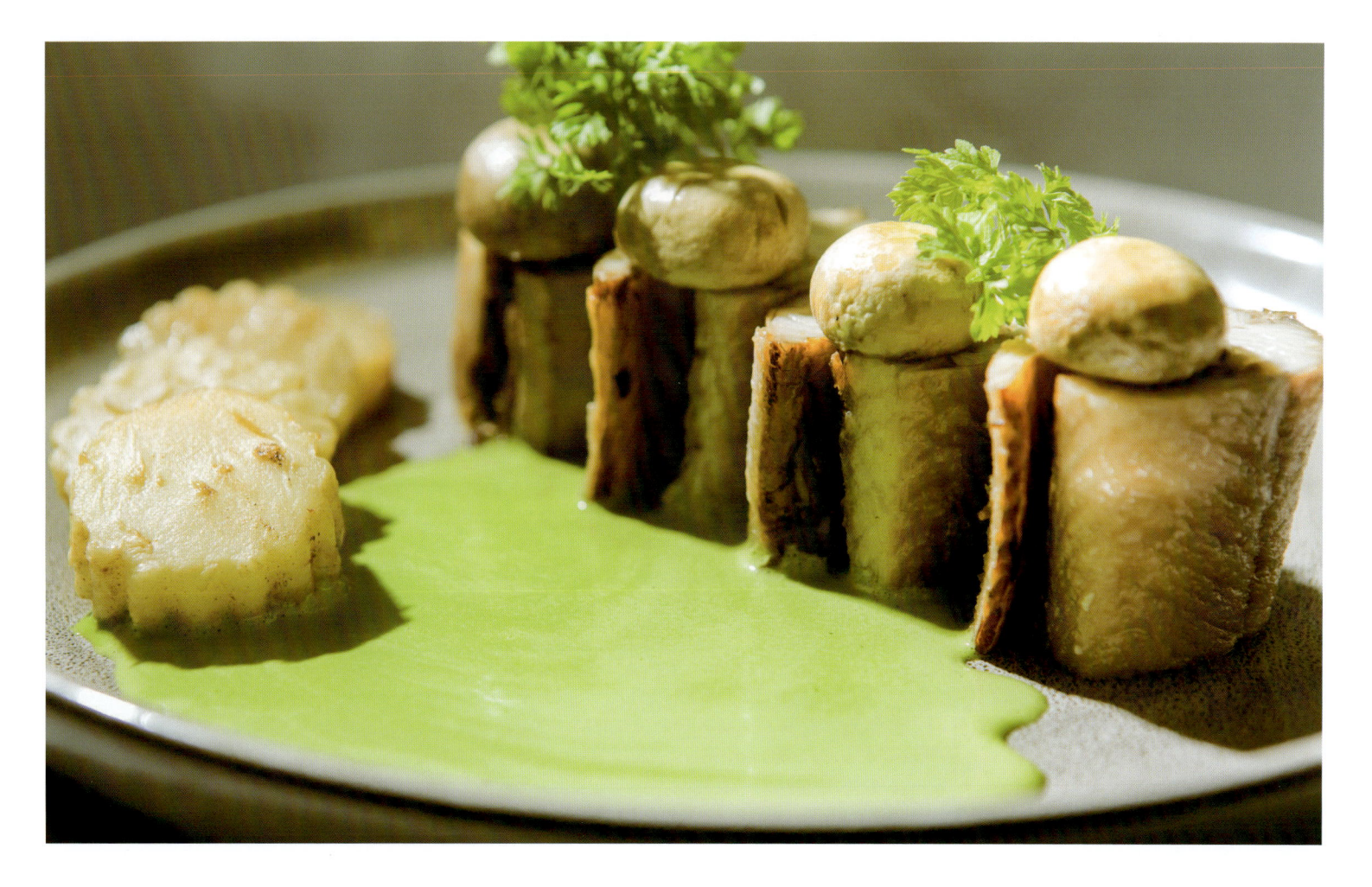

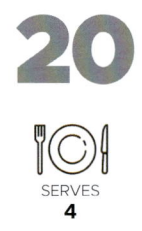

Smoked Eel with Green Sauce

SERVES 4

This recipe takes inspiration from the traditional Flemish dish, anguilles au vert, which literally means eels in green. The vibrantly verdant sauce is made with herbs and greens often found on the banks of the rivers where eels are caught. In my version, I use all the traditional green components: spinach, chervil, flat-leaf parsley, tarragon, watercress, chives, and thyme. Smoked eel is available at some high-end fishmongers. You're looking for fatty fillets with a creamy pinkish color and glistening skin. Do yourself a favor and ask the fishmonger to debone the eels; it can be a tricky process for the uninitiated.

INGREDIENTS

Spinach sauce
1. 4 tablespoons (1/2 stick/57 grams) unsalted butter
2. 3 tablespoons (28 grams) finely chopped shallots
3. 1 tablespoon + 2 teaspoons (14 grams) finely chopped garlic
4. 8 ounces (225 grams) baby spinach, washed well and dried
5. 2 ounces (57 grams) finely chopped chervil
6. 2 ounces (57 grams) finely chopped flat-leaf parsley
7. 2 ounces (57 grams) finely chopped tarragon
8. 2 ounces (57 grams) finely chopped watercress
9. 2 ounces (57 grams) finely chopped chives
10. 2 ounces (57 grams) finely chopped thyme
11. 3/4 teaspoon (3 grams) kosher salt
12. 1/4 cup + 1 tablespoon (65 grams) dry vermouth
13. 1 1/2 cups (350 grams) heavy cream

To assemble
1. 24 medium white mushrooms (about 1 pound/450
2. grams)
3. 1/4 cup (65 grams) dry white wine
4. 2 tablespoons (33 grams) unsalted butter
5. 3/4 teaspoon (3 grams) kosher salt
6. Four 4-ounce (125 gram) portions skin-on smoked eel
7. fillet
8. 4 sprigs fresh chervi

DIRECTIONS

To make the spinach sauce, in a medium saucepan over medium heat melt the butter. Add the shallots, garlic, spinach, chervil, flat-leaf parsley, tarragon, watercress, chives, thyme

 and salt, and cook it until the spinach is wilted but not mushy, about 3 minutes. Add the vermouth and cook until it has completely evaporated, 5 to 8 minutes. Add the heavy cream and simmer until it has thickened and reduced by half, about 15 minutes. Take the spinach off the heat and let it cool. Place in a blender and blend until smooth, about 1 to 2 minutes. Strain the sauce through a fine-mesh strainer and set aside.

Clean the mushrooms and place them in a large bowl filled with cold water for 5 minutes. Drain them and remove their stems. In a large saucepan over medium heat, place the mushrooms, wine, butter, and salt. Cover with a lid and cook until the mushrooms have softened and taken on a gray tone, about 10 minutes. Remove from the heat and set aside.

 Preheat the oven to 350°F (175°F).

 Cover a sheet pan with parchment paper, place the eel on it and place it in the oven for 10 minutes to warm it up.

To assemble the dish. Reheat the mushrooms and spinach sauce if necessary. Place a portion of the eel on each plate, spoon on spinach sauce, and surround it with 6 mushrooms. Garnish each with a sprig of chervil.

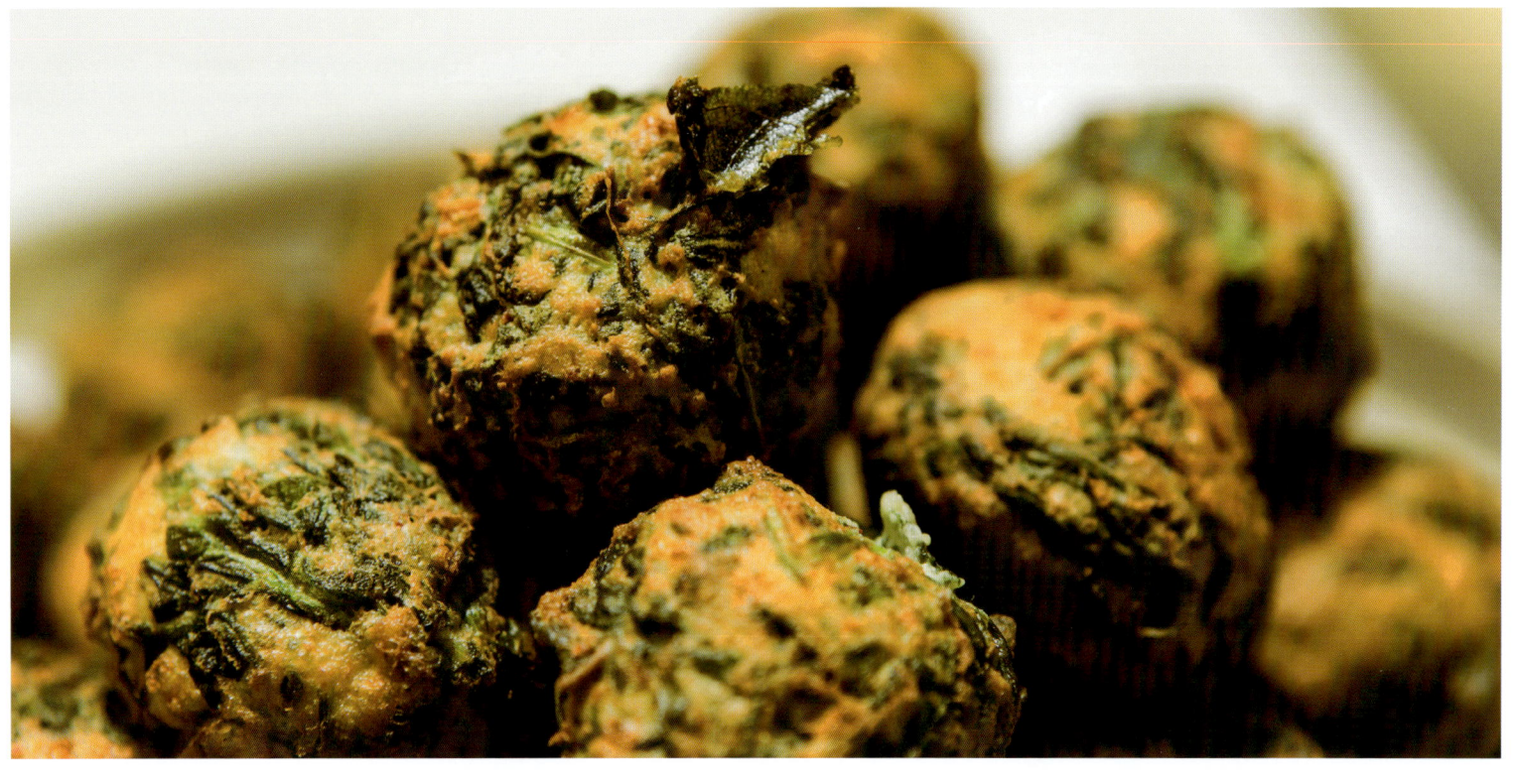

Ricotta-Spinach Gnocchi Fritters

with Marinara Sauce (Step By Step)

This recipe was a happy accident. I was making ricotta gnocchi, but messed up the dough, so I threw plug-shaped pasta into the deep-fryer. The results were phenomenal. Crispy on the outside, they were tender on the inside—and even better when dunked in warm marinara sauce. They're a great appetizer or an excellent side dish for the Cherry Beer–Braised Rabbit (page 142), Sole à l'Ostendaise (page 98), or Pork Chops with Blackwell Sauce (page 130). For the best flavor, use a high-quality buffalo mozzarella, which you can buy at good grocery stores and Italian import stores.

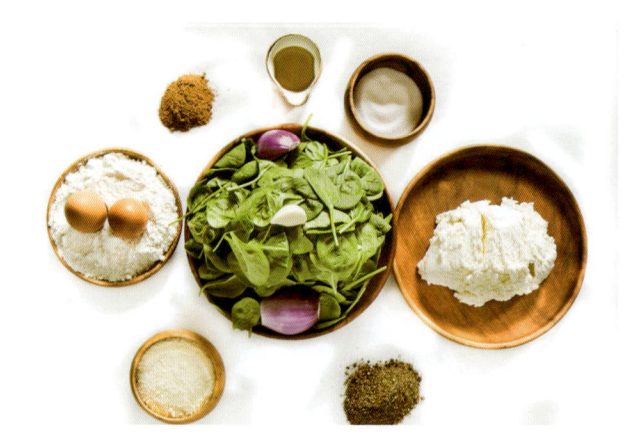

INGREDIENTS

1. 1 teaspoon (5 grams) canola oil, plus more for frying
2. 1/2 pound (5 cups/225 grams) fresh spinach, washed well
3. 1 medium shallot, finely diced
4. 2 cloves garlic, finely diced
5. 1 3/4 cup (400 grams) ricotta cheese
6. 1 cup + 1 tablespoon (140 grams) 00 flour
7. 2 large eggs (100 grams)
8. 3/4 cup (80 grams) grated Grana Padano cheese
9. 1 1/2 teaspoons (7 grams) kosher salt
10. 1 3/4 teaspoons (4 grams) freshly ground black pepper
11. 3/4 teaspoon (2 grams) freshly ground nutmeg
12. 1 3/4 teaspoons (4 grams) Espelette pepper
13. Coarse sea salt

DIRECTIONS

In large pot over high heat, heat the canola oil until shimmering. Add the spinach. Stir with a wooden spoon until the leaves have wilted, then add the shallot and garlic and mix until the ingredients are well combined and the garlic is fragrant, 30 to 60 seconds. Transfer the spinach mixture to a strainer set in the sink and drain. Press down on the spinach with the back of a spoon to remove as much moisture as possible[Image 1 through 8].

In a medium bowl, using a wooden spoon, mix together the ricotta, flour, eggs, cheese, kosher salt, black pepper, nutmeg, and Espelette pepper[Image 9].

Roughly chop the spinach leaves and add them to the ricotta mixture, mixing thoroughly with the wooden spoon. Cover and let sit for 1 hour at room temperature[Image 10].

To make the gnocchi, take 2-tablespoon (30 milliliter) scoops of the ricotta and spinach mixture and roll them by hand into balls about the size of ping pong balls. Cover a sheet pan with parchment paper, place the gnocchi on it, and store, covered, in the refrigerator for 2 hours[Image 11 and 12].

Cover a sheet pan with paper towels and set aside. Following the manufacturer's instructions, fill a deep-fryer with oil and heat it to 350°F (175°C). Using a slotted wooden spoon and working in batches, gently place the gnocchi in the oil and fry until deep golden brown, 3 to 5 minutes. Using the slotted spoon, remove them from the oil and place them on the prepared sheet pan. Sprinkle with sea salt while they are still warm and serve once all are cooked[image 13].

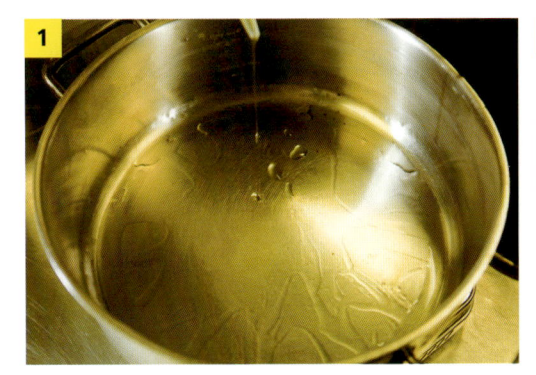

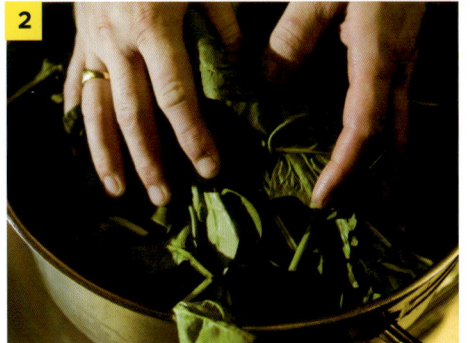

Stepwise Instructions

PAGE 80

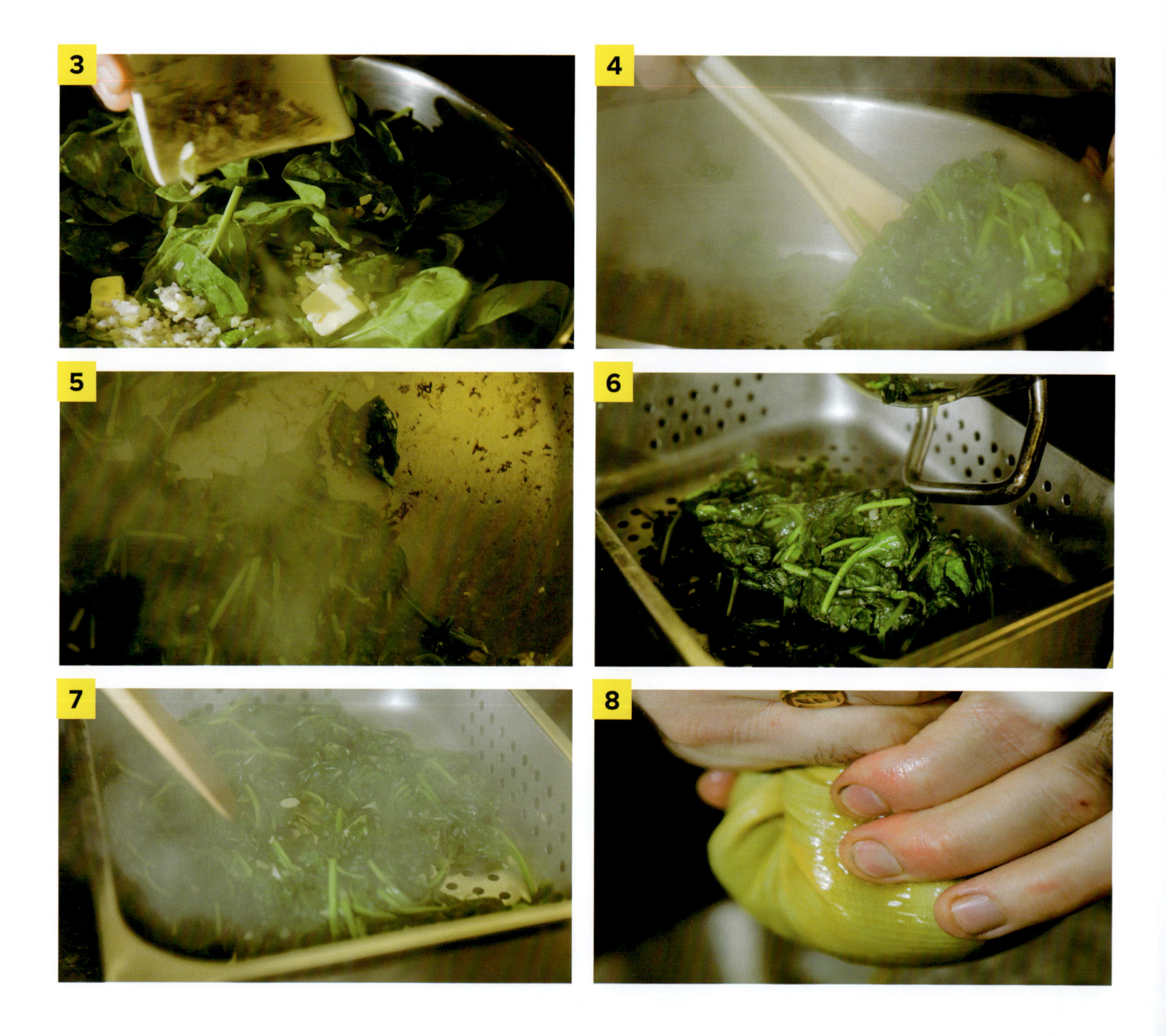

PAGE 81

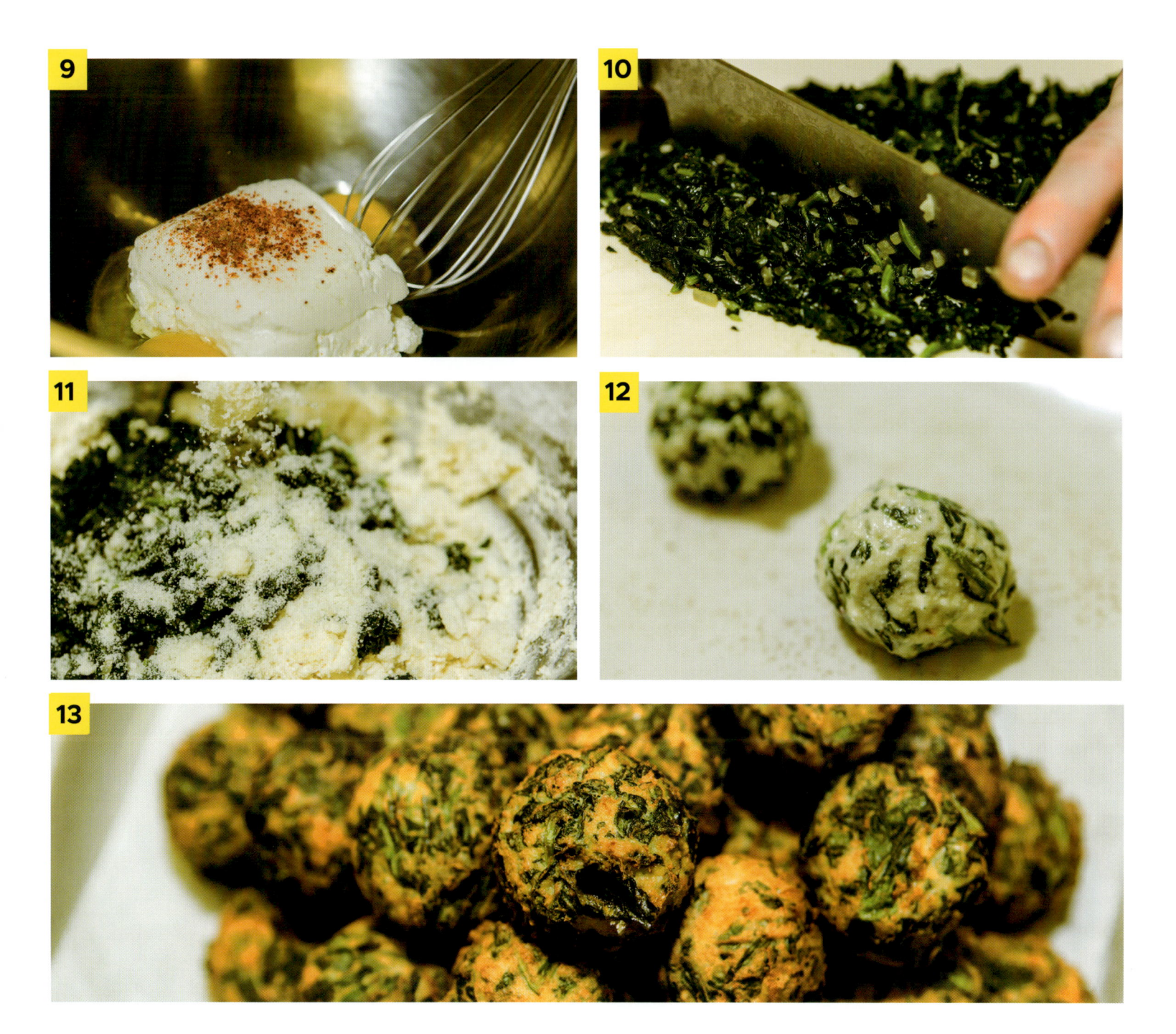

PAGE 82

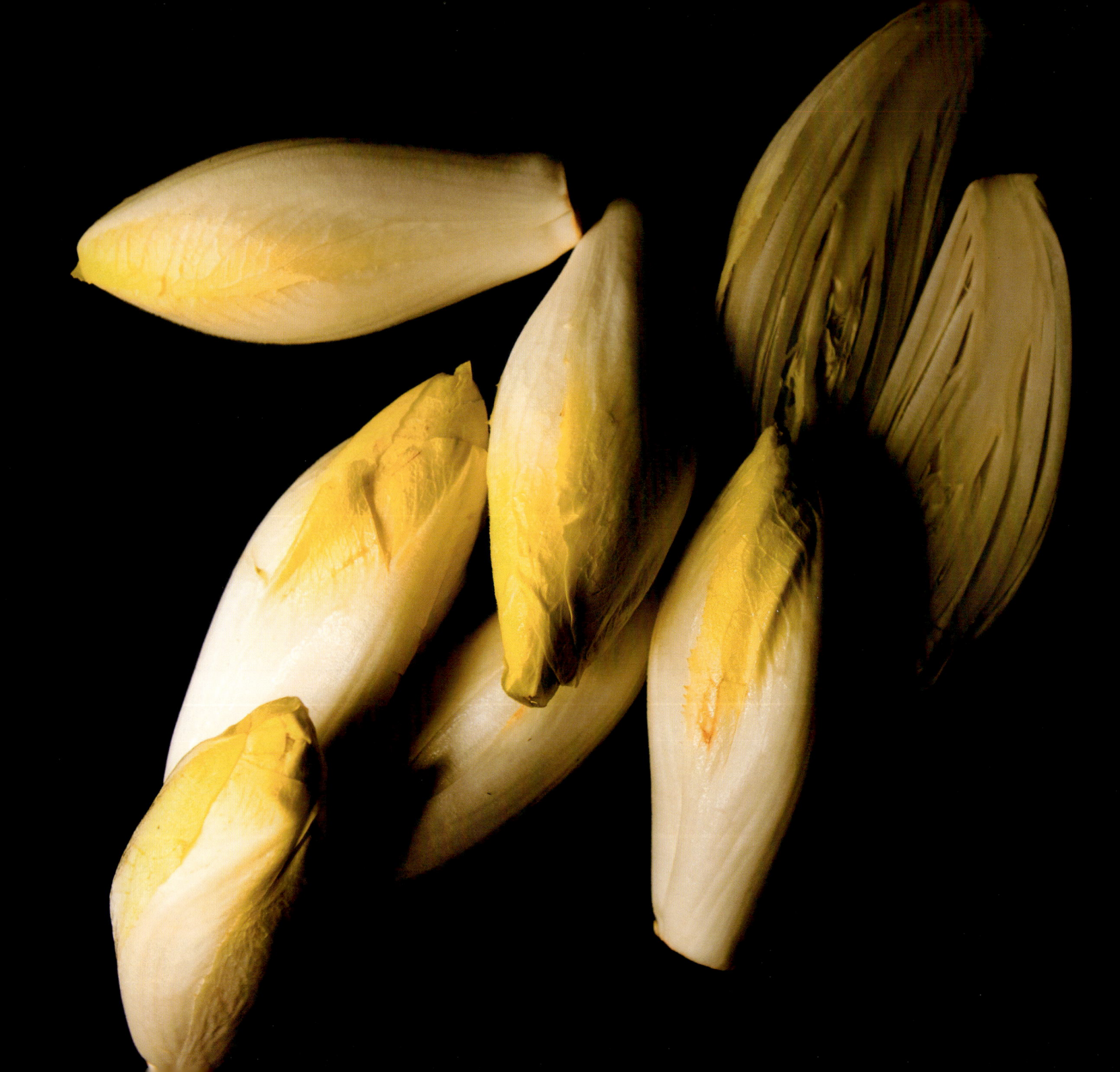

BELGIAN ENDIVE

Endive is practically the national vegetable of Belgium. Walloons (French speaking Belgians) call it chicon, while the Flemish word for it is witloof. It's a popular salad green, though it needs to be a paired with a sweet component to balance out its biting bitterness. When purchasing them, you want heads that aren't too big, but approximately the size of a pinecone. Inspect the leaves to ensure they're pure white with no brown speckles, and tightly packed. Buy them in season at a farmers' market. Imported varieties from Holland or Belgium are available year-round from good grocers.

22

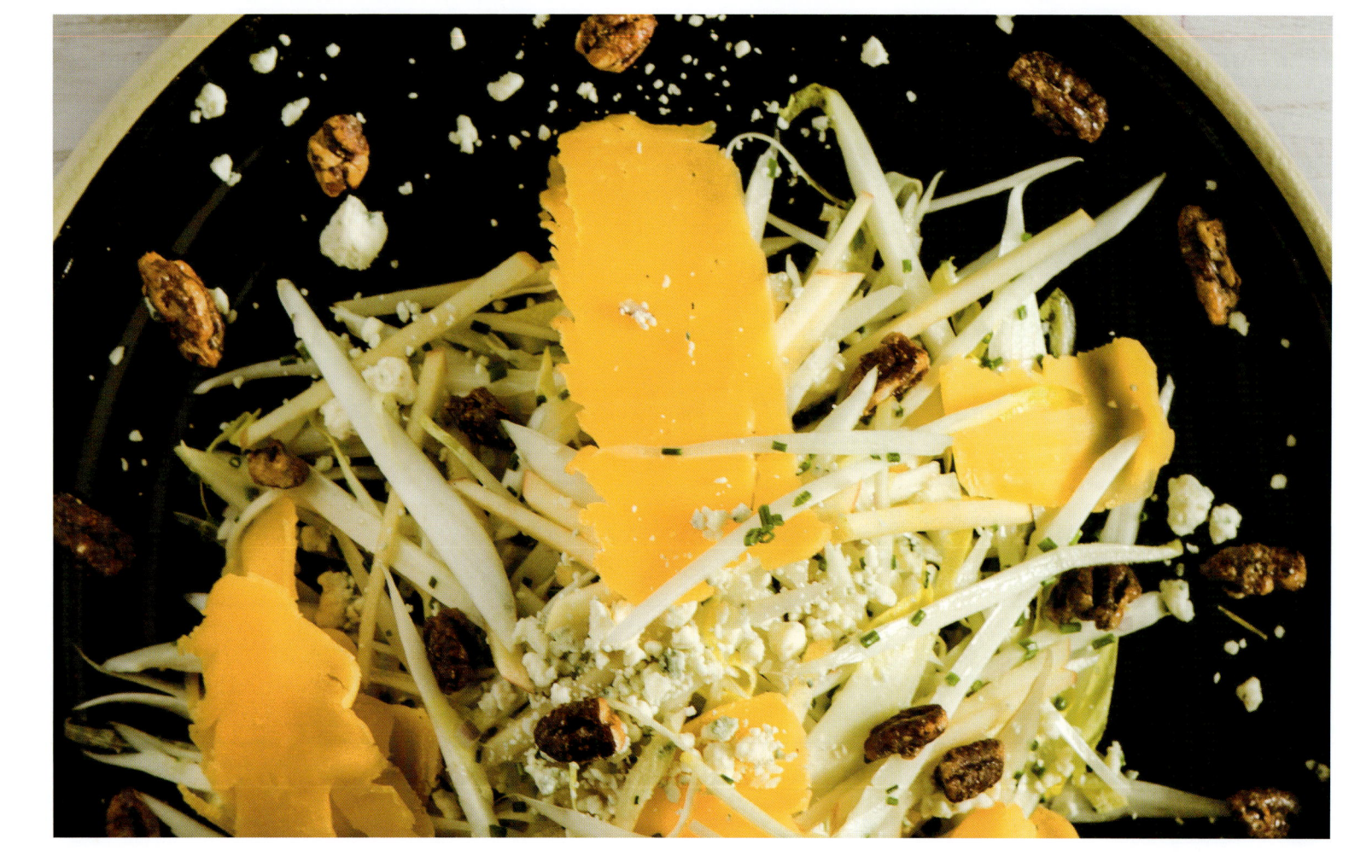

SERVES 4

Endive Salad with Chimay Cheese and Pecans

Endive shines in this stripped down, flavor-forward salad. The crunchy canoe-shaped leaves are lavished with garlicky vinaigrette, supremely creamy slices of Chimay Grand Classique cheese, and candied pecans. You can purchase Chimay at any grocery store with a respectable cheese section or a cheese specialty shop. If none is available, Gruyère is a good alternative.

INGREDIENTS

Dressing

1. 2 1/2 teaspoons (12 grams) Dijon mustard
2. 2 1/4 teaspoons (16 grams) honey
3. 2 1/4 teaspoons (6 grams) finely chopped garlic
4. 3 tablespoons (40 grams) mayonnaise (store-bought, or page 204)
5. 2 tablespoons (30 grams) extra virgin olive oil
6. 1 tablespoon (16 grams) freshly squeezed lemon juice

Salad

1. 6 large Belgian endives, cut in half lengthwise, centers removed, and cut into 1 1/2-inch (4 cm) pieces
2. 1/4 cup (36 grams) diced shallots
3. 1/4 cup (12 grams) chopped fresh chives
4. 3/4 teaspoon (3 grams) granulated sugar
5. 1 1/4 teaspoons (6 grams) kosher salt
6. 1/2 Gala apple or similar, peeled, cored, and diced
7. 3/4 cup (100 grams) diced Chimay cheese
8. 1/2 cup (60 grams) crumbled blue cheese
9. 1/2 cup (60 grams) candied pecan halves (store-bought)

DIRECTIONS

To make the dressing, in a medium bowl, gently whisk together the mustard, honey, garlic, and mayonnaise until well combined. Add the olive oil, whisking vigorously, until well combined. Add the lemon juice and whisk vigorously until well combined. Set aside.

In another medium bowl, using salad tongs toss together the endive, shallots, chives, sugar, salt, apples, and cheese. Pour half the dressing over the salad and gently toss again. Divide the salad between plates, drizzle with the remaining dressing, and garnish with blue cheese and pecans.
from the oil and place them on the prepared sheet pan. Sprinkle with sea salt while they are still warm and serve once all are cooked

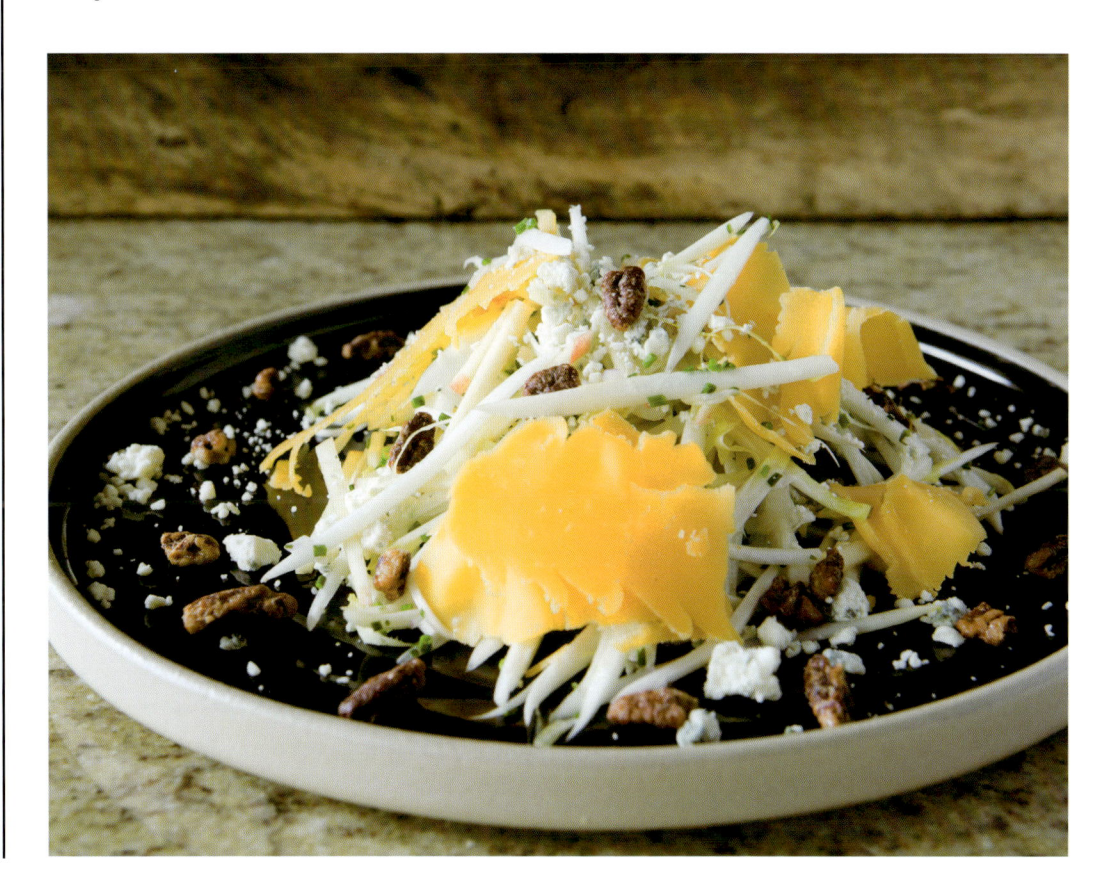

23

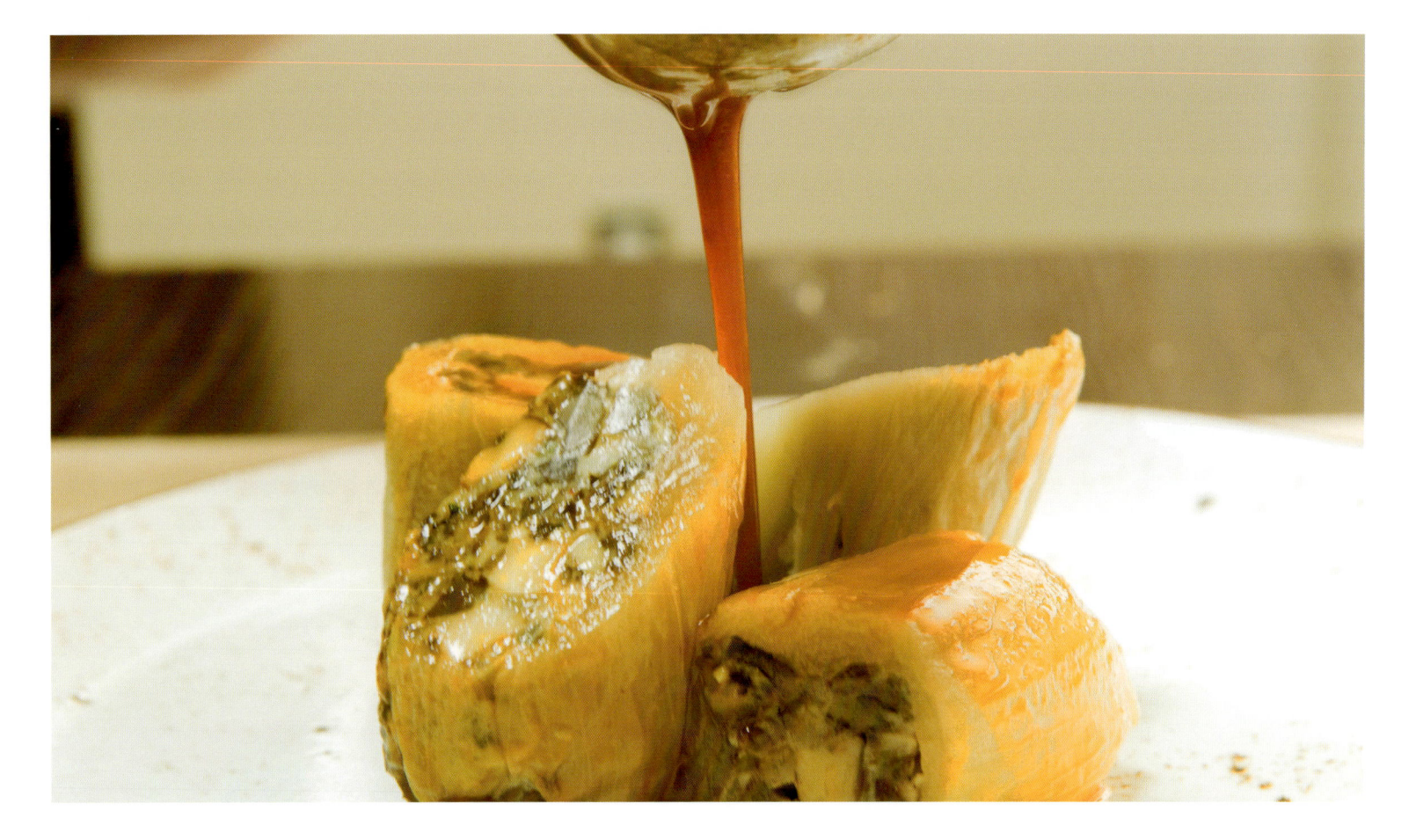

SERVES 2

Escargot-Stuffed Endive

When I was working in Belgium, I saw a chef reimagine an endive gratin by gently parting its leaves to stuff in the cheese and sauce. That gave me the idea for this preparation, which involves poaching the endive and opening it up like a flower. The folds are filled with an escargot-studded scallop mousse, then closed back up and poached a second time. I love the contrast between the toothsome leaves with their slightly bitter bite, the sweet brininess of the scallops, and the meaty chunks of snail coated with plenty of sautéed garlic and shallots. It's complemented by a honey-sweetened orange sauce that brightens everything up. I prefer to use Burgundy snails, which you can buy at some specialty grocers and online; CaviarLover.com has a good selection. Just make sure you buy unseasoned snails out of their shells.

INGREDIENTS

Endives
1. 8 tablespoons (1 stick/125 grams) unsalted butter
2. 1/2 teaspoon (3 grams) flaky sea salt
3. 1 1/2 teaspoons (6 grams) granulated sugar
4. 2 pinches of freshly grated nutmeg
5. 1 cup (200 grams) chicken stock (store-bought, or page 208)
6. 4 large Belgian endives

Scallop mousse
1. 7 ounces (200 grams) fresh sea scallops, trimmed
2. 1/2 teaspoon (3 grams) kosher salt
3. 1/4 teaspoon (2 grams) freshly ground black pepper
4. 1 large egg white (30 grams)
5. 1/4 cup + 1 tablespoon (65 grams) heavy cream

Snails
1. 1 1/2 cups (250 grams) shelled snails, drained
2. 4 tablespoons (1/2 stick/60 grams) unsalted butter, divided
3. 1/2 cup (50 grams) chopped shallots
4. 1 clove garlic, chopped

DIRECTIONS

To make the endives, in a medium pot with a tight-fitting lid, place the butter, sea salt, sugar, nutmeg, chicken stock, and endives. Bring to boil over high heat, then cover and reduce the heat to medium. Cook until the endives are tender and the tip of a knife goes through easily, approximately 40 minutes. Remove them from the liquid and place them on paper towel–lined plate. Set aside to cool.

Meanwhile, prepare the scallop mousse. In a food processor, mix the scallops with the salt and pepper until smooth, about 3 minutes. Add the egg white and mix again for 1 minute until combined. Add the cream and mix for another 2 minutes until everything is well combined. Place in a small bowl and keep it refrigerated while preparing the snails.

Rinse the snails under cold water and drain thoroughly. In a medium sauté pan over medium heat, melt the butter. Add the shallots and garlic and cook until fragrant, about 1 minute. Add the snails, mushrooms, and salt to taste. Cook until the mushrooms are slightly caramelized, 4 to 5 minutes. Carefully pour in the liqueur and stir, scraping the bottom of the pan to deglaze. Cook until the liquid is reduced by half, then stir in the chives. Place everything in a small container to cool to room temperature.

When the snail mixture is cool, chop all of it into small pieces. Incorporate this mixture into the scallop mousse, gently folding them together with a whisk or spatula. Season with salt and pepper to taste. Set aside.

Gently open the cooked endives leaf by leaf without cutting the bottom, as if you are peeling a banana. Carefully remove the center of the endive, being sure not to break the leaves. Working on a flat surface, place a 10-inch (25 cm) square of plastic wrap under each endive. Open an endive widely and gently spoon about 1/4 cups (60 milliliters) of the snail mixture in the middle. Cover the stuffing with the leaves, as if you are recomposing a flower. Roll the plastic around the endive and tightly close both ends by knotting them. Repeat with the remaining endives and snail mixture. Freeze any leftover snail mixture for next time or use it to fill small sausages or make little patties.

Fill a medium stew pot with a tight-fitting lid halfway with water and set over medium heat. Place in a metal strainer in the pot so the bottom of the strainer remains above the water. Bring the water to a boil. Place the wrapped endives in the strainer, cover with the lid, and cook until you can feel resistance from the cooked meat inside when you press the endives, about 25 minutes.

5. 1 cup (120 grams) cleaned, stemmed, and diced shiitake
6. mushrooms
   Kosher salt
7. 2 tablespoons + 1 teaspoon (30 grams) anise liqueur
8. 3 tablespoons (10 grams) chopped fresh chives
9. Flaky sea salt for garnish

To serve
1. 1/2 cup (200 grams) red wine sauce (page 210)

Using tongs, remove the endives from the pot and place them on sheet pan lined with a kitchen towel. Cut the knots off both ends and gently remove the plastic wrap. Let them drain for a few seconds on the towel. Cut them in half vertically and place them on a serving platter.

In a small pot over medium heat, warm the red wine sauce until just hot. Spoon about 2 tablespoons of the sauce on each endive and serve immediately.

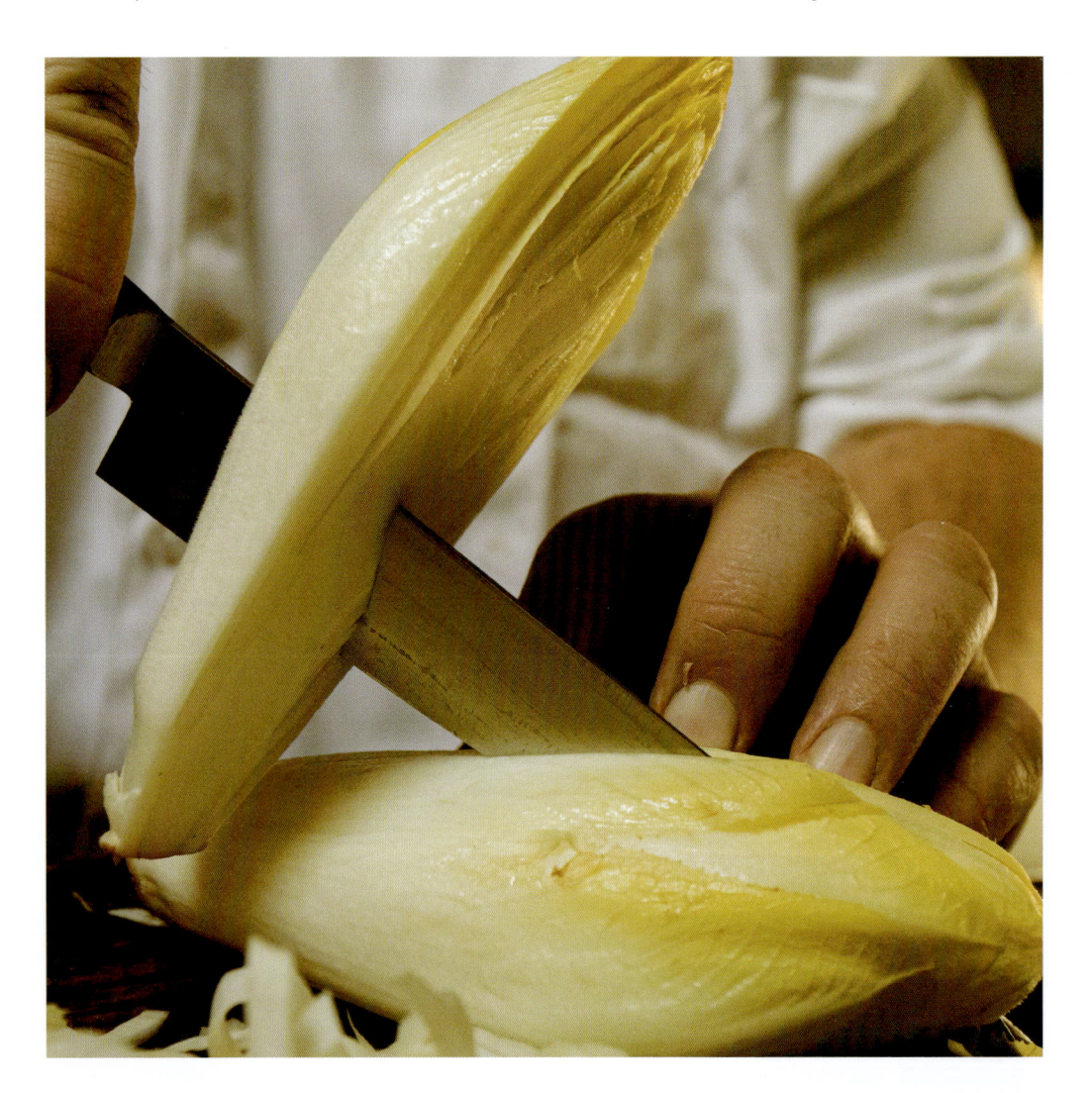

24

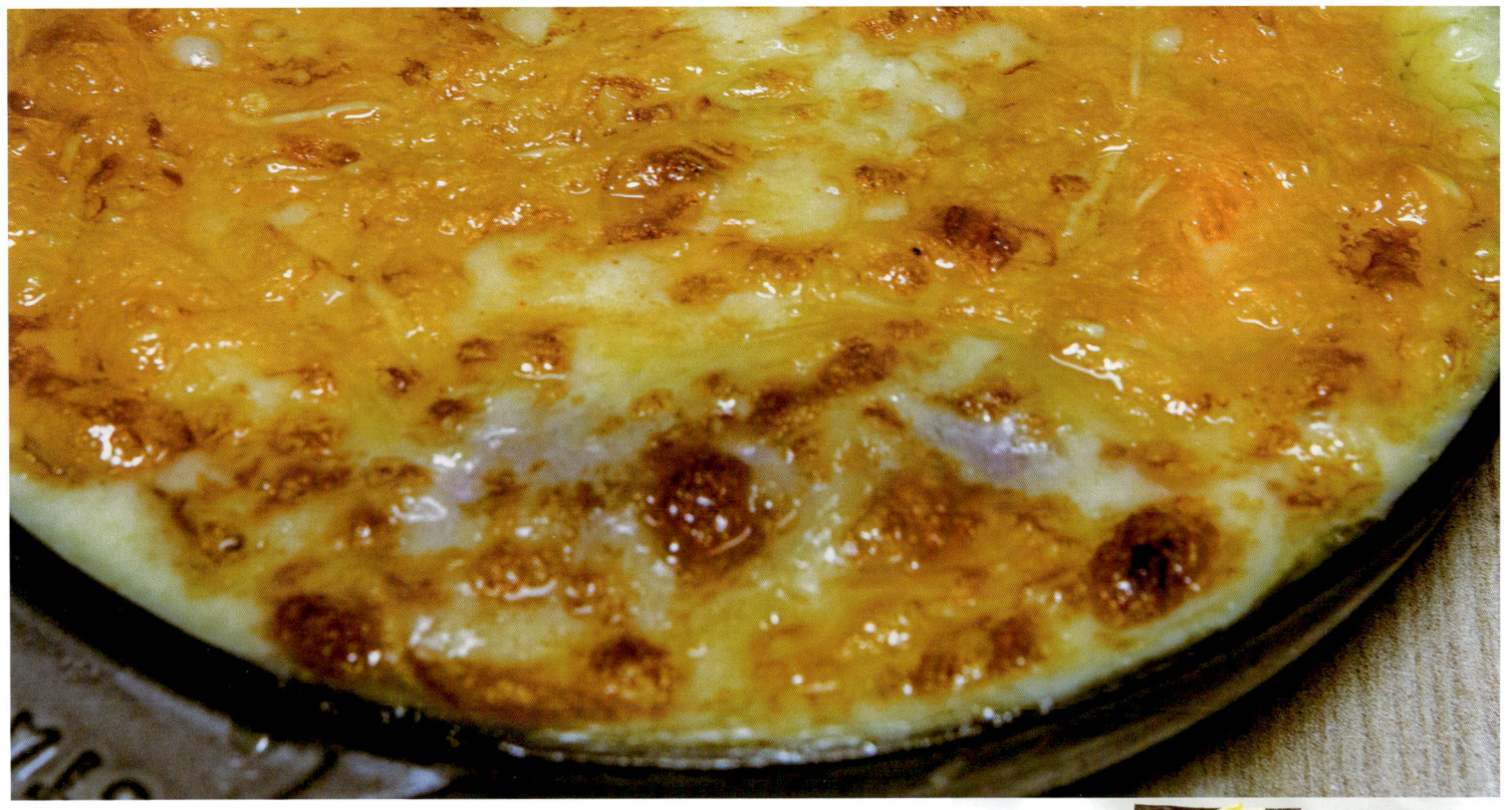

SERVES 4

Endive Gratin

(Step By Step)

Growing up, this dish would always be on the menu when friends invited us over for Sunday supper during the winter. It's very rich, packed with well-aged Gruyère, an ocean of béchamel, and lots of thin-sliced deli ham. I like leaving it under the under the broiler until the cheesy top is bubbling, while its edges are caramelized and crispy.

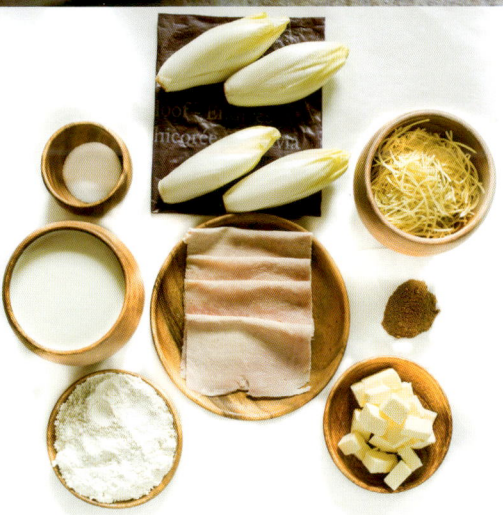

PAGE 89

INGREDIENTS

1. 4 large Belgium endives
2. 8 tablespoons (1 stick/125 grams) unsalted butter, divided
3. 1 1/2 teaspoons (8 grams) granulated sugar
4. 2 pinches of freshly grated nutmeg, divided
5. 1 1/2 teaspoons (8 grams) kosher salt, divided
6. 1 quart (1 liter) whole milk
7. 2 teaspoons (4 grams) Espelette pepper
8. 1/2 cup + 2 tablespoons (80 grams) all-purpose flour
9. 2 3/4 cups (300 grams) grated Gruyère

DIRECTIONS

- Cut out a circle of parchment paper to fit inside a large stew pot.
- In the pot, over medium heat, place the endives, 4 tablespoons (60 grams) of the butter, 1/2 cup (125 grams) water, the sugar, 1 pinch of the nutmeg, and 1/2 teaspoon (3 grams) of the salt. Cover with the parchment and cook until the endives are tender and a knife passes through them without any resistance, about 30 minutes. Remove the endives from the pot and drain them in a colander set in the sink, discarding the liquid in the pot.[Images 1, 2 & 10]
- While the endives are cooking, place a large saucepan over high heat and add the milk, the remaining salt, remaining nutmeg, and the Espelette pepper and bring to a boil. As soon as the mixture is boiling, take the saucepan off the heat.[Image 7]
- In another large saucepan over medium heat, melt the remaining 4 tablespoons (60 grams) butter, then add the flour. Mix with a whisk until the mixture is completely smooth without any clumps. [Image 3 & 4]
- Add the milk mixture to the butter mixture and whisk until thoroughly combined. Let the mixture cook until it is thickened and clings to a spoon, about 20 minutes. [Image 5 & 6]
- Remove saucepan from the stove and add 1/2 cup (55 grams) of the Gruyère. Mix with a wood spatula until the cheese is totally melted and the sauce is smooth. Set aside. [Image 8 & 9]
- Preheat the oven to 375°F (190°C). Place a slice of ham on a clean work surface and position an endive along one short edge. Roll it up so the ham completely covers the endive. Repeat with the remaining endives. [Image 11 & 12]
- In a 9-inch (23 cm) square metal baking pan, spread a generous spoonful of the sauce at the bottom.
- Lay the endives in the pan. Pour the remaining sauce on top, ensuring they are completely covered. [Image 13]
- Sprinkle the remaining Gruyère evenly across the surface. [Image 14]
- Bake the gratin until it bubbles and the surface is pale gold, about 30 minutes. Turn on the broiler and broil until the top is crisp and golden, 5 to 10 minutes. Let cool for 10 minutes before serving.

PAGE 91

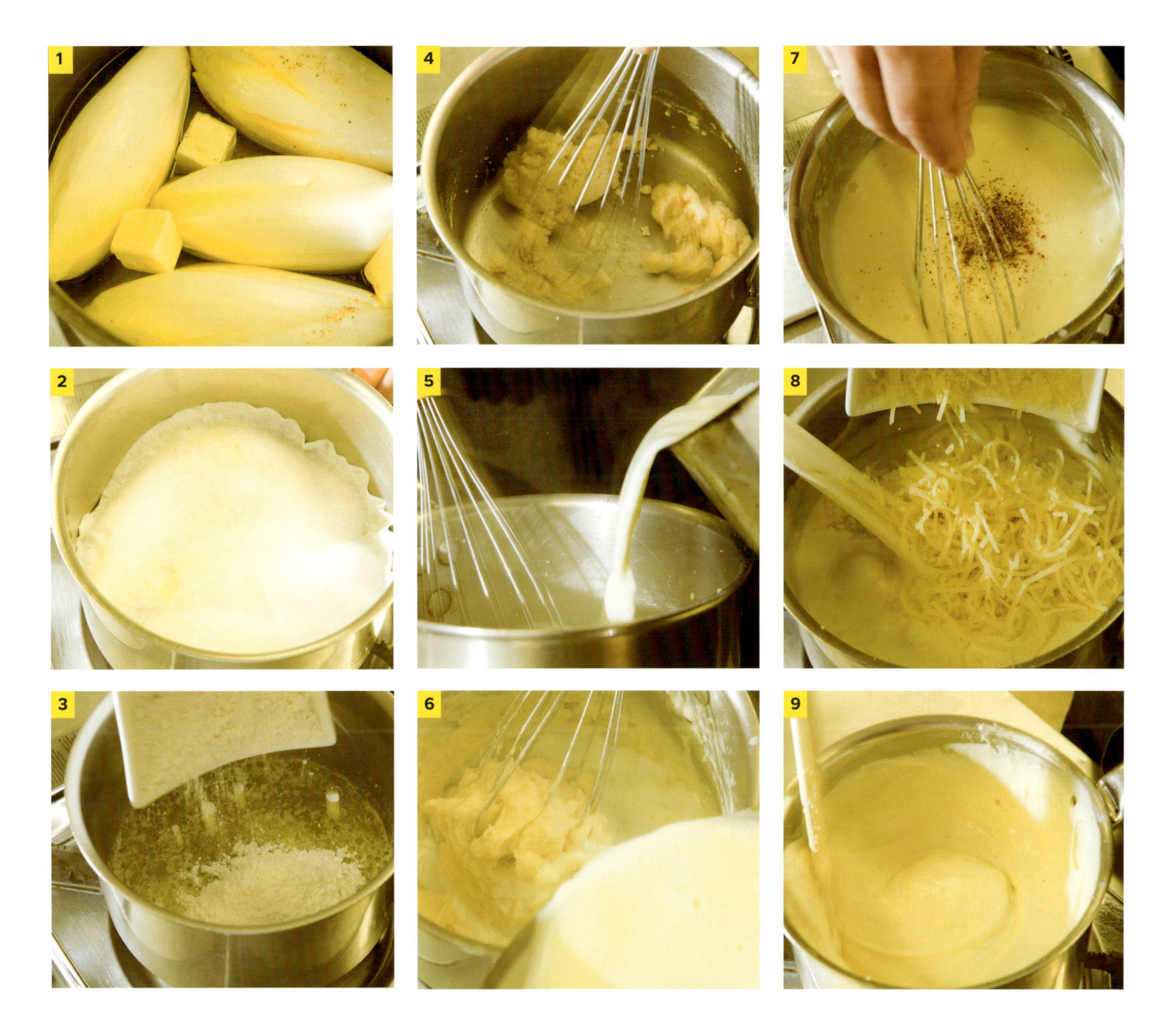

PAGE 92

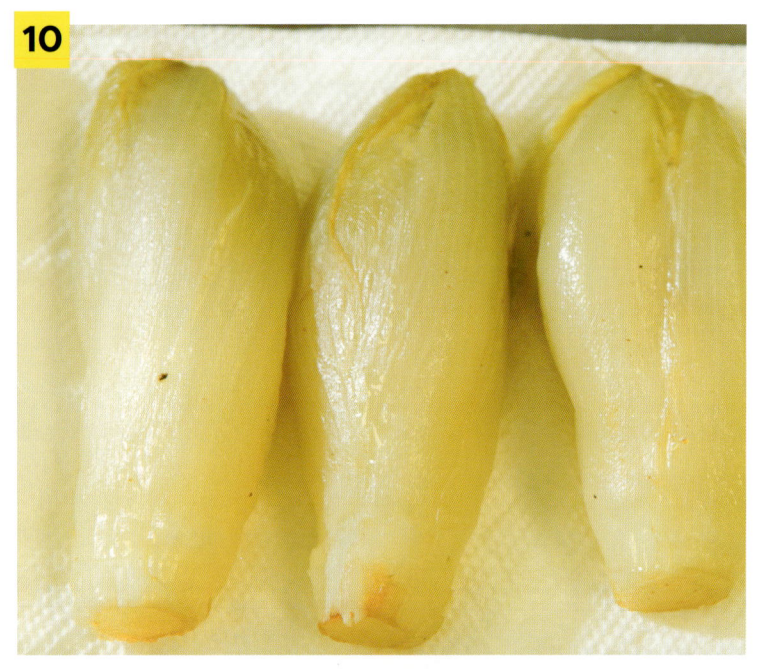

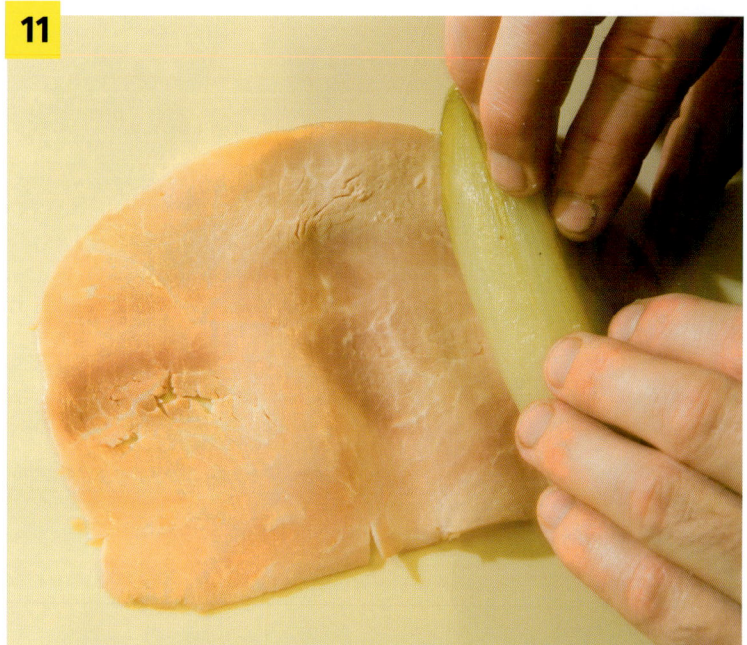

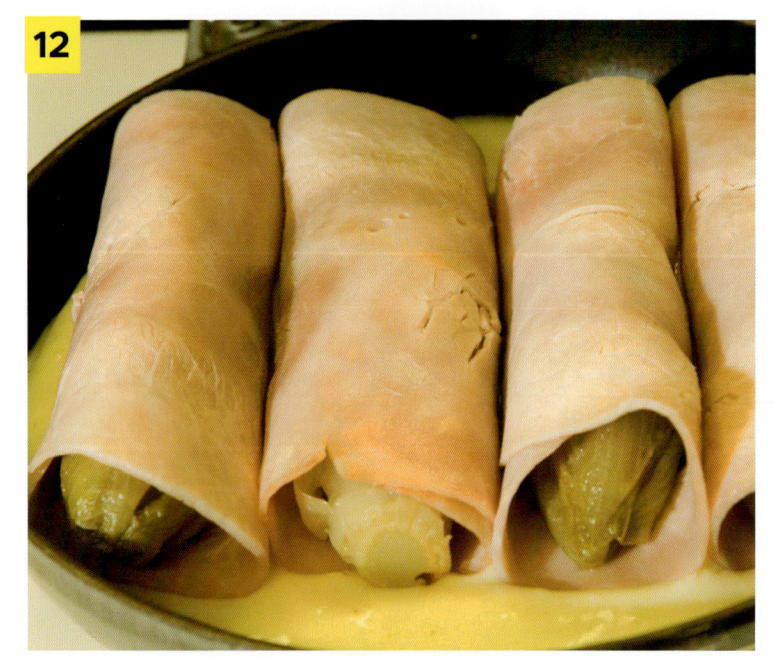

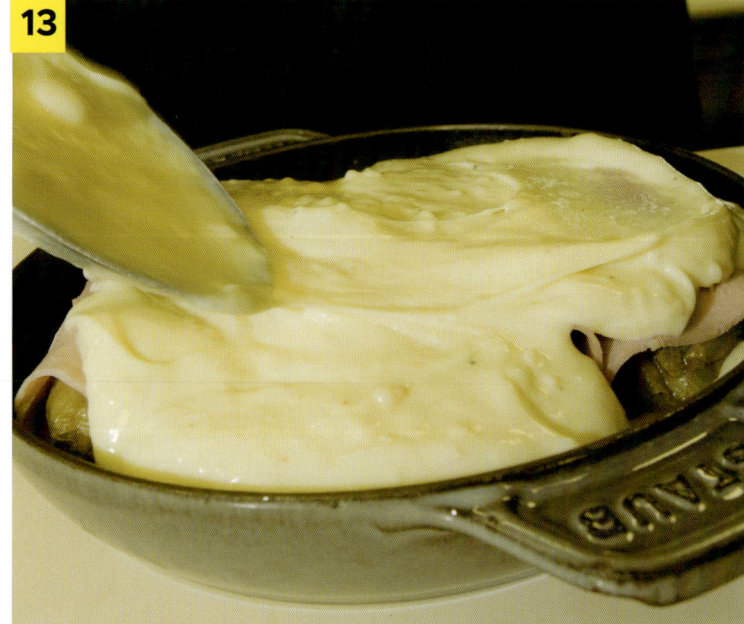

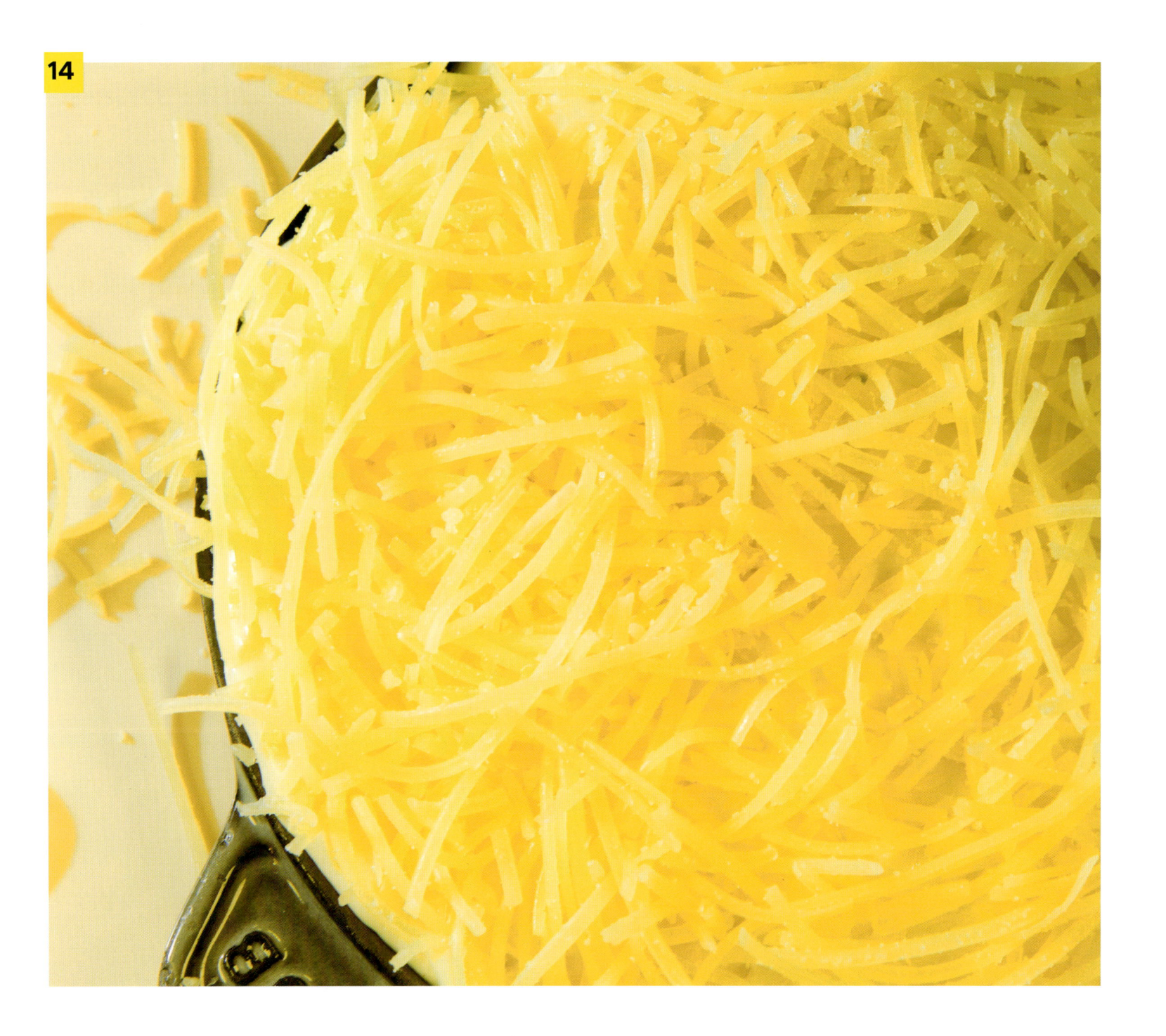

14

PAGE 94

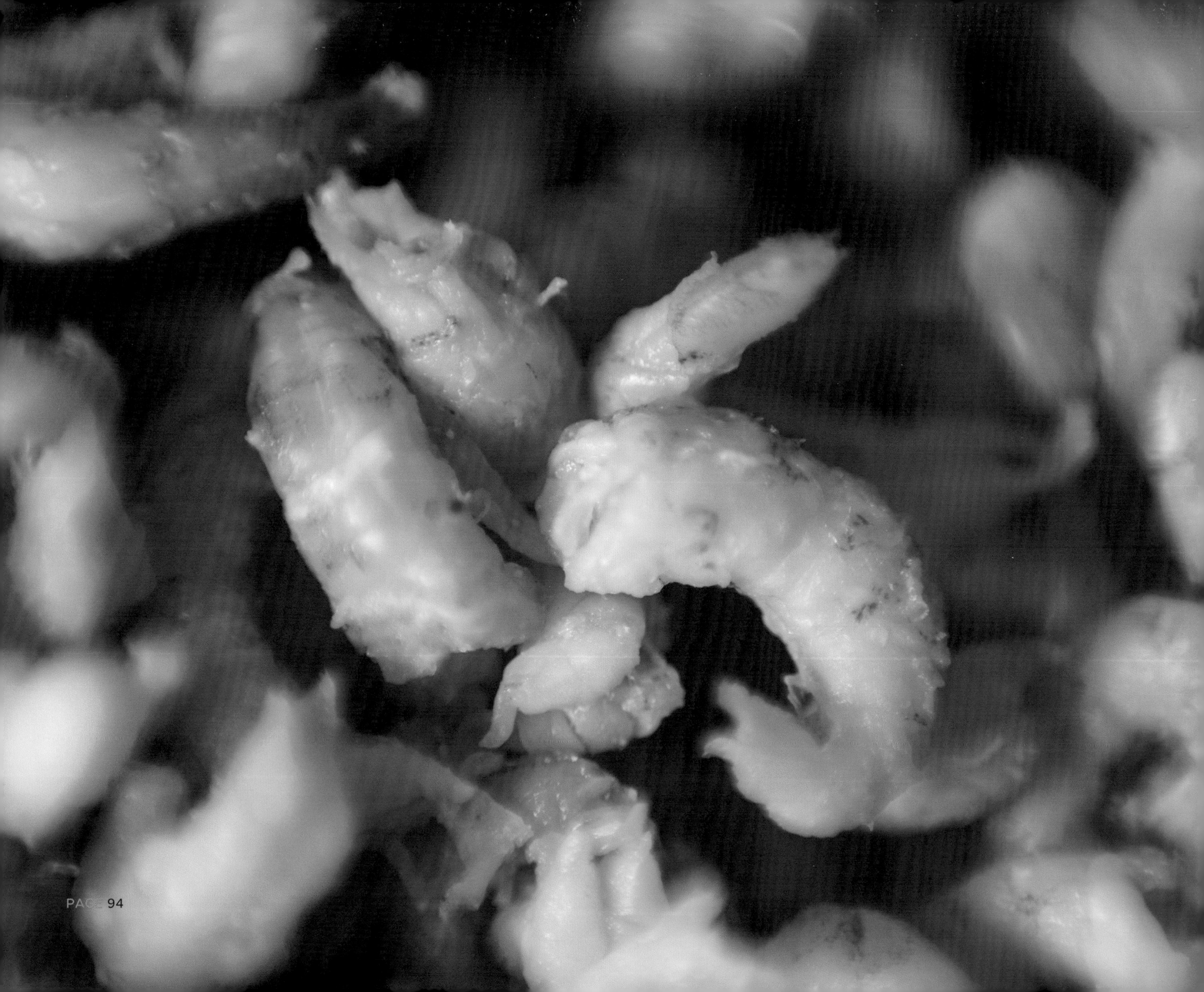

GRAY SHRIMP

Harvested from the North Sea, gray shrimp are smaller than those pulled out of the Gulf of Mexico. They're also a little sweeter and more flavorful than their Atlantic brethren. You can eat them raw right out of their shells; they go down well with a Hoegaarden. They are difficult to source in the States, though some upper-crust seafood counters stock them.

25

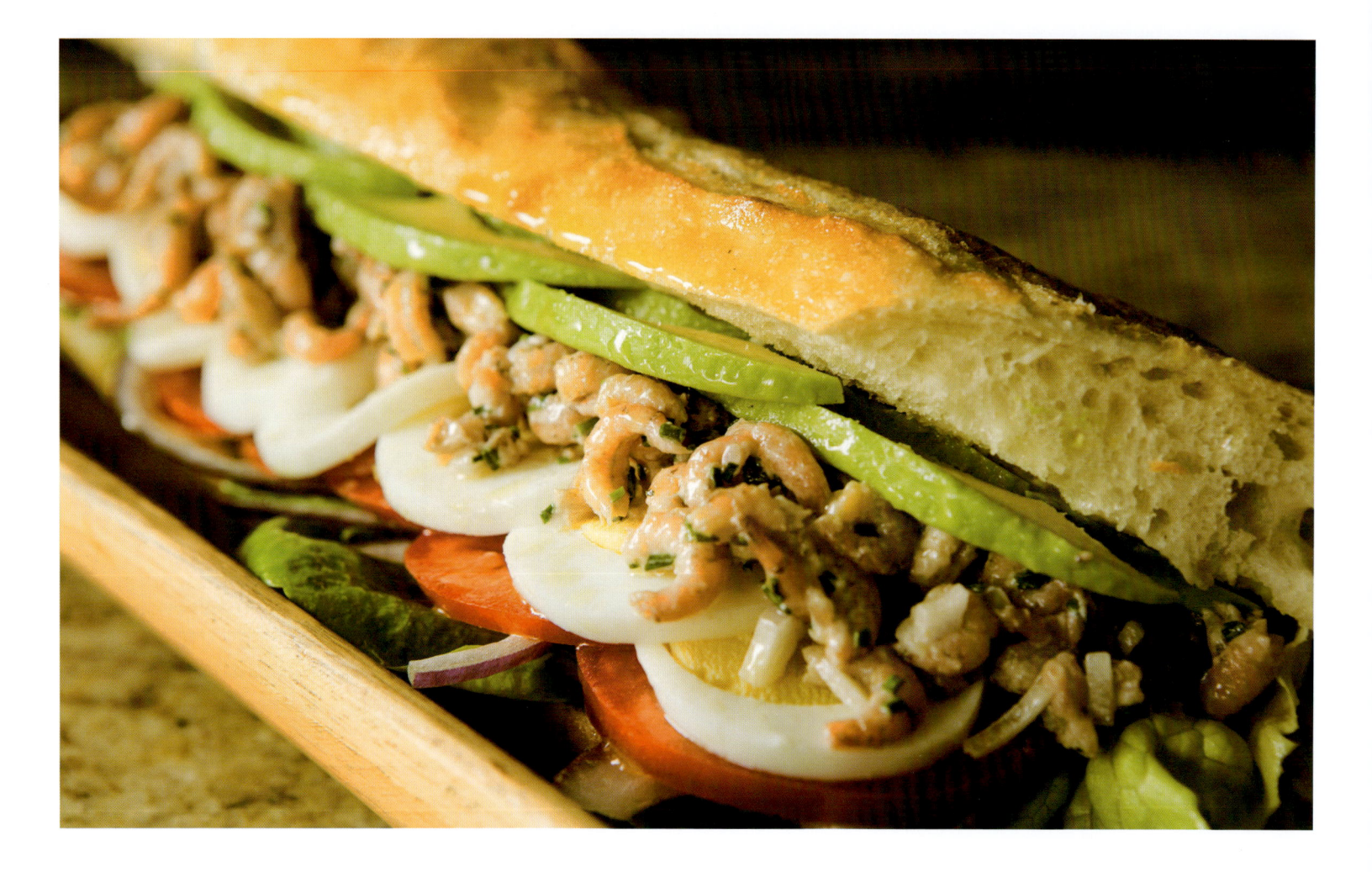

SERVES 2

Shrimp Club Sandwich

The club sandwich has endured since it was created in the late 19th century at the Saratoga Club House in Saratoga Springs, New York. I love the classic, but I wanted to give it a Belgian bent. My version features shrimp salad accented with parsley, lemon juice, and shallots. The sandwich is filled out with hard-boiled eggs, red onions, avocado, and fresh tomato rounds. Serve it at brunch, afternoon tea, or a summertime picnic, with a side salad if you like. Gray shrimp come peeled and are small enough you don't need to dice them.

INGREDIENTS

1. 1 cup (100 grams) gray shrimp, cooked and peeled
2. 1 medium shallot, finely diced
3. 2 tablespoons (7 grams) chopped curly parsley
4. 1/4 cup (32 grams) mayonnaise (store-bought, or page 204)
5. 1/4 teaspoon (1.5 grams) kosher salt
6. Juice of 1/2 lemon
7. 2 large eggs (100 grams)
8. 1 baguette, cut in half horizontally, then crosswise
9. 6-8 leaves from the heart of a head of Boston lettuce, leaves separated, washed, and dried
10. 1 large tomato (preferably on the vine), sliced into rounds
11. 1 avocado, pitted, peeled, and cut lengthwise into slices
12. 1/2 medium red onion, sliced into thin rounds

DIRECTIONS

In a medium bowl, using a spatula, mix together the shrimp, shallots, parsley, mayonnaise, salt, and lemon juice. Set aside.

In a medium saucepan over high heat, place the eggs and cover them completely with cold water. Bring the water to a boil and then cook them for 13 minutes. Remove the saucepan from the heat and run the eggs under cold water. Peel the eggs and cut them into 1/4-inch (6 mm) slices.

To make the sandwich, use the two flat bottom halves of the baguette. Place several lettuce leaves on the bottom, pile half of the shrimp salad on each, and then top them with tomato, avocado, onion, and eggs. Complete each sandwich with the remaining baguette pieces.

26

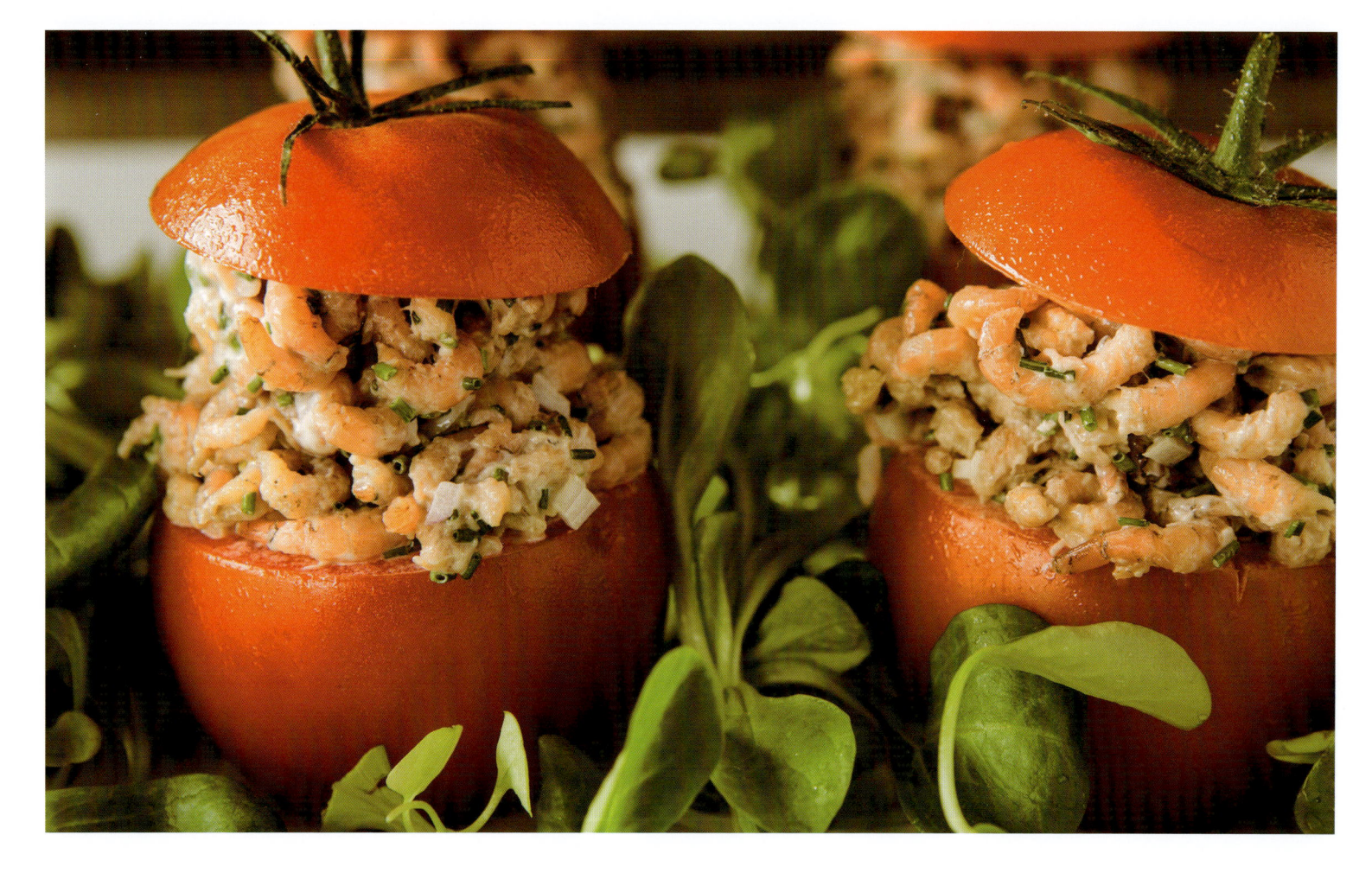

SERVES 4

Stuffed Tomato with Shrimp Salad

My mother used to make tomates farcies (tomatoes stuffed with beef, pork, or veal) based on a recipe she learned from the family for whom she worked. I fell hard for the dish, and my love has endured. When I return home in the summertime and tomatoes are in season, I always ask her to make them for me. If I ever come across stuffed tomatoes at a brasserie or bistro in Belgium, I always order them—but they never compare to my mother's version. This rendition switches in a gray shrimp and egg salad for the usual ground beef, giving it a summery sensibility

INGREDIENTS

1. 8 medium tomatoes (preferably on the vine)
2. Kosher salt
3. 2 large eggs (100 grams)
4. 1 pound (450 grams) gray shrimp, cooked and peeled
5. 1/4 cup + 1 tablespoon (50 grams) diced shallots
6. 1/4 + 3 tablespoons (20 grams) chopped fresh chives
7. Grated zest of 2 limes
8. 2 tablespoons (30 grams) freshly squeezed lemon juice
9. 3/4 cup (150 grams) mayonnaise
10. One 5-ounce (150 gram) container mixed salad greens, washed and dried
11. 3 tablespoons (45 grams) balsamic dressing (store-bought, or page 201)

DIRECTIONS

Cut off the top of each tomato off, about 1/2 inch (1 cm) down from the top. Using a spoon, scoop out the seeds and core, leaving the exterior intact to create a bowl inside. Salt the interior of the tomatoes and place them upside down on a paper towel–covered plate to allow the juices to drain out. Let sit for about 10 minutes.

Put the eggs in a small pot filled with cold water, bring them to a boil over medium-high heat, and cook for 13 minutes. Pour off the water and run cold water over the eggs until they are cool. Peel the eggs and place them in a large bowl. Cut them in half, then crush them with a fork until crumbled. Add the gray shrimp, shallots, chives, lime zest, lemon juice, and mayonnaise and fold the ingredients together using a spatula. Add salt to taste.

Gently toss the salad greens with the balsamic dressing.

To assemble, fill each tomato with gray shrimp salad. Plate each one on a small mound of dressed salad.

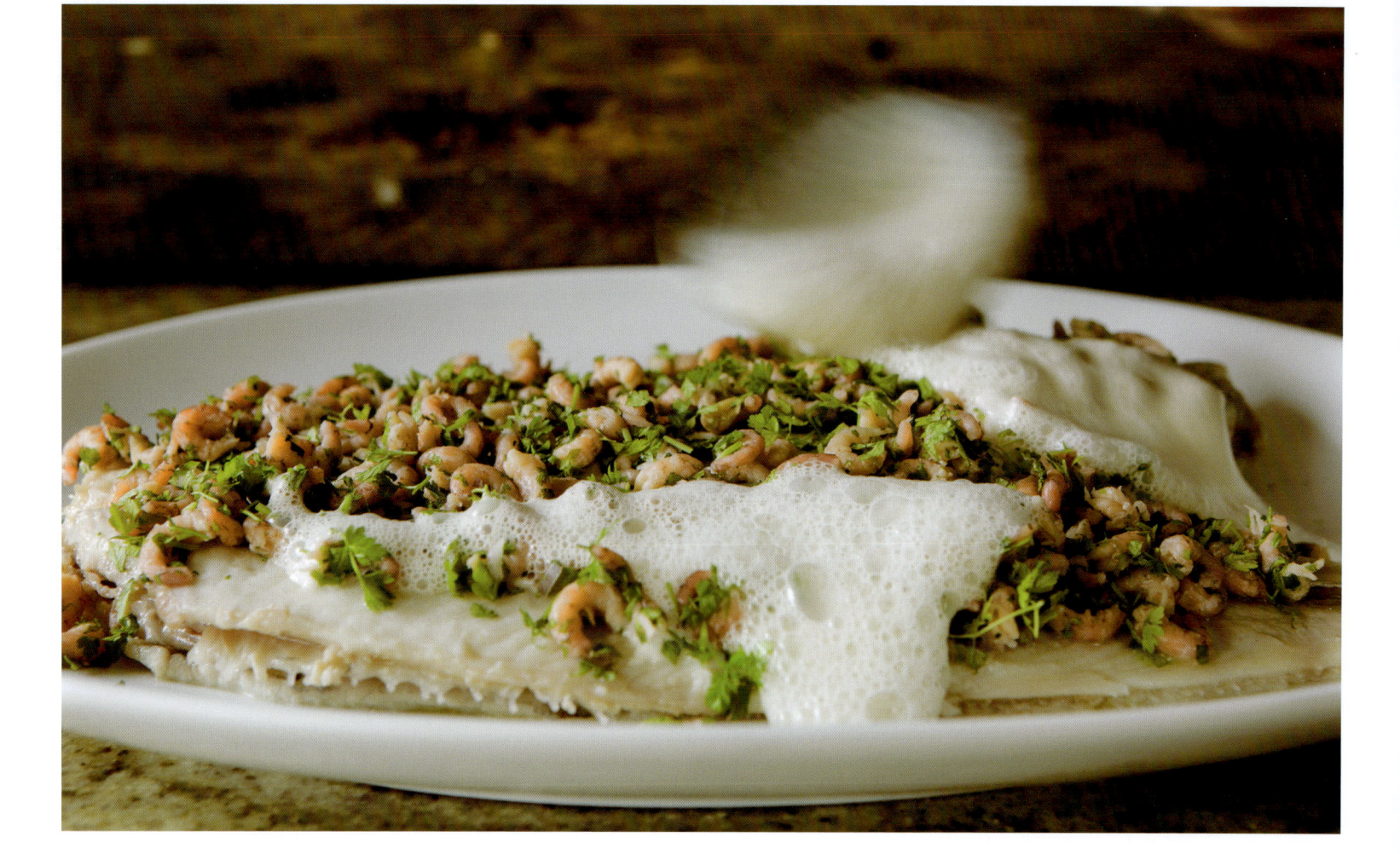

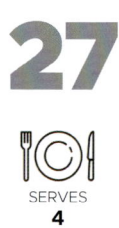

Sole à l'Ostendaise

(Step By Step)

27

SERVES 4

This is one of those dishes that looks impressive but requires impressively little work. Simply poach the sole in white wine and butter. Once the fish is cooked, you reduce the cooking liquid before adding cream and gray shrimp. After the mixture generously coats the back of a spoon, pour it over the fish. Dover sole is widely available at fishmongers and grocery store seafood counters. I prefer Norwegian sole, because the flesh has a sweet edge to it.

INGREDIENTS

1. 2 large whole sole (approximately 1 1/2 pounds/700 grams each)
2. Kosher salt and freshly ground black pepper
3. 8 tablespoons (1 stick/125 grams) unsalted butter, divided
4. 2 medium shallots, finely chopped
5. 3/4 cup (150 grams) dry white wine
6. 2 cups (500 milliliters) mussel juice (page 205)
7. 3/4 cup (200 grams) heavy cream
8. Juice of 1 lemon, strained
9. 1 tablespoon (3 grams) chopped fresh chervil
10. 1 cup (100 grams) gray shrimp, cooked and peeled

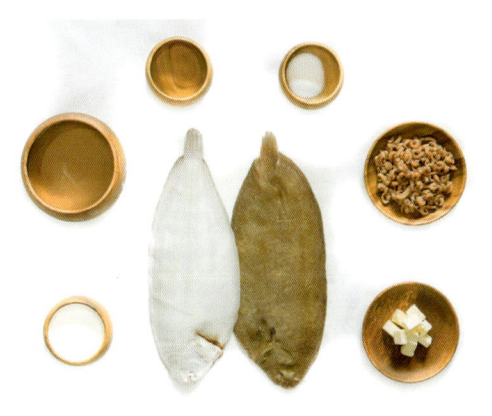

DIRECTIONS

Clean the sole by removing the skin on both sides. Remove all the organs and the eggs (if any), then cut off the head. Keep all the trimming, except the gills and eggs, to make fish stock (page 206).

Preheat the oven to 350°F (175°C). Season the sole on both sides with salt and pepper.
In large cast-iron skillet over medium heat, melt 4 tablespoons (60 grams) of the butter. Add the shallots and sauté until translucent, about 5 minutes. Add the wine and bring it to a boil. Turn off the heat, place the sole in the pan and cover with parchment paper, so it is pressed down against the fish.

Place the skillet in the oven and cook the sole for 7 minutes. To check if they are cooked, press your finger into the middle of the sole. If the meat easily separates, it's done. Remove the sole from the skillet, place them on a sheet pan, and cover them with the same parchment paper. Set aside.
Strain the juices from the skillet into a medium saucepan set over medium heat. Add the mussel juice, bring to a simmer, and let the liquid reduce by half, 10 to 12 minutes. Add the heavy cream and reduce it again by half, 10 to 12 minutes more. Cut the remaining 4 tablespoons (60 grams) butter into small cubes and add them one at a time, whisking thoroughly in between each addition. Use an immersion blender to mix vigorously until the sauce is frothy, about 1 minute. Add the lemon juice and mix again for 1 minute, until fully incorporated. Using a wooden spoon, fold in the chervil and gray shrimp. Remove from heat and set aside.

To bone the fish, run a spoon along the center of the fillet. Push both sides off the bones using a fork. This will expose the spine. Slide the spoon under the bones and gently lift up. Place fillets in a large casserole dish.

To warm the sole fillets, heat them in the oven at 250°F (120°C) for 5 minutes. Plate the fillets and cover each one with the sauce and shrimp. Serve immediately.

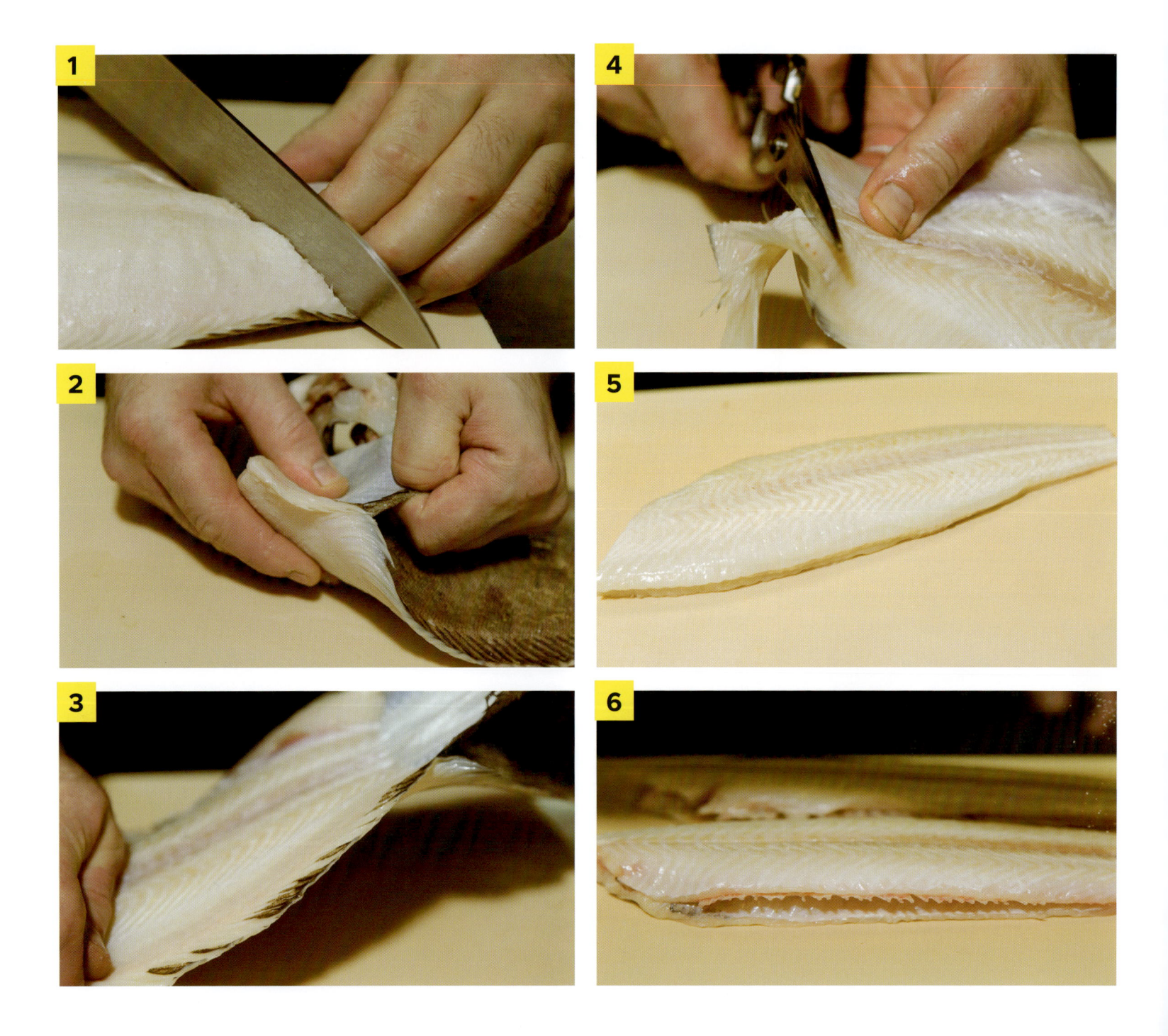

PAGE 103

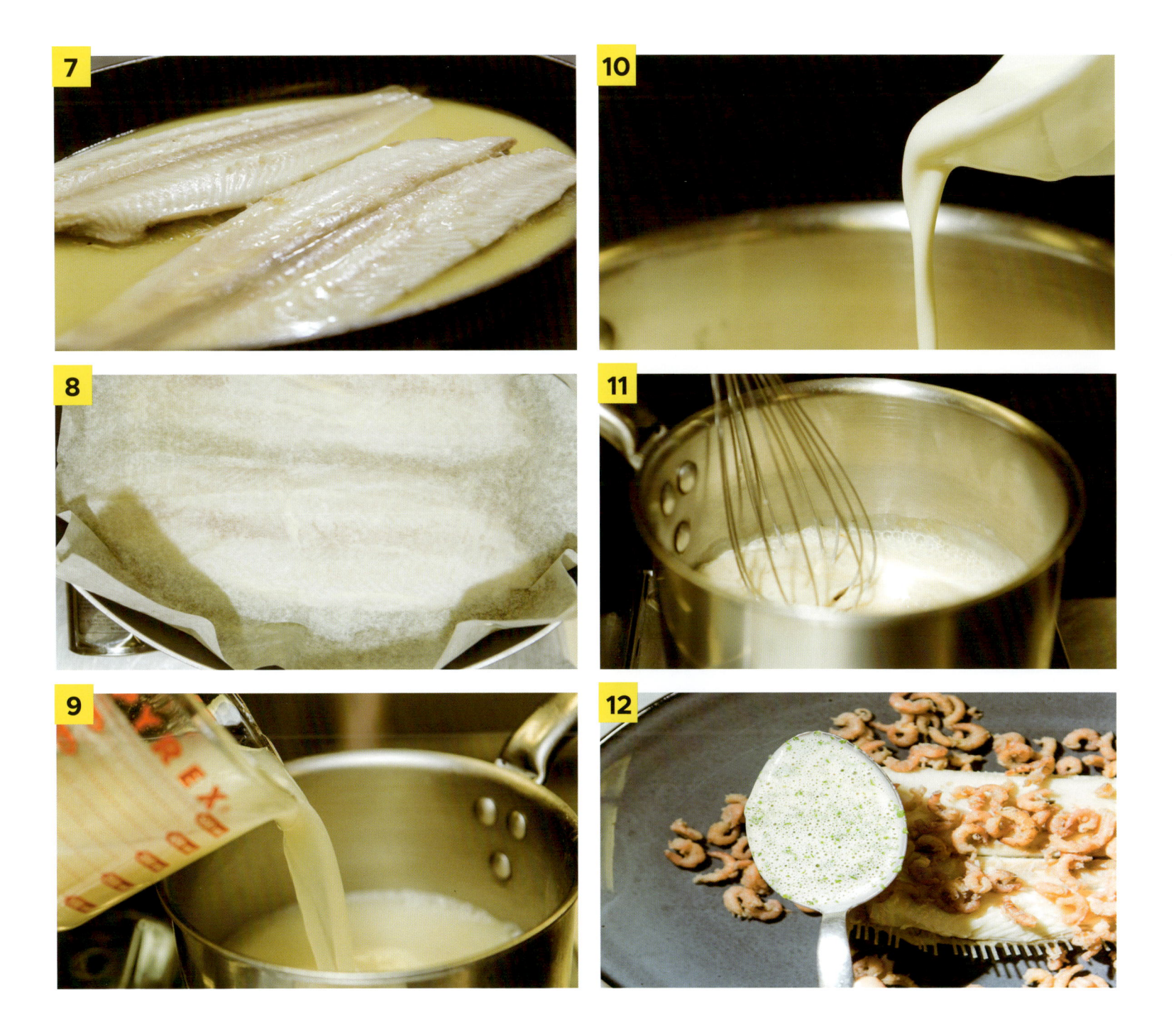

Steps to Debone the fish

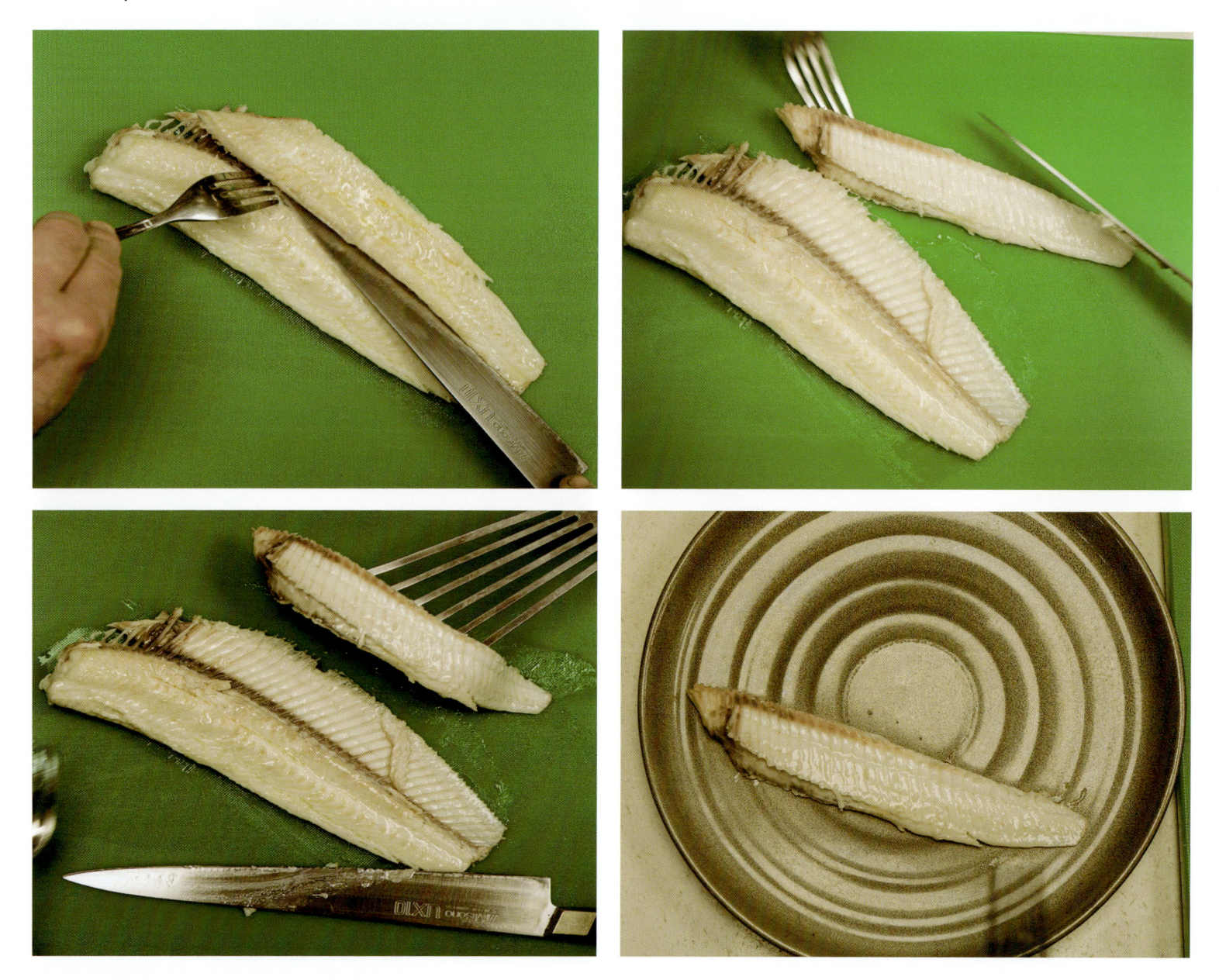

PAGE 105

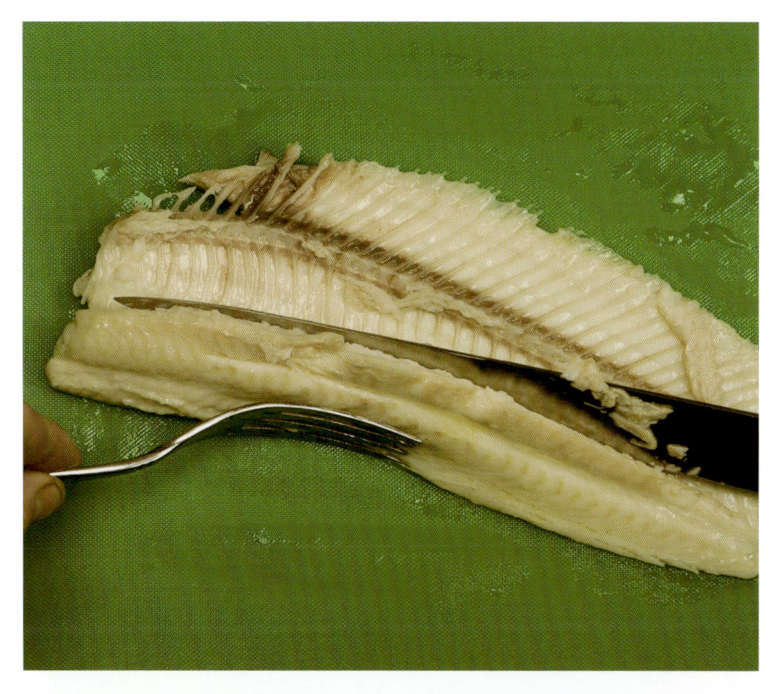

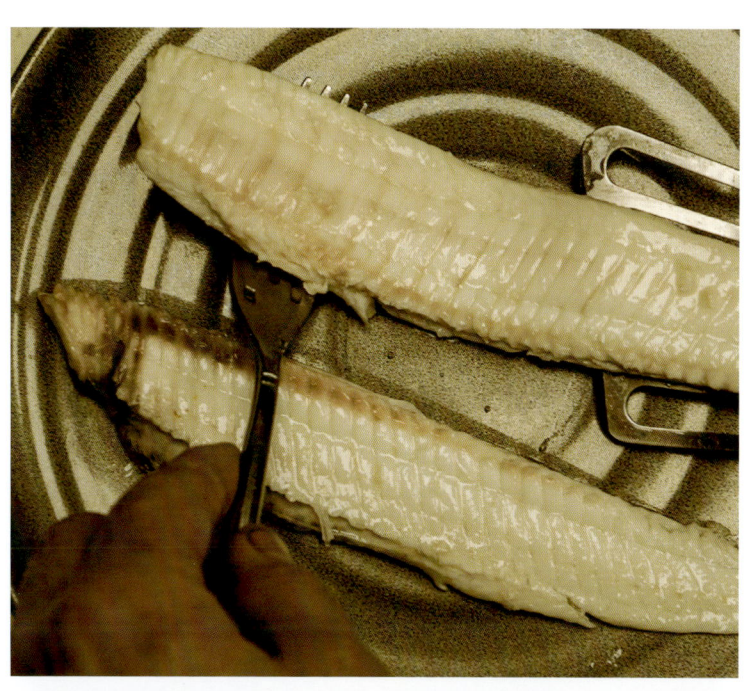

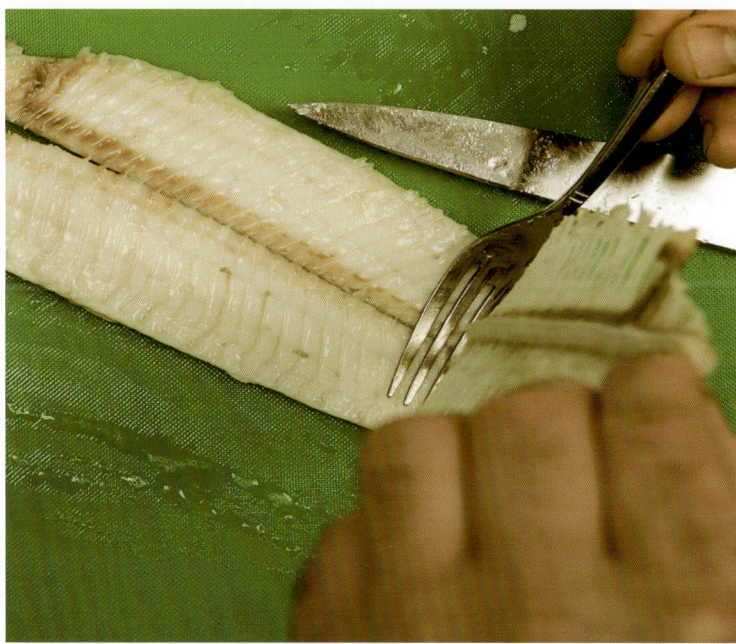

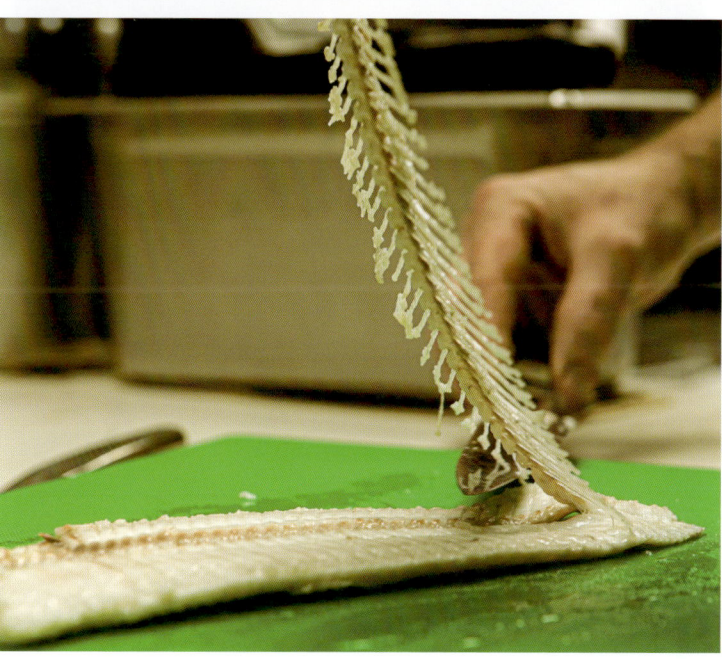

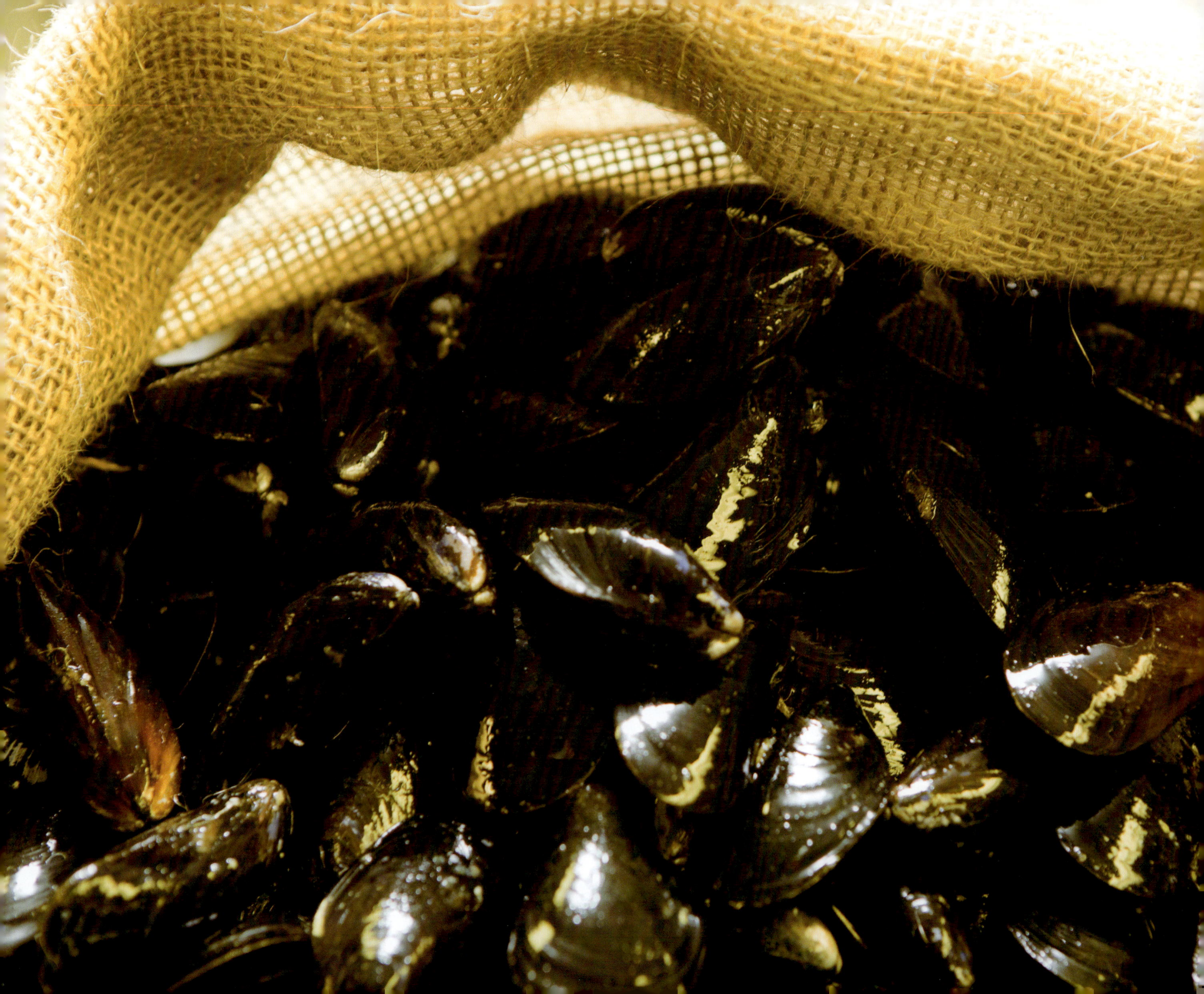

MUSSELS

Mussels are revered in Belgian cuisine. Whether you're at a small bistro or a high-end Michelin-starred restaurant, you'll find them on the menu. That's because they work just as well in humble presentations as they do in more refined fare. I prefer mussels from Blue Bay on Prince Edward Island, which you can find at many good fishmongers

28

SERVES 4

Mussel Gratin

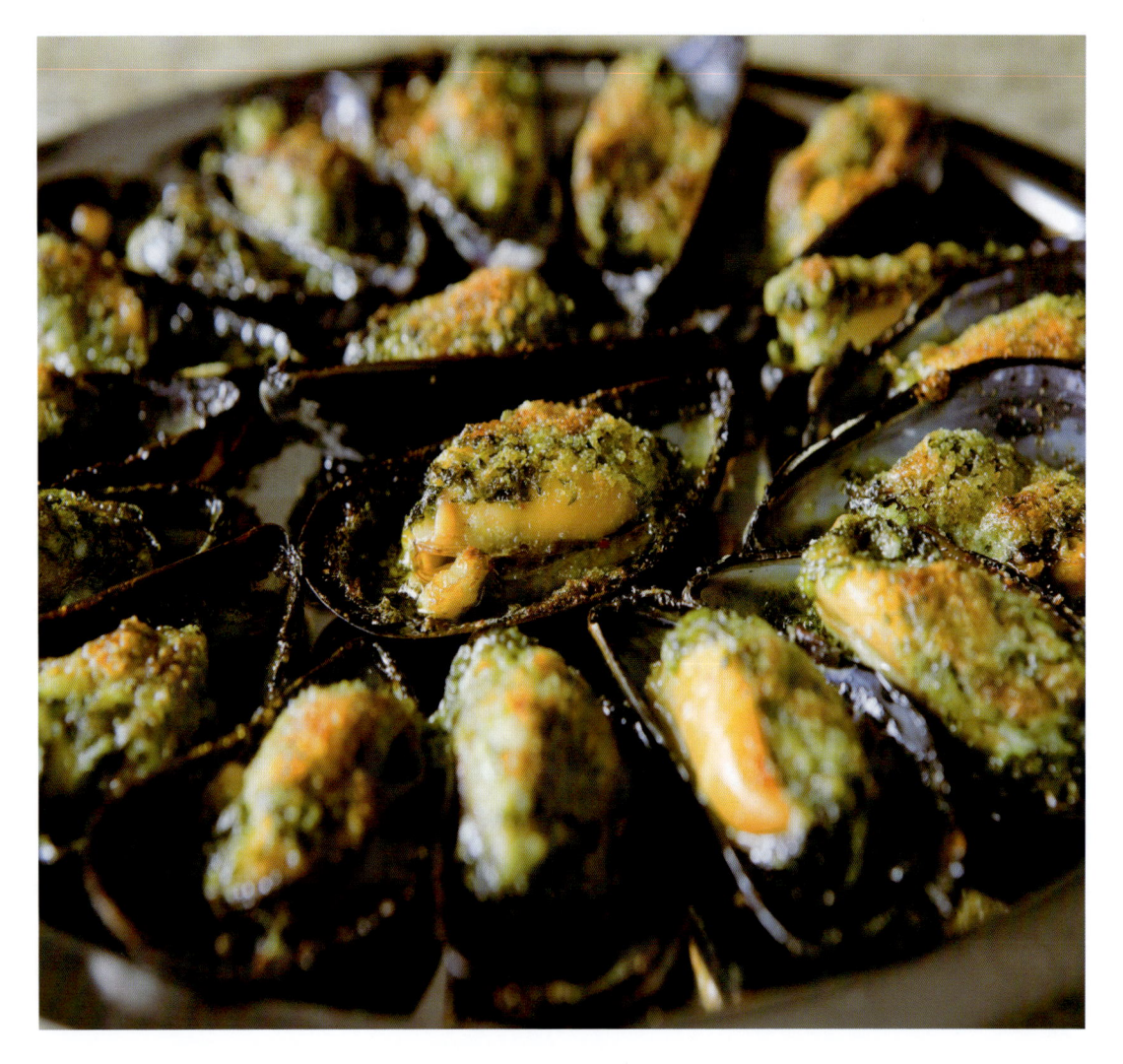

INGREDIENTS

1. 8 tablespoons (1 stick/125 grams) unsalted butter
2. 1 large yellow onion, diced
3. 2 stalks celery, diced
4. 1 medium leek, white and light green parts), washed and diced
5. 1 clove garlic, roughly chopped
6. 3 pounds (1.35 kilograms) mussels, cleaned in a cold-water bath
7. 1 sprig fresh thyme
8. 1 dried bay leaf
9. 1 1/4 cups (250 milliliters) dry white wine
10. 1 teaspoon (4 grams) flaky sea salt

This is one of the most popular dishes at the restaurant. A crunchy crust of Grana Padano cheese–tossed breadcrumbs conceals tender mussels swimming in a sea of melted garlic butter. I love enjoying it in the winter when there's a steady snowfall, the sidewalks are slick with ice, and the wind comes whipping off the Potomac. On those cold days, this dish never fails to comfort to the core. I prefer mussels from Prince Edward Island, especially from Blue Bay, but whatever is freshest from your local fishmonger or the seafood counter at the grocery store will work just as well. To clean the leeks, cut them lengthwise, then wash them thoroughly.

Garlic butter

1. 1/2 pound (2 sticks/250 grams) unsalted butter, room temperature
2. 5 cloves garlic, finely diced
3. 1 bunch curly parsley, thoroughly rinsed, stems removed, leaves finely diced
4. 1 tablespoon (15 milliliters) freshly squeezed lemon juice
5. 1 3/4 teaspoons (4 grams) Espelette pepper
6. 3/4 teaspoon (4 grams) flaky

To assemble

1. 1 1/2 cups (250 grams) shelled snails, drained
2. 4 tablespoons (1/2 stick/60 grams) unsalted butter, divided
3. 1/2 cup (50 grams) chopped shallots
4. 1 clove garlic, chopped
5. 1 cup (120 grams) cleaned, stemmed, and diced shiitake mushrooms
6. Kosher salt
7. 2 tablespoons + 1 teaspoon (30 grams) anise liqueur
8. 3 tablespoons (10 grams) chopped fresh chives
9. Flaky sea salt for garnish

DIRECTIONS

To make the mussels, in a large stew pot over medium heat, melt the butter. Add the onion, celery, leek, and garlic and cook, stirring occasionally with a wooden spoon, until the vegetables have softened, about 10 minutes. Add the mussels, thyme, bay leaf, wine, and salt. Cover, turn the heat up to high and cook until all the mussels open up, about 8 minutes. Remove from heat and drain out the liquid; reserve the liquid for future projects.

To make the garlic butter, in a food processor fitted with the stainless-steel blade, pulse together the butter, garlic, parsley, lemon juice, Espelette pepper, and salt until thoroughly combined and the butter takes on a greenish hue. Set aside at room temperature.

Preheat the broiler.

To assemble, remove the mussels from their shells, keep the better-looking half of each shell. Place the shells on a sheet pan, insides facing up and each shell supporting the shell on either side of it. Place a mussel in each shell. Place the garlic butter in a pastry bag and pipe some onto each mussel, just enough to cover it. Sprinkle each mussel with a pinch of Espelette pepper, then cover them with cheese and breadcrumbs. Place the mussels under the broiler as close to the heat as possible and broil until the cheese has melted, about 10 minutes.

Brush the bread slices with olive oil. In the broiler or a toaster oven, toast the bread until golden.

To serve, place coarse sea salt on four plates. Balance the mussels on top of the salt in a circular pattern. Serve each portion with a piece of toasted bread.

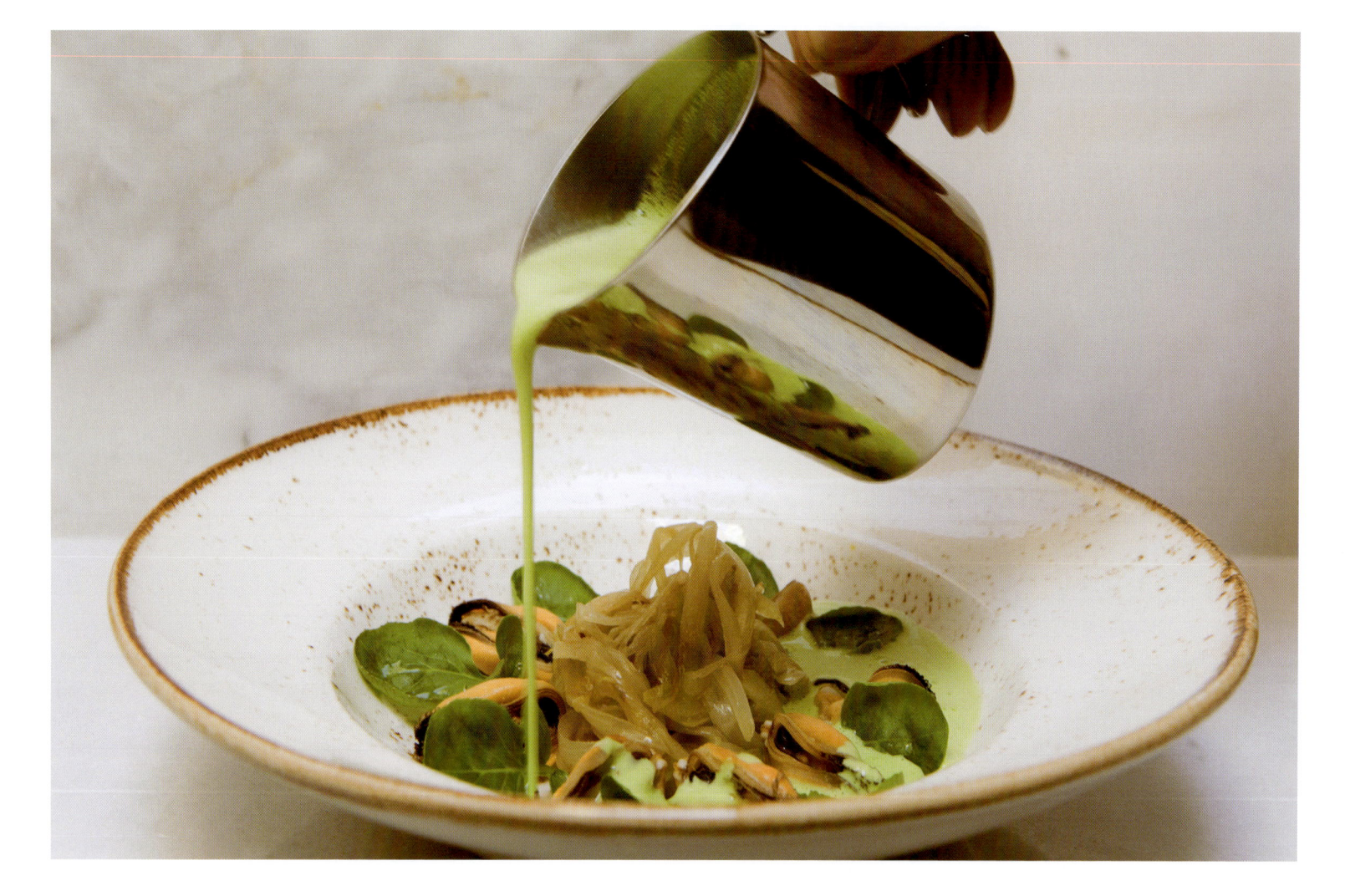

29

SERVES 6

Cream of Mussel Soup

I love watercress because of its slightly bitter bite. For this recipe, I sauté the green leaves with sugar, salt, and butter to slightly caramelize them, giving them a sweet note. That goes in the bottom of the bowl along with steamed mussels. Both are covered with a creamy soup made with both components. It feels like you've discovered hidden treasure when you dig your spoon in to discover those plump mussels wrapped in strands of watercress. When it comes to mussels, I prefer those from Blue Bay on Prince Edward Island, which you can find at many good fishmongers.

INGREDIENTS

1. 12 tablespoons (1 1/2 sticks/180 grams) unsalted butter, divided
2. 2 medium shallots, finely diced
3. 1/2 medium leek (white and light green parts), cut lengthwise, chopped
4. 2 stalks celery, diced
5. 4 cloves garlic, roughly chopped
6. 2 sprigs fresh thyme
7. 2 dried bay leaves
8. 1 tablespoon + 1 teaspoon (18 grams) kosher salt, divided
9. 2 1/4 cups (500 milliliters) dry white wine
10. 4 pounds (2 kilograms) mussels
11. 1 quart (1 liter) heavy cream
12. 3/4 teaspoon (1.6 grams) Espelette pepper
13. 1 tablespoon + 1 teaspoon (16 grams) vegetable oil
14. 6 Belgian endives, cut in half lengthwise, centers removed, and thinly sliced crosswise
15. 1 tablespoon (12 grams) granulated sugar
16. Leaves from 2 large bunches watercress, washed and dried

DIRECTIONS

In a large stew pot over high heat, melt 8 tablespoons (125 grams) of the butter until bubbling slightly, then add the shallots, leek, celery, garlic, thyme, and bay leaves. Cook, stirring occasionally, until the vegetables are translucent and softened, about 10 minutes. Add the mussels and 2 teaspoons (9 grams) of the salt and cook for 5 minutes uncovered. Add the white wine, cover, and let the mussels cook until all the shells have opened, about 10 minutes. Remove the mussels from the pot, let cool briefly, and remove them from their shells. Set the mussels aside in a medium bowl.

Strain the remaining liquid through a fine-mesh strainer into a medium saucepan over medium heat. Reduce the liquid by half, 5 to 8 minutes. Add the cream and Espelette pepper and reduce by half, about 20 minutes. Set aside.

In a large sauté pan over medium-high heat, heat the oil until smoking slightly, then add the endive and cook until light brown, stirring occasionally, 5 to 8 minutes. Add the sugar, remaining salt, and the remaining 4 tablespoons (60 grams) butter and cook until caramelized, stirring occasionally, 5 to 10 minutes.

Over medium-high heat, bring the cream and mussel juice mixture to a boil; let it simmer for 10 minutes, until it has thickened. Take it off the heat and let cool. Pour it into a blender, add the watercress leaves (leaving 60 to the side for the garnish), and blend until it's a rich green color and the watercress is thoroughly mixed in, about 5 minutes.

To reheat the mussels, in a medium sauté pan over medium heat, warm 1 cup (240 milliliters) of the soup and add the mussels. Let them warm for 3 to 5 minutes.

To assemble, divide the mussels and endive between four bowls, then pour the soup on top. Garnish each bowl with 15 watercress leaves. Serve immediately.

Our Famous Mussel Burger

(Step By Step)

SERVES 4

We have gotten more press for this burger than any other item on our menu. I was inspired to create it after watching Michel Richard craft premium patties out of lobster and tuna. Those are great burgers, but I wanted to do one that was closer to Belgian cuisine. It took only two tries before we nailed it. Fried onions on top add crunch factor, while the saffron-garlic aïoli is a nice complement to the smooth brininess of the mussels. Don't worry, it's not too difficult to make—and it's guaranteed to make a big impression. I prefer Blue Bay mussels from Prince Edward Island, but you should use whatever is freshest at your fishmonger

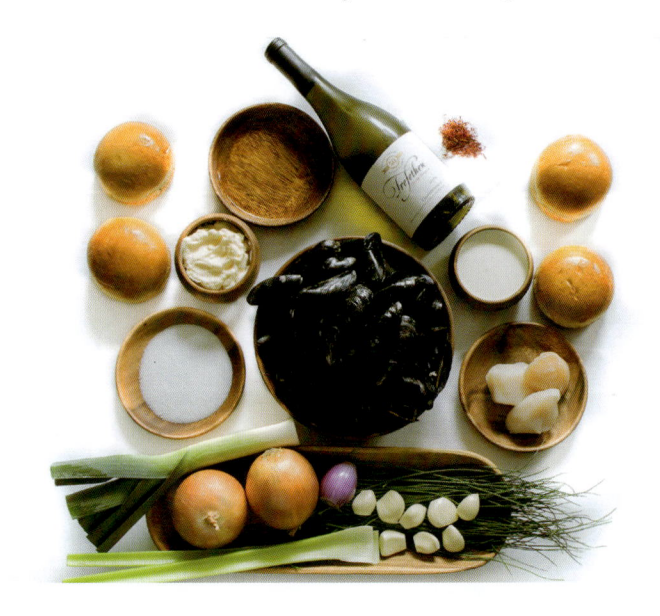

INGREDIENTS

Scallop mousse
1. 4 large sea scallops (about 5 ounces/160 grams total), trimmed
2. 1 large egg white (30 grams)
3. 1 1/4 teaspoons (6 grams) kosher salt
4. Pinch of Espelette pepper
5. 3 tablespoons + 1 teaspoon (50 grams) heavy cream
6. 1/4 cup (40 grams) chopped shallots
7. 1/4 cup + 1 tablespoon (15 grams) chopped fresh chives

Mussels
1. 1/2 pound (2 sticks/250 grams) unsalted butter
2. 2 stalks celery, diced
3. 1 medium leek (white and light green parts), diced
4. 1 medium yellow onion, diced
5. 5 cloves garlic, smashed
6. 2 sprigs fresh thyme
7. 2 dried bay leaves
8. 5 1/2 pounds (2.5 kilograms) mussels
9. 1 1/4 teaspoons (6 grams) kosher salt
10. 2 cups (375 milliliters) dry white wine

Saffron aïoli
1. 1 cup (200 grams) mayonnaise (store-bought, or page 204)
2. 5 cloves garlic, finely chopped
3. Large pinch of saffron

To assemble
1. 1 tablespoon (13 grams) canola oil
2. 4 hamburger buns

DIRECTIONS

For the scallop mousse, in a food processor fitted with the stainless-steel blade place the scallops, egg white, the salt, and the Espelette pepper. Process until mixture is fully combined and smooth, about 1 to 2 minutes. Add the heavy cream and process on high speed until mixture is fully combined and smooth, about 2 minutes. Remove the mixture from the food processor and place it in a large bowl. Using a spatula, fold in the shallots and chives. Cover and refrigerate until ready to use.

To prepare the mussels, melt the butter in a large pot over high heat. Add the celery, leek, onion, garlic, thyme, and bay leaves. Stir to combine, then reduce the heat to medium and cook until the vegetables are softened, about 10 minutes. [Image 1 and 2]

Add the mussels, the salt, and wine and stir to combine. [Image 3]

Cover and cook until the mussels are open, about 12 minutes. Remove the mussels and set them aside to cool. Reserve the liquid for future projects. [Image 4]

When the mussels are cool enough to handle, remove them from their shells and place them on a cutting board. [Image 5 and 6]

Using a large chef's knife, chop the mussels into small pieces. [Image 7]

Gently fold the chopped mussels into the scallop mousse. [Image 8]

Divide the mousse into four equal portions and form into burgers using a 4-inch (10 cm) ring mold. Refrigerate until ready to cook. [Image 9 and 10]

To make the saffron aïoli, in small bowl whisk together mayonnaise, garlic, and saffron. After you're finished making the burgers, you can store any excess aïoli in an airtight container in the refrigerator for 10 days or so. [Image 11]

Preheat the oven to 350°F (175°C). Place canola oil in a cast-iron skillet over medium-high heat and heat it until it is just beginning to smoke. [Image 12]

To cook the burgers, sear them until each side is golden brown. Place the skillet in the oven and cook until feel resistance when you press the center, about 6 minutes. [Image 13]

To assemble, toast the hamburger buns. Schmear both top and bottom with saffron aïoli before slipping in the burgers.

Stepwise Instructions

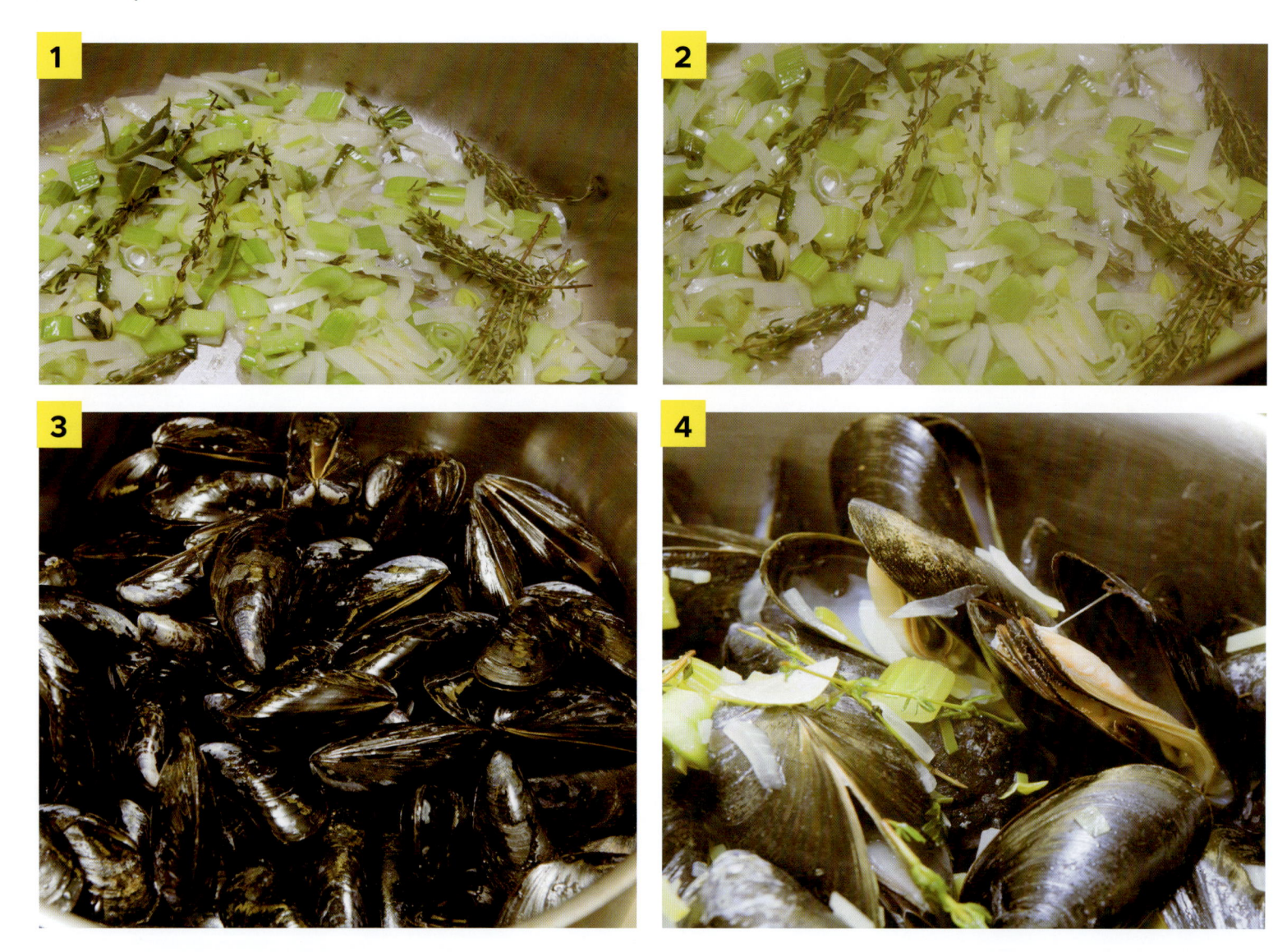

1

2

3

4

PAGE 115

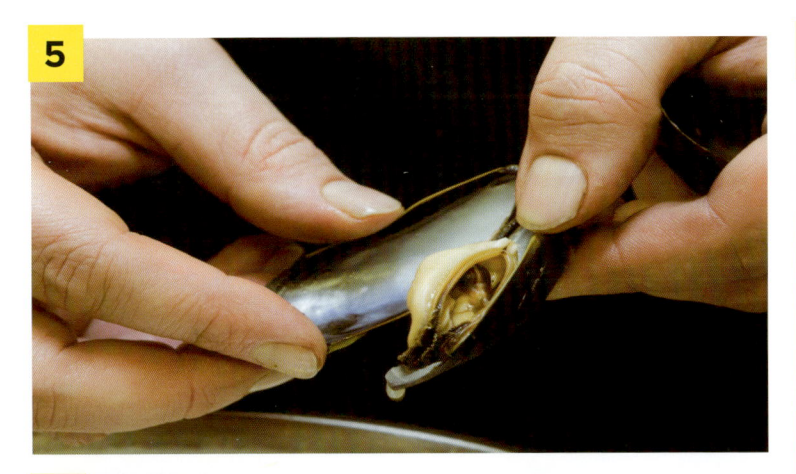

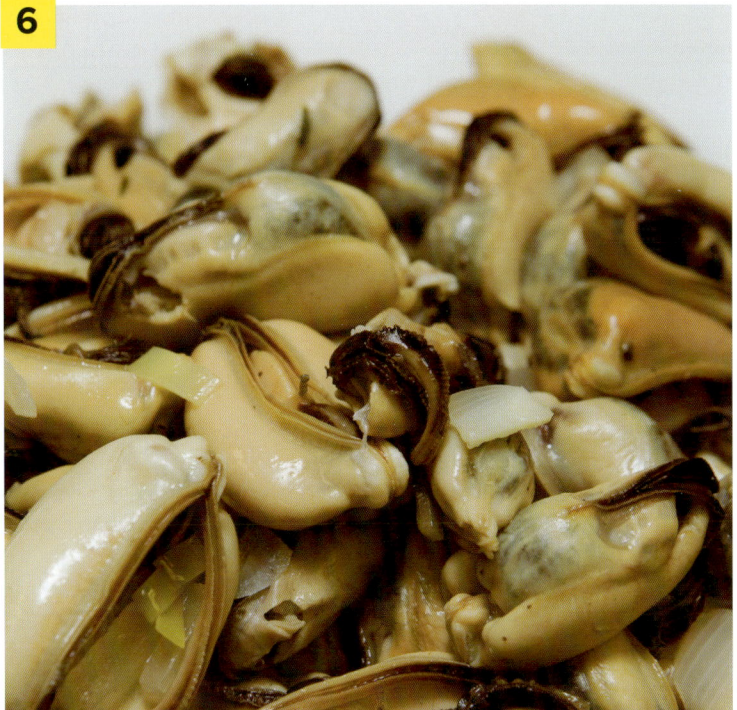

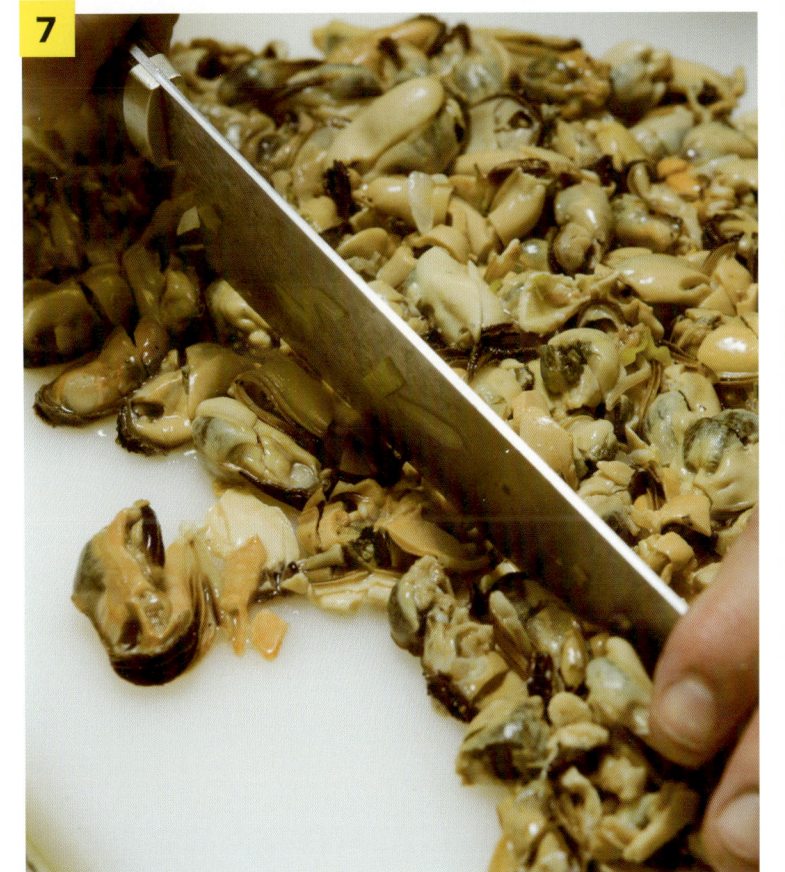

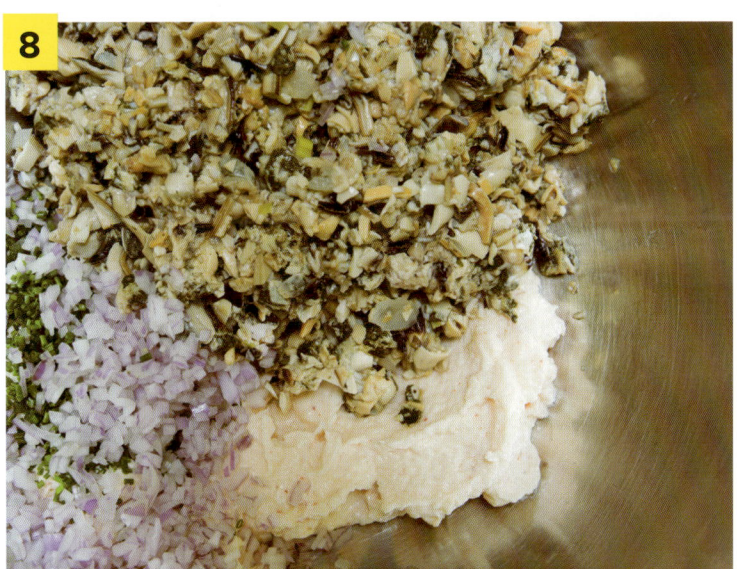

PAGE 116

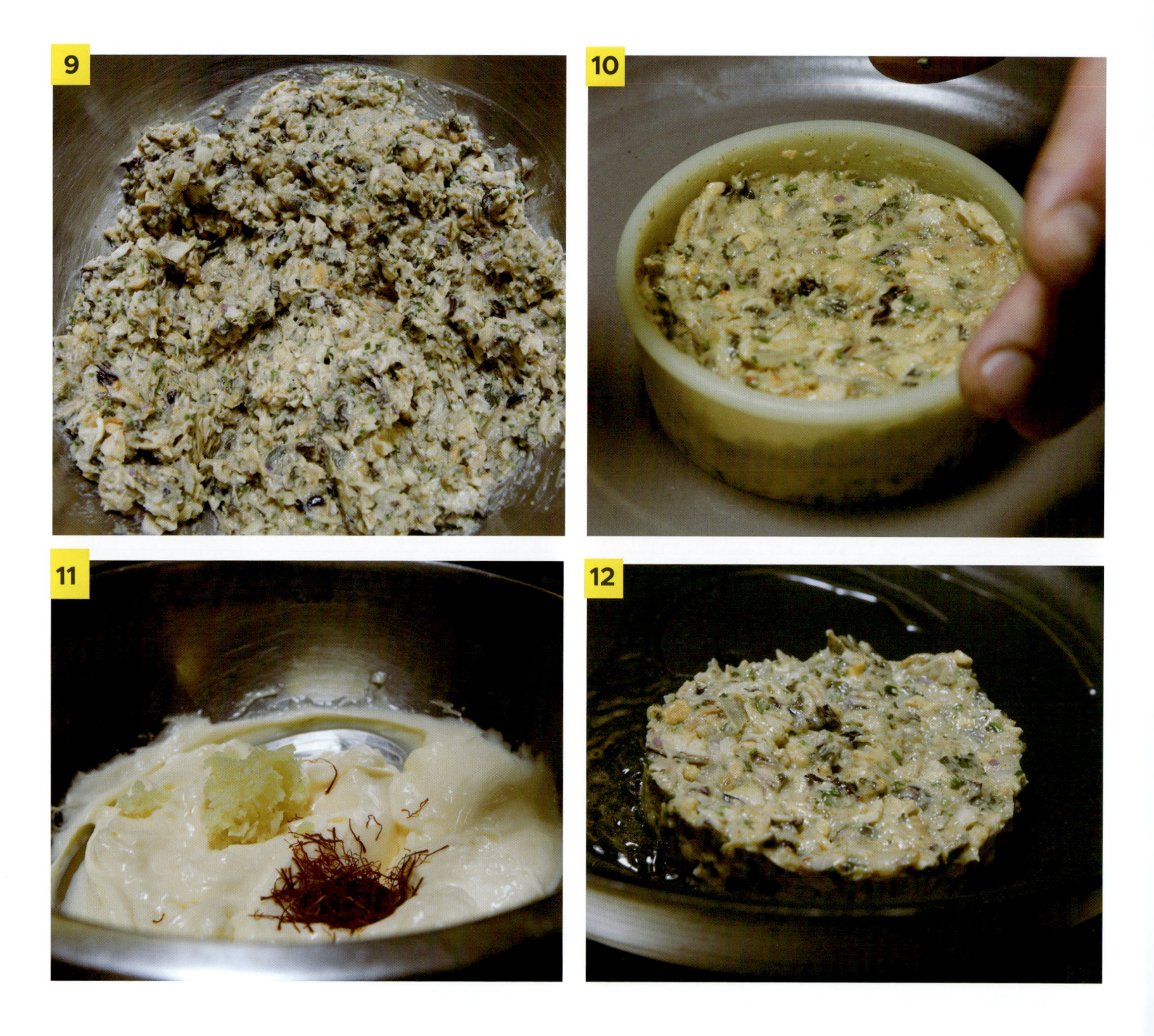

PAGE 117

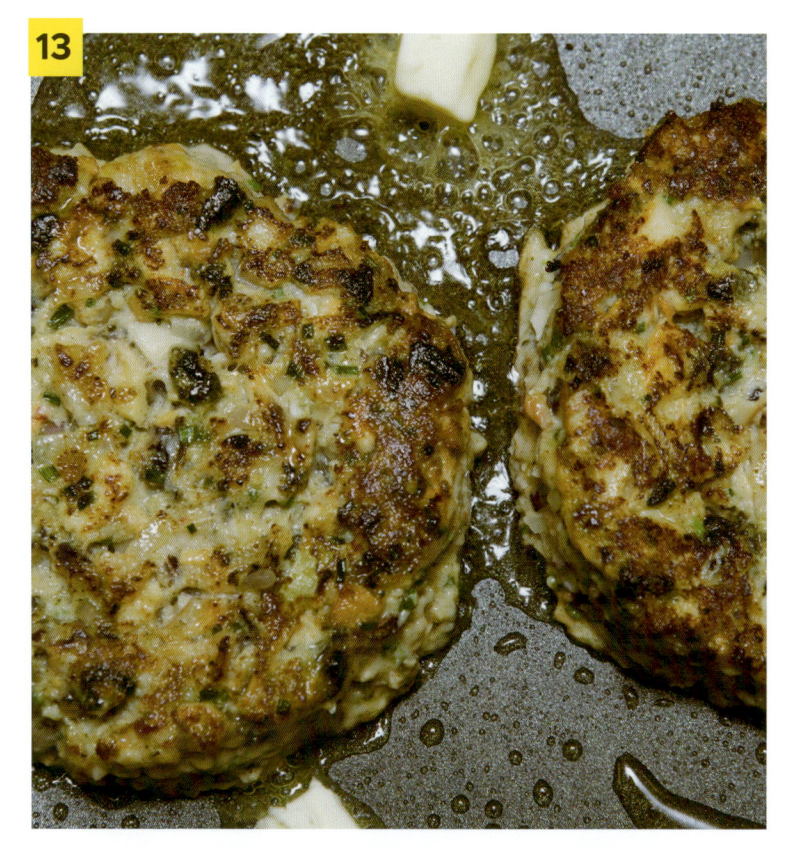

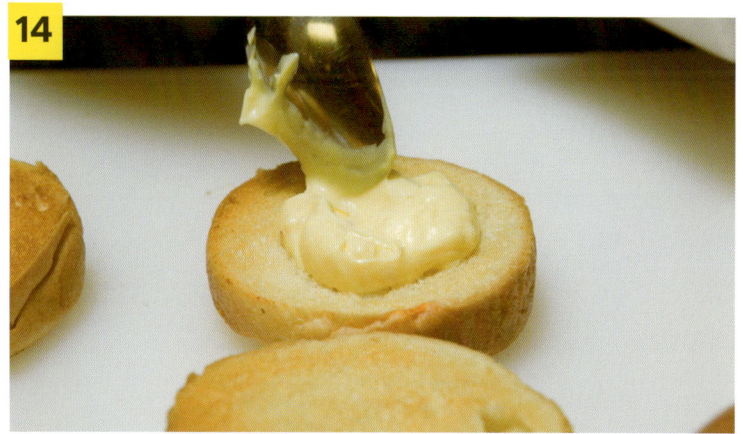

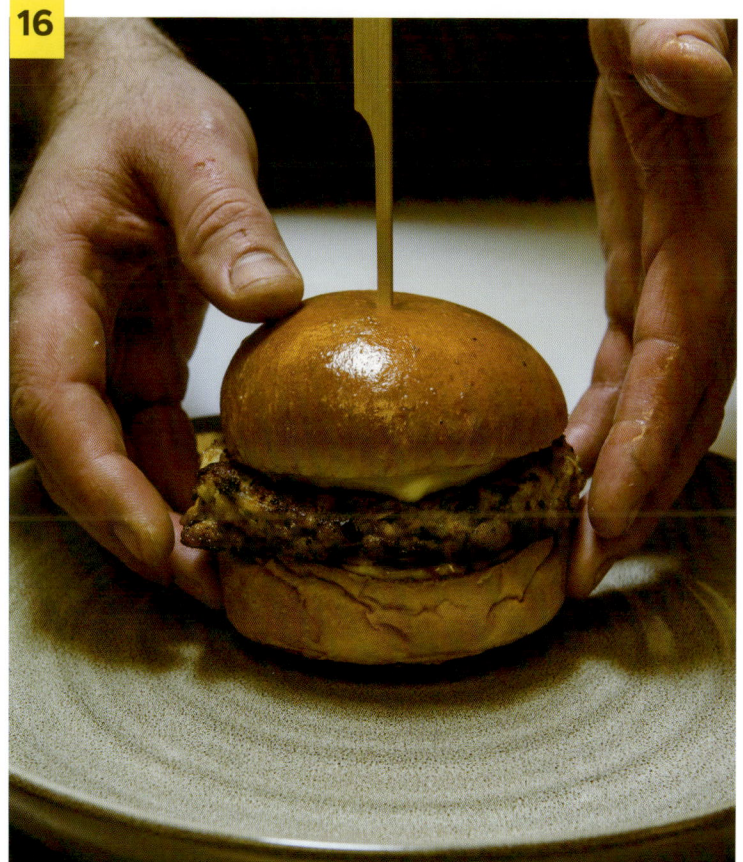

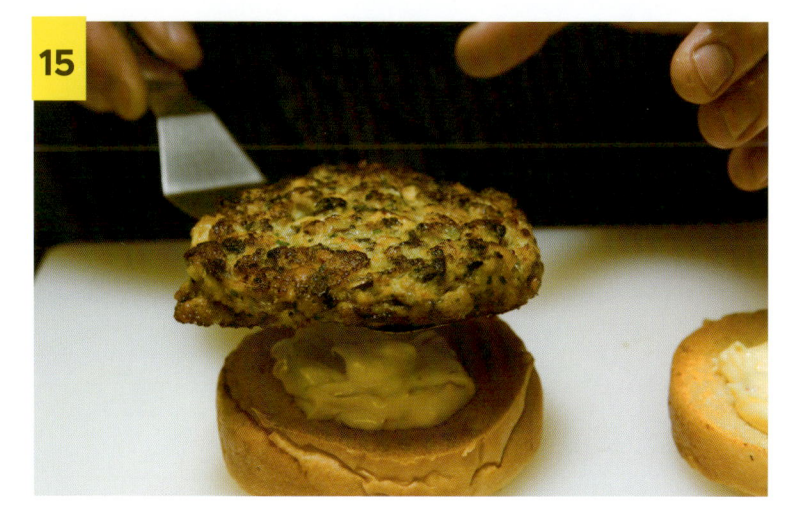

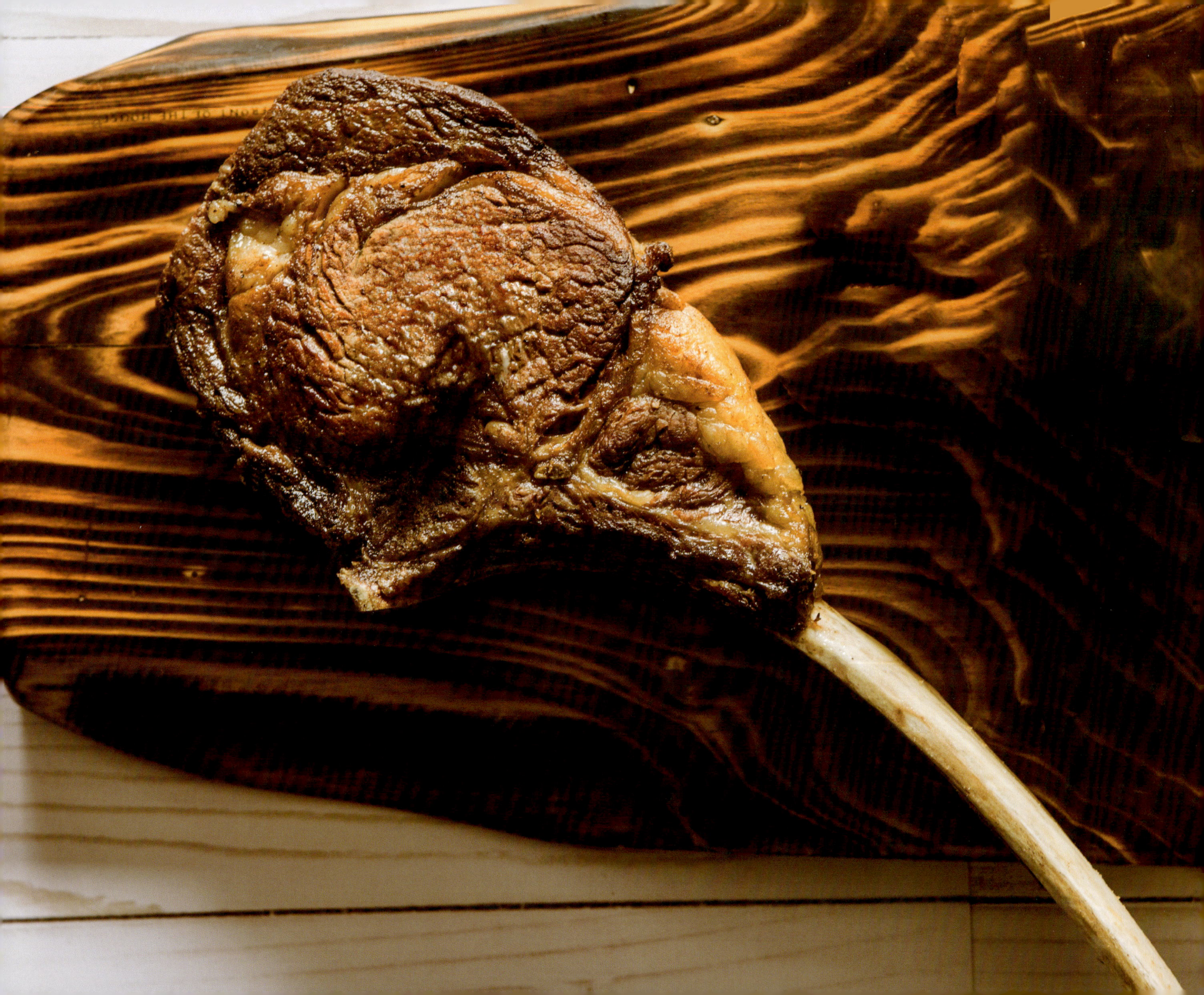

BEEF

We eat a lot of beef in Belgium, but Americans make us look like vegetarians by comparison. All three of the beefy recipes in this chapter are strong sellers at Et Voila!. I love working with beef, because it can be prepared in myriad ways to reflect the needs of the season. I source our meat from Creekstone Farms and Foods In Season, but home cooks can get high-quality cuts from their butcher, farmers' market, or the counter at a good grocery store. When possible, opt for organic. I personally like grass-fed beef's leaner and more herbaceous qualities, but that's a matter of preference.

Steak Frites with Green Peppercorn Sauce

31

SERVES 4

When I went out with friends as a teenager, I'd always order steak frites. I can still eat it twice a week and never get bored. To give the steak a good crust with a perfectly cooked center, sear it in a cast-iron pan with butter before finishing it in the oven. When it's finished cooking, let it rest for at least 5 minutes before eating it. This ensures the meat's juices stay locked in and don't run out when you cut into it. A hanger steak works best for this recipe, though it can also be made with ribeye, flank, or skirt steak. Brined green peppercorns can be found at good grocery stores and online; I like those made by Moulin. I recommend serving each steak with a side of Belgian Frites (page 58) and small green salad with Balsamic Dressing (page 201).

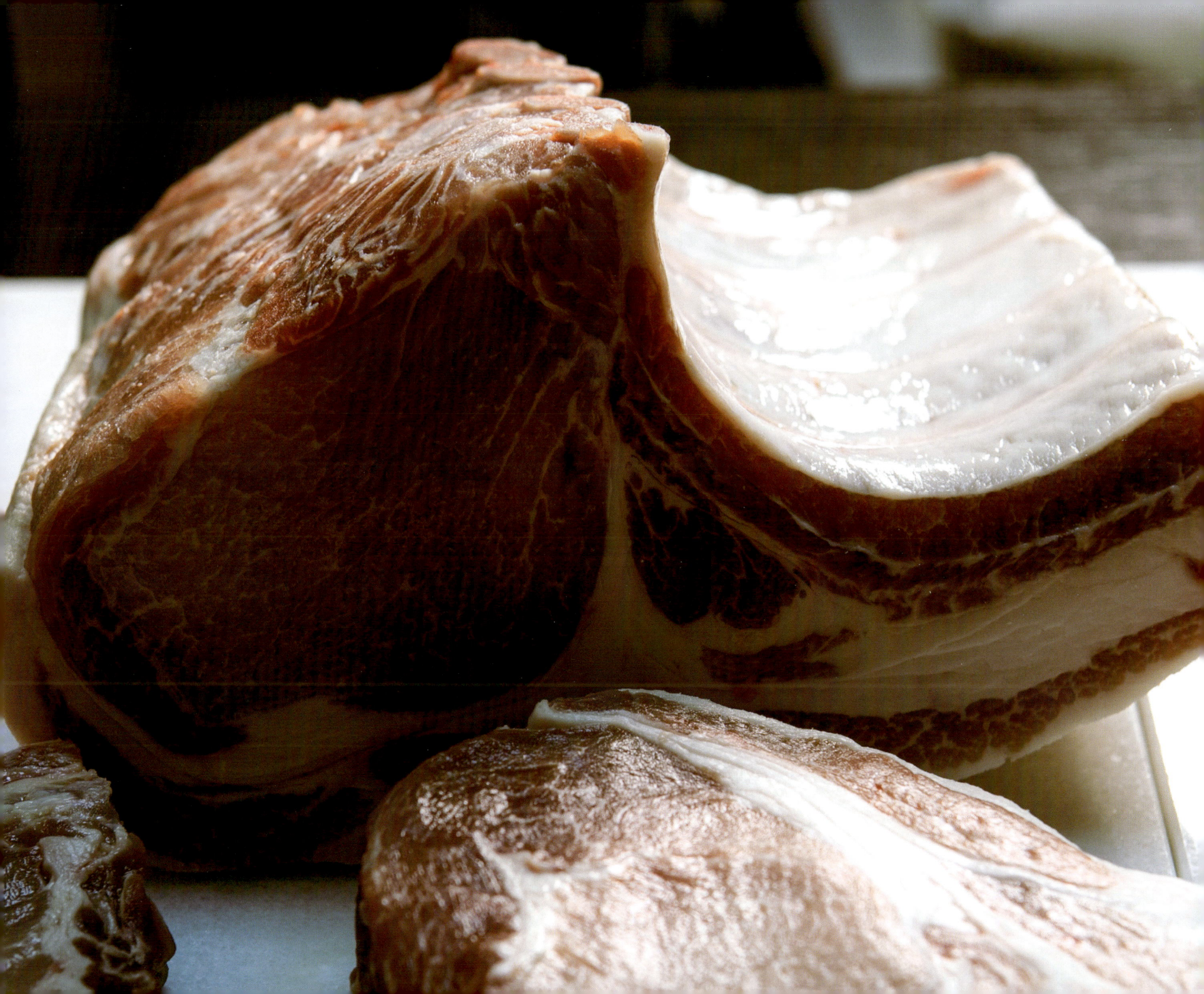

PAGE 127

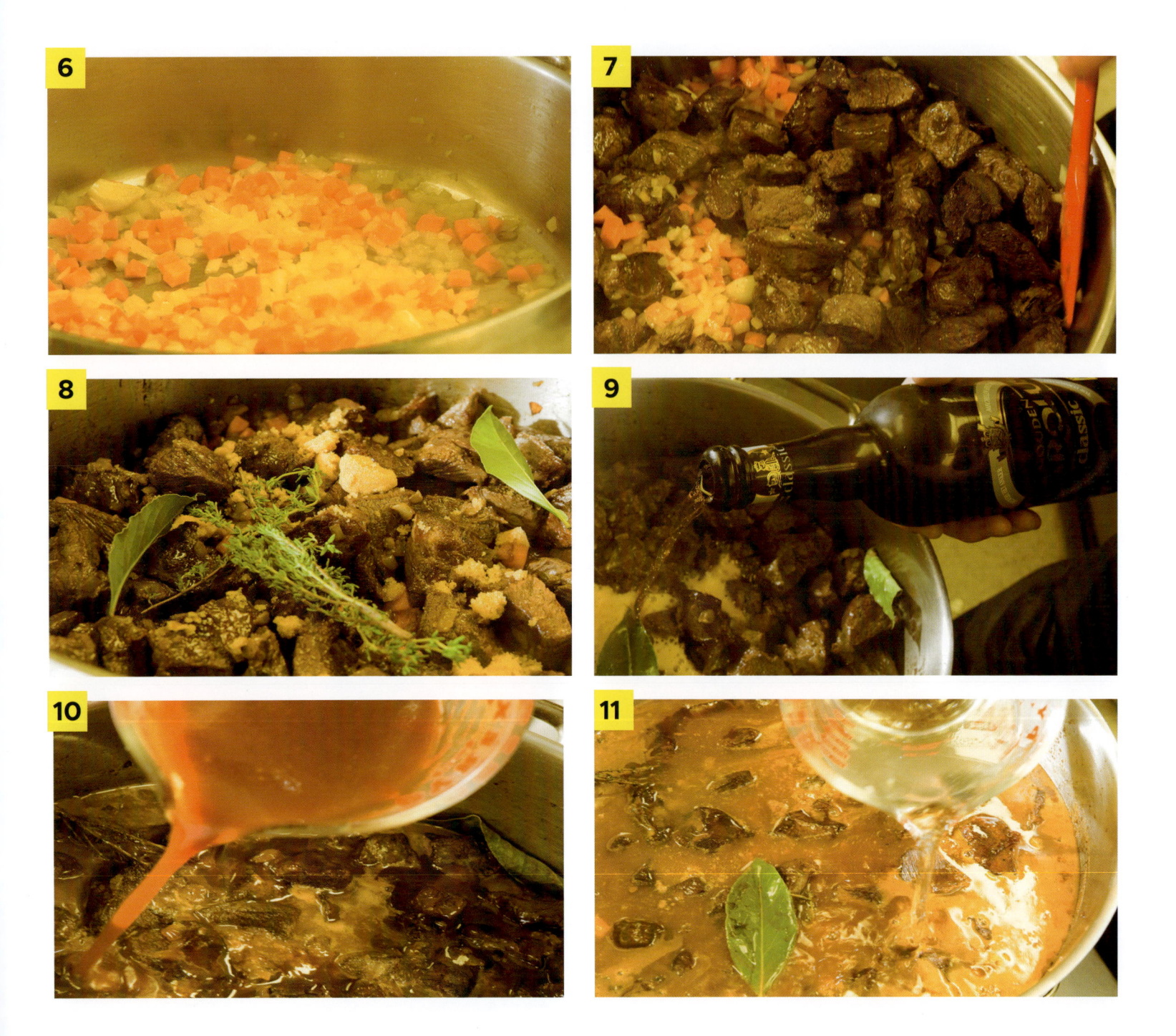

Stepwise Instructions

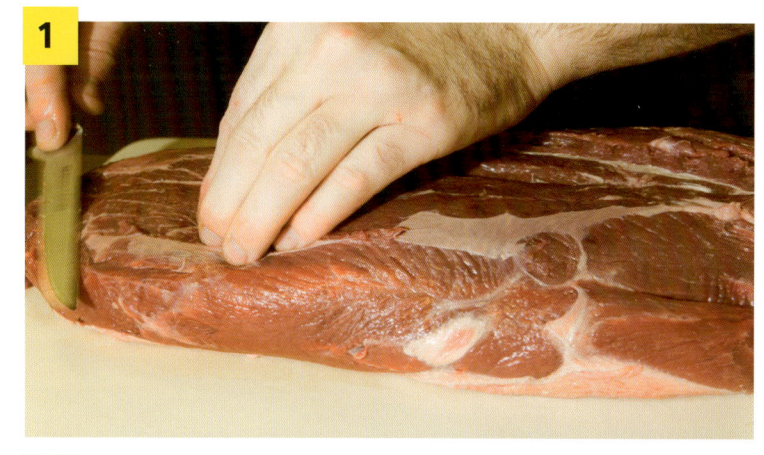

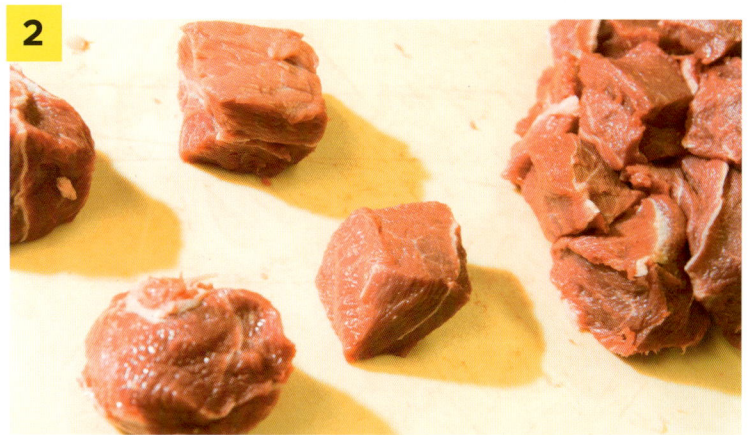

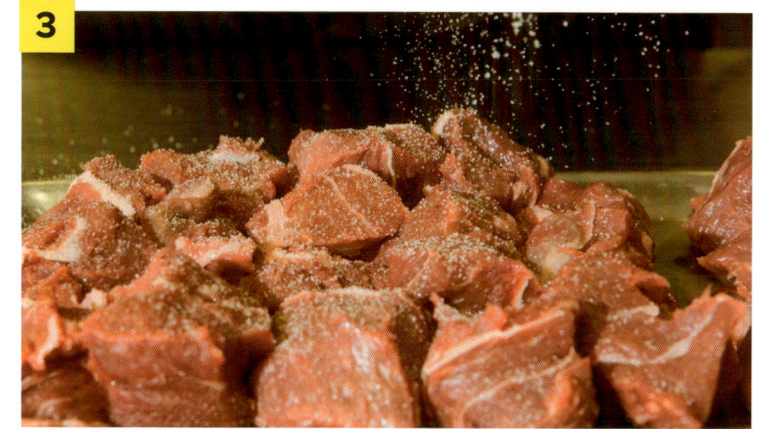

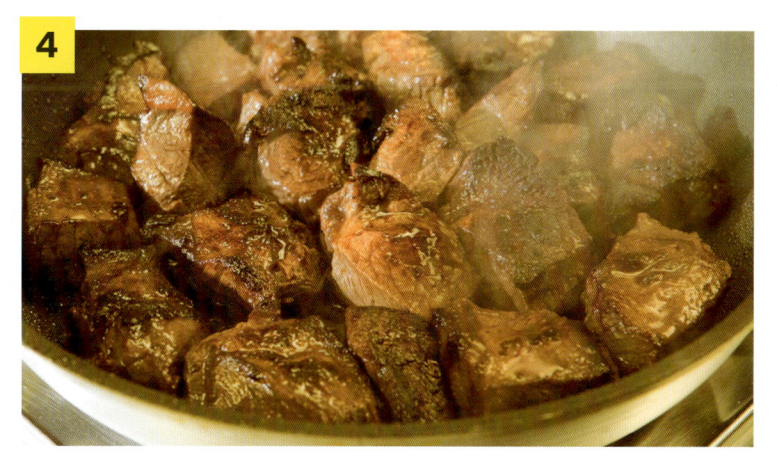

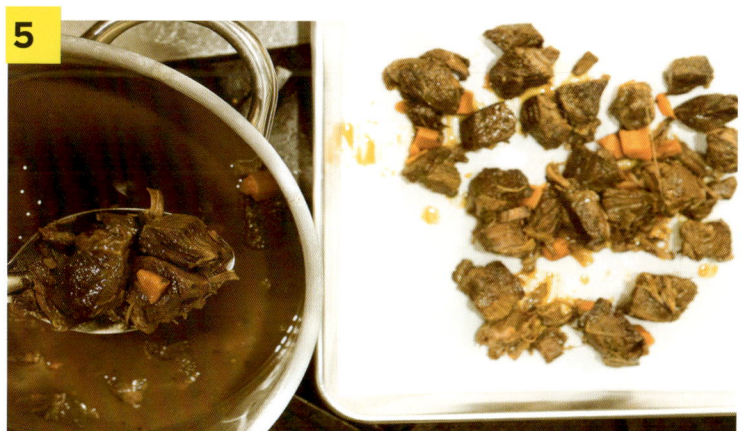

INGREDIENTS

1. 6 1/2 pounds (3 kilograms) flat-iron steak
2. 1 tablespoon + 2 teaspoons (30 grams) flaky sea salt
3. 1/4 cup + 1 tablespoon (65 grams) canola oil, divided
4. 2 large onions, diced
5. 3 large carrots, diced
6. 1/4 cup + 1 tablespoon (70 grams) light brown sugar
7. 1 bottle (26 ounces/750 milliliters) Gouden Carolus Classic beer
8. 1 quart (1 kilogram) veal stock (store-bought, or page 207)
9. 2 large Gala apples
10. 1/2 baguette
11. 2 tablespoons (30 grams) Dijon mustard

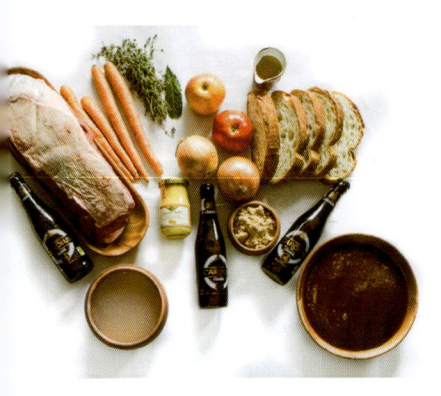

DIRECTIONS

Using a boning knife, remove the white membrane on the top of the flat-iron steak and remove half of the fat on the bottom, leaving a layer of fat half as deep as it was originally. Cut the beef into cubes approximately 1 1/2 inches (4 cm) square. Place beef on a sheet pan and season all over with sea salt. [Image 1, 2 and 3]

Place a large sauté pan over medium heat and add 1 tablespoon (15 milliliters) of the canola oil. Warm the oil until smoking slightly, then add cubes of beef, being careful not to overcrowd the pan. (You will probably have to do this in 3 batches, adding 1 tablespoon of canola oil before each batch). Once the beef is dark brown on all sides, remove it from the pan and place it in a strainer resting in the sink. [Image 4]

In a large stew pot over medium heat, heat 2 tablespoons (30 milliliters) of the canola oil until shimmering, then add the onion and carrots. Cook, stirring occasionally, until softened, about 10 minutes. [Image 5 and 6]

Add the beef and let it cook for 10 minutes uncovered, until the onions have begun to caramelize. [Image 7]

Add the sugar and beer and cook until the liquid is reduced by half, 15 to 20 minutes. Add the veal stock and 6 quarts (5 1/2 liters) water. Let the mixture simmer for about 3 hours, until the beef is soft. To test the meat's readiness, press down on it with your finger. If there's no resistance and starts to come apart, it's cooked. Let the meat cool in the pot. [Image 8 and 9]

Once the liquid has cooled, use a mesh skimmer or slotted spoon to remove the beef and vegetables from the sauce. Place the sauce back on the stove over medium heat and bring to a simmer. Cut the apples into 4 pieces each, leaving the skin on and the seeds in, and put them in the sauce. Cook until the apples are completely soft, about 30 minutes. With an immersion blender, mix until the apples, core, and seeds are completely pureed and fully incorporated into the sauce. Pour the sauce through a fine-mesh strainer back into the large stew pot over medium-high heat and add the beef and vegetables. Bring the stew to a boil for 5 minutes, then set it aside. [Image 10, 11 and 12]

Cut the baguette half on the diagonal into 8 slices. Toast until golden and crispy on both sides. With a small brush, spread each slice with mustard on one side.

Divide the stew into bowls and top each with a piece of baguette with the mustard side up.

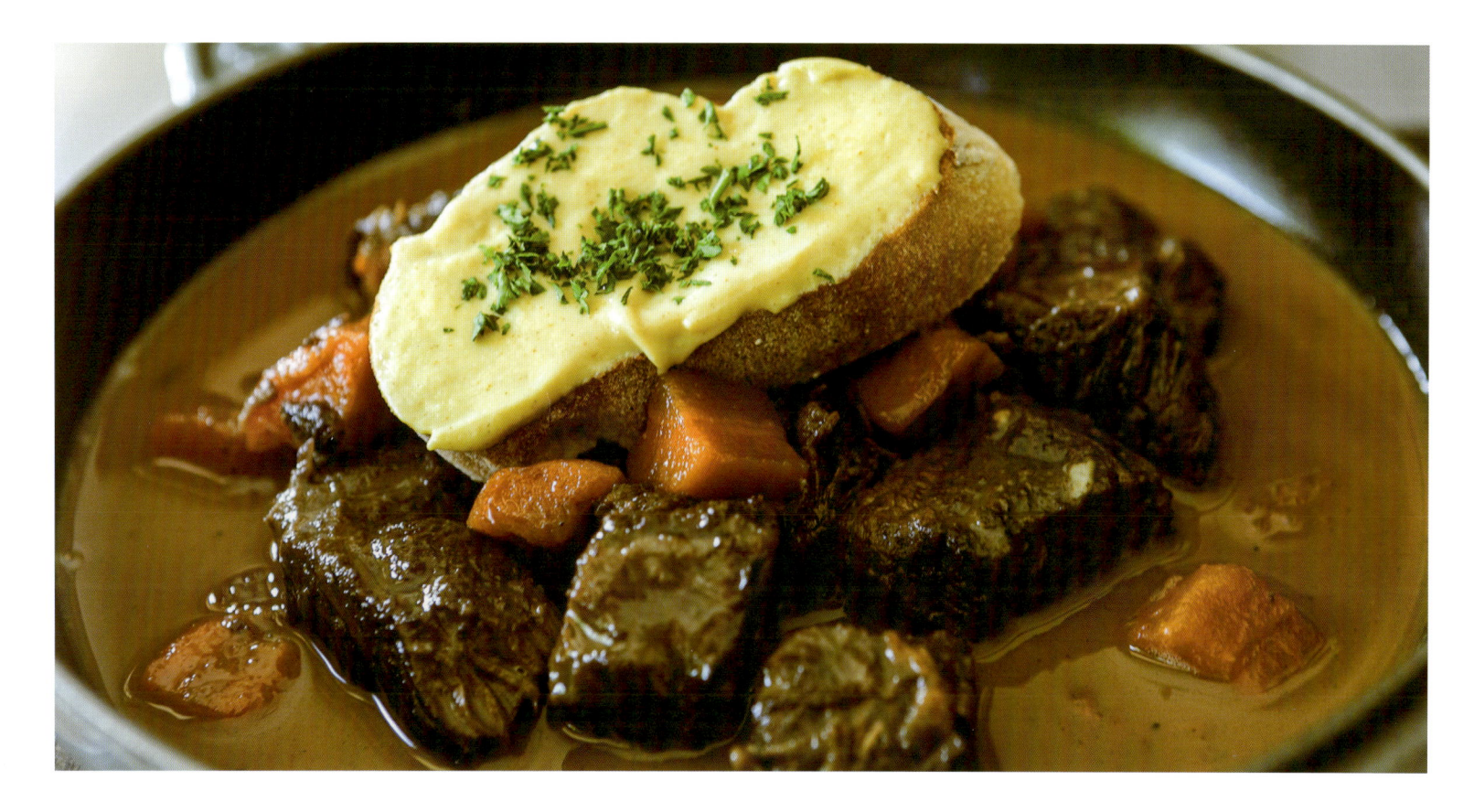

Flemish Beef Stew

(Carbonnade à la Flamande) | Step By Step

Whether it's raining, snowing, or just one of those grayish overcast days that drags you down with its dreariness, this traditional Belgian favorite possesses the power to comfort. In his first review of the restaurant, the Washington Post's Tom Sietsema called it "Comfort food, sexed up." Packed with chunks of tender beef, the gravy-like stew is enriched with brown beer and thickened with blended apples (Gala apples are best, and most varietals will work, but Granny Smiths are too tart.). Top it with a slice of baguette brushed with Dijon mustard or serve it with a side of Belgian Frites (page 58). This dish works best with a flat-iron steak, which is sometimes known as a boneless top chuck steak, book steak, or butler steak. You will need a heavy-bottomed stewpot or Dutch oven. You can purchase Gouden Carolus Classic beer at some liquor stores and online at TotalWine.com

INGREDIENTS

1. 1 1/4 pounds (560 grams) beef tenderloin, trimmed and finely diced
2. 2 tablespoons (20 grams) chopped shallots
3. 3 tablespoons (10 grams) chopped fresh chives
4. 1 tablespoon + 2 teaspoons (12 grams) small capers
5. 1 tablespoon + 2 teaspoons (25 grams) chopped small sour gherkins
6. 2 teaspoons (12 grams) flaky sea salt
7. 3/4 teaspoon (3 grams) freshly ground black pepper
8. 1/4 cup (50 grams) extra virgin olive oil
9. 1/4 cup + 1 tablespoon (80 grams) cocktail sauce (store-bought, or page 203)
10. 1/4 teaspoon (1 gram) Tabasco sauce
11. 2 1/4 teaspoons (6 grams) Worcestershire sauce

DIRECTIONS

Place medium bowl in the refrigerator to chill for 30 minutes.

In the chilled bowl, using a spatula, mix together the beef, shallots, chives, capers, gherkins, salt, and pepper until thoroughly combined. Add the olive oil, cocktail sauce, Tabasco, and Worcestershire sauces and mix until thoroughly incorporated. Cover and place in the refrigerator to chill for 30 minutes.

Using a 3-inch-wide (8 cm) ring mold placed at the center of plate, place a quarter of the meat. Press down gently to ensure an attractive round circle and a level top is created. Repeat 3 more times.

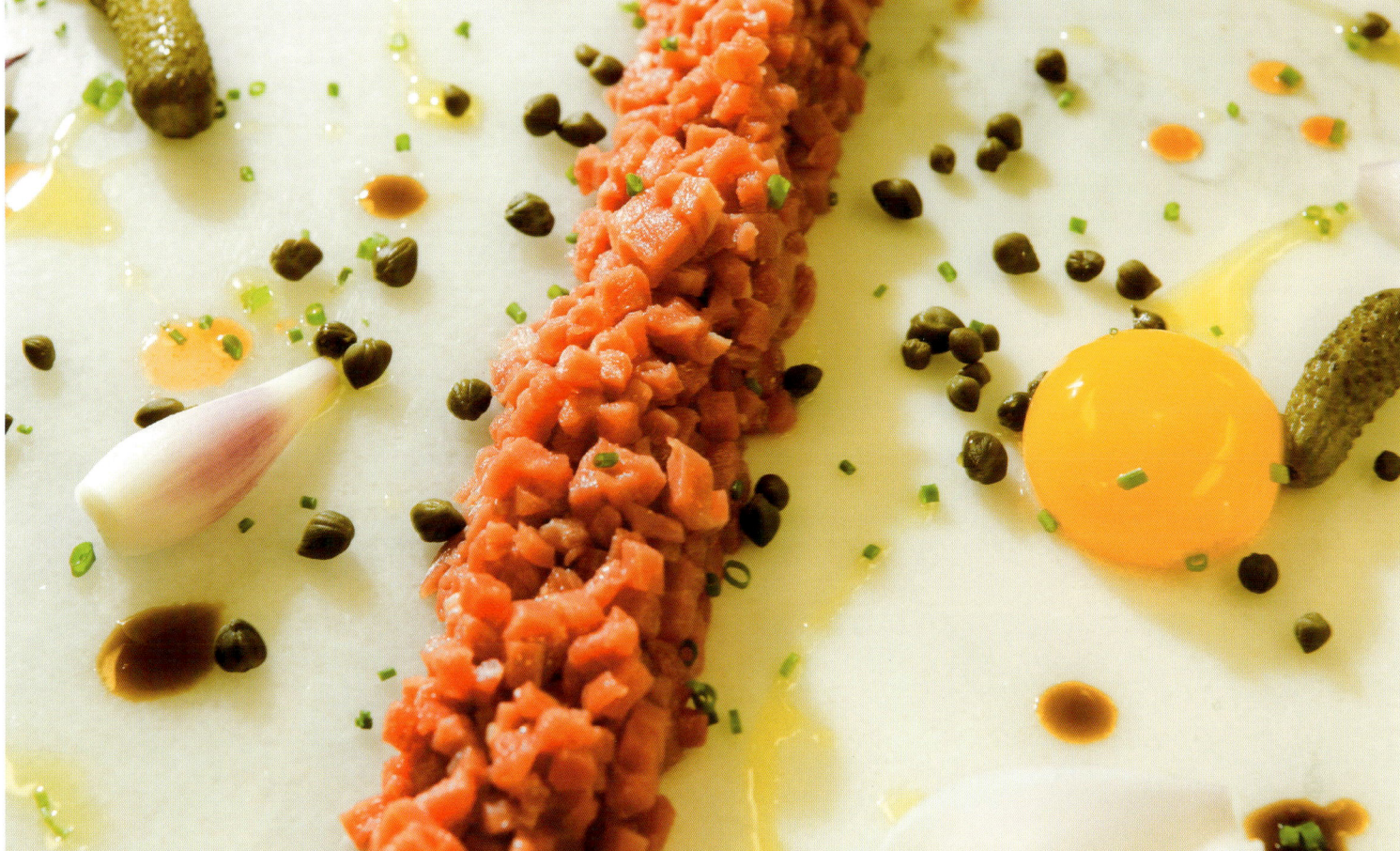

Beef Tartare

32

SERVES 4

Back in Belgium, beef tartare is called filet américain. That's because the raw ground beef is dressed with sauce américaine, an iconic French condiment featuring ketchup, mayonnaise, Tabasco sauce, Worcestershire sauce, cornichons, and capers. Think of it as a fancy Thousand Island dressing. We always top the beef with a sunny raw egg yolk and a drizzle of good olive oil. Serve it with a salad or a pile of Belgian Frites (page 58) and it makes for a good meal. It's best to use tenderloin for this recipe, though top round is a satisfying substitute—and costs a little less. You will also need a 3-inch (8 cm) ring mold, which can be purchased at any good cookware supply store or online.

INGREDIENTS

1. 1/4 cup + 2 tablespoons (40 grams) drained green peppercorns (packed in brine)
2. 2 tablespoons (30 grams) brandy
3. 1 cup + 2 tablespoons (250 grams) heavy cream
4. 1/2 cup (125 grams) veal stock (store-bought, or page 207)
5. Four 8-ounce (250 gram) hanger steaks
6. Kosher salt
7. 2 tablespoons + 1 teaspoon (30 grams) vegetable oil, divided
8. 1/4 pound (1 stick/125 grams) unsalted butter
9. 4 servings Belgian Frites (page 58), freshly cooked

DIRECTIONS

Place a medium sauté pan over medium heat. Add the peppercorns and brandy and cook until the brandy has evaporated, about 10 minutes. Add the cream and veal stock and cook until the sauce has thickened and coats a spoon, 10 to 20 minutes. Set aside.

Season both sides of the steaks with salt and set aside.

Preheat the oven to 400°F (205°C).

In a large sauté pan over medium heat, warm 2 scant teaspoons (8 milliliters) of the oil until it just starts to smoke. One a time, place each steak in the pan with 2 tablespoons (30 grams) of the butter and cook, basting the meat with the melted butter constantly, until the meat is a rich brown, 2 to 5 minutes per side. In between cooking the steaks, wipe out the pan. Place the steaks on a cooling rack set in a rimmed sheet pan. Move the steaks, still on the rack in the pan, into the oven and cook to desired temperature, 5 to 10 minutes for medium-rare.

Let the steaks rest for 5 minutes before topping with the green peppercorn sauce. Serve with the frites.

PORK

Pork may be the most versatile of proteins, lending itself to a variety of preparations ranging from quickly cooked chops and easy-to-execute meatballs to slow-cooked barbeque and well-aged charcuterie. I love its unctuous, umami-rich flavor, which is unlike anything else out there, and I appreciate the fact that you can use every part of the animal, from the snout to the tail and all points in between. High-quality heritage pork can be purchased through specialty retailers such as D'Artagnan, as well as at your local butcher, farmers' market, or the meat counter of a good grocery store.

34

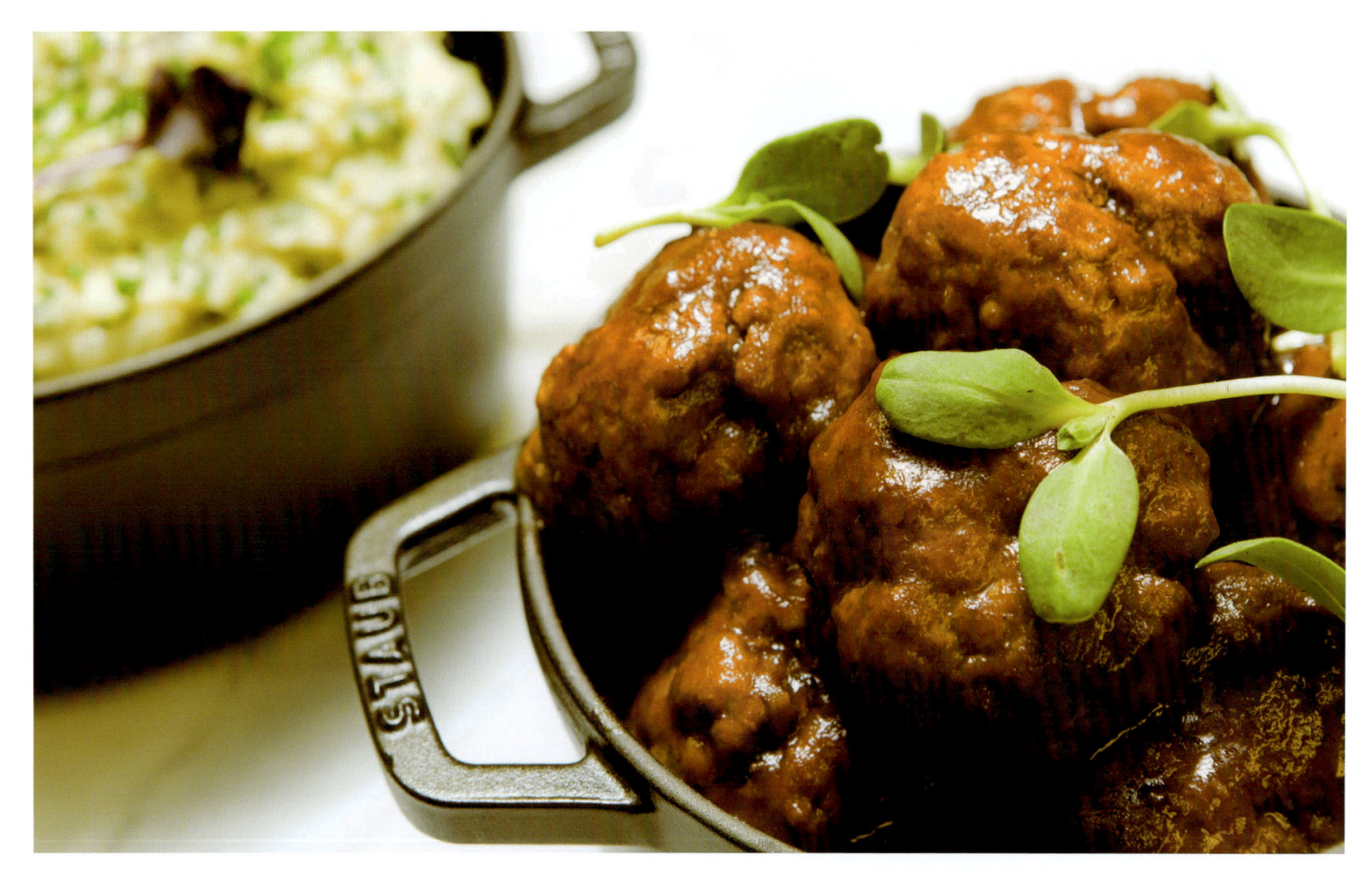

SERVES 8

Liège Meatballs

These memorable meatballs are forged from a mix of veal, pork, and mild Italian sausage and seasoned with garlic, onion, and thyme. Eggs are the binder, while milk-soaked bread creates tenderness and juiciness. After giving them a quick sear, they are cooked in an aromatic broth sweetened with sirop de Liège, which adds a subtle fruitiness. Serve with Leek Stoemp (page 217) or Mashed Potatoes (page 56).

INGREDIENTS

1. 1 pound (450 grams) ground lean veal
2. 1 1/2 pounds (675 grams) bulk Italian sausage
3. 1 pound (450 grams) ground pork shoulder
4. 1 tablespoon + 1 teaspoon (18 grams) kosher salt
5. 1 pound (450 grams) white bread, sliced and torn into pieces
6. 2 cups + 2 tablespoons (500 milliliters) whole milk
7. 8 tablespoons (1 stick/125 grams) unsalted butter
8. 3 medium yellow onions, diced, divided
9. 5 cloves garlic, diced
10. 6 large eggs (300 grams)
11. 1 cup (250 milliliters) canola oil, divided
12. 1/4 cup + 1 tablespoon (15 grams) chopped fresh thyme
13. 4 sprigs fresh thyme
14. 2 dried bay leaves
15. 1 cup (250 milliliters) dry white wine
16. 1 quart (1 liter) veal stock (store-bought, or page 207)
17. 1 quart (1 liter) chicken stock (store-bought, or page 208)
18. 2 tablespoons + 1 1/2 teaspoons (50 grams) sirop de Liège (see page 12)

DIRECTIONS

In a large bowl, mix by hand the veal, sausage, pork, and salt. Cover and refrigerate.

In another large bowl, place the bread and cover with the milk. Let sit for 15 minutes. Drain off the milk and using your hands, squeeze out the excess milk from the bread. Discard the milk.

In a medium sauté pan over medium heat, melt the butter. Add half of the onions and all the garlic and cook until translucent but not browned, about 10 minutes. Place in small bowl and set aside.

Use your hands to thoroughly mix the bread, eggs, chopped thyme, and the sautéed onions and garlic into the meat mixture.

In a large stew pot over medium heat, place 3 tablespoons (45 milliliters) of the canola oil, the remaining onions, the thyme sprigs, and bay leaves and cook until the onions are translucent but not browned, about 10 minutes. Add the wine and let it reduce by half, about 5 minutes. Add the veal and chicken stocks and cook for 10 minutes, until fully incorporated and there is no gelatin remaining. Turn off the heat and leave the pot on the stove.

Using your hands, form meatballs roughly the size of tennis balls, about 3 ounces (90 grams) each. In a large sauté pan over medium heat, heat the remaining 13 tablespoons (205 milliliters) oil until it smoke slightly. Place the meatballs in the pan, making sure to not overcrowd it, and sear on all sides until golden brown. Place the meatballs on a sheet pan covered in paper towels to drain.

Pass the sauce through a fine-mesh strainer and return it to the stew pot over medium heat. Add the sirop de Liège and the meatballs, cover, and cook until the meatball is tender (you can also a fork to pry one open slightly; it is done if the meat's color inside is uniformly gray), about 45 minutes. Let them cool for 15 minutes before serving.

35

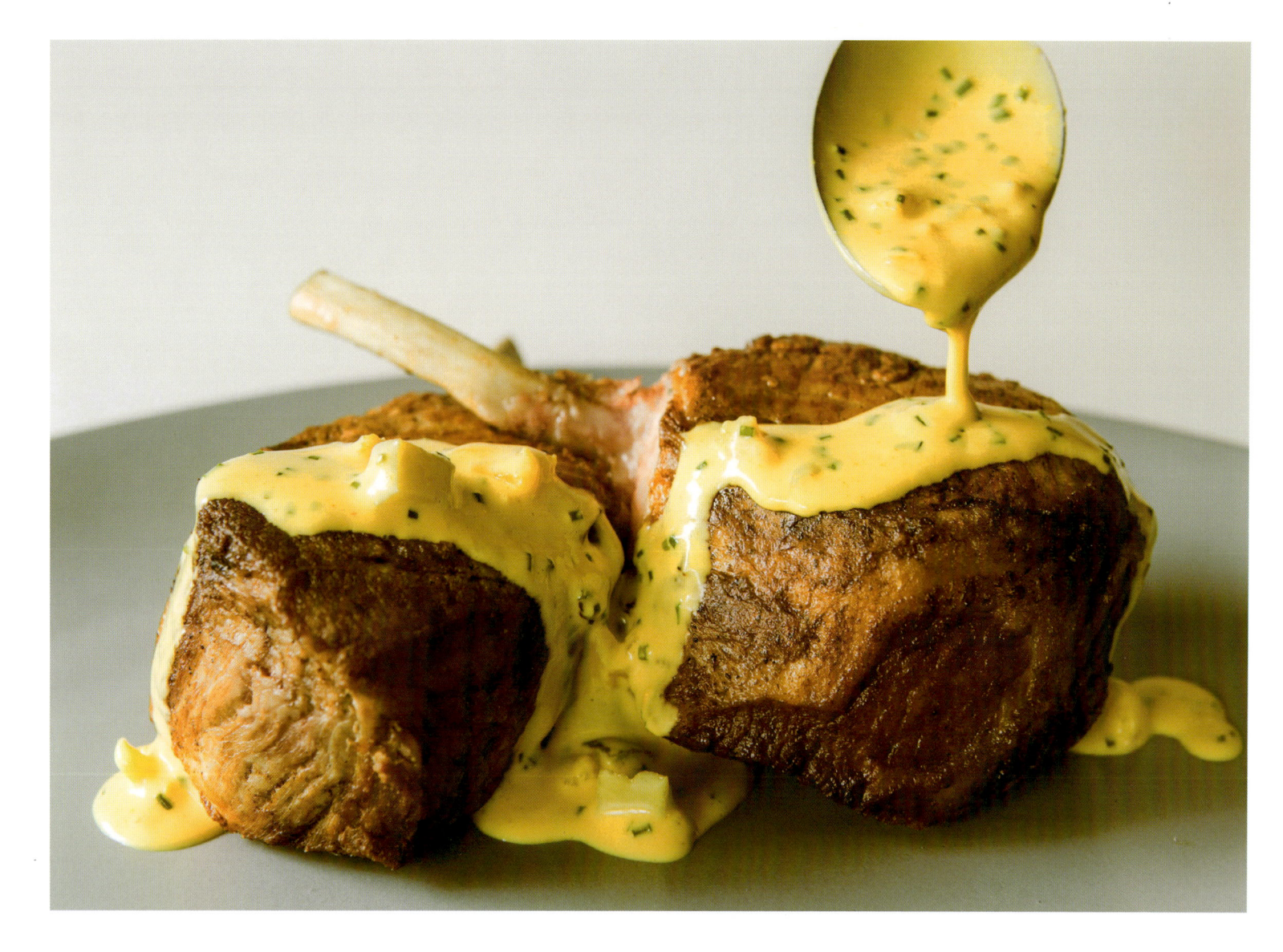

SERVES 4

Pork Chops with Blackwell Sauce

Packed with big flavors, this dish only requires a little work. The hardest part may be finding the Belgian pickles for the Blackwell sauce. I'm fond of those made by Devos & Lemmens, which can be purchased online or at some import stores.

INGREDIENTS

blackwell sauce

1. 2 1/4 cups (500 milliliters) heavy cream
2. 2 sprigs fresh thyme
3. 3 cloves garlic, smashed
4. 2 dried bay leaves
5. 1/4 cup + 2 tablespoons (100 grams) veal stock (store-bought, or page 207)
6. 1 cup (160 grams) finely diced Belgian pickles

Pork chops

1. 4 bone-in pork chops (10 to 12 ounces/about 280 grams each)
2. 1 tablespoon + 1 teaspoon (18 grams) kosher salt
3. 8 tablespoons (1 stick/125 grams) unsalted butter
4. 3 tablespoons (40 grams) canola oil

To assemble

1. 4 servings (about 4 cups/800 grams) Mashed Potatoes (page 56)

DIRECTIONS

To make the Blackwell sauce, in a medium saucepan over medium heat, place the cream, thyme, garlic, and bay leaves and cook until the cream has reduced and thickened slightly, about 20 minutes. Add the veal stock and cook until reduced by half, 10 to 15 minutes. Remove from the heat and pass the mixture through a fine-mesh strainer to remove the solids. Return it to the pot, add the pickles to the sauce, mix, and set aside.

Preheat the oven to 350°F (175°C).

Place the pork chops on a sheet pan and season both sides with salt. In a sauté pan over medium heat, warm the butter and canola oil. When the butter has melted completely and foaming lightly, cook the pork chops one at a time, until each side is golden brown, about 4 to 5 minutes per side. As each is done, place the pork chops on a clean sheet pan. Bake the chops in the oven for 8 to 10 minutes for medium-rare/medium doneness. Let the chops rest for 10 minutes.

To assemble, rewarm the sauce if necessary. Place mashed potatoes and a pork chop on each of four plates and ladle sauce over both.

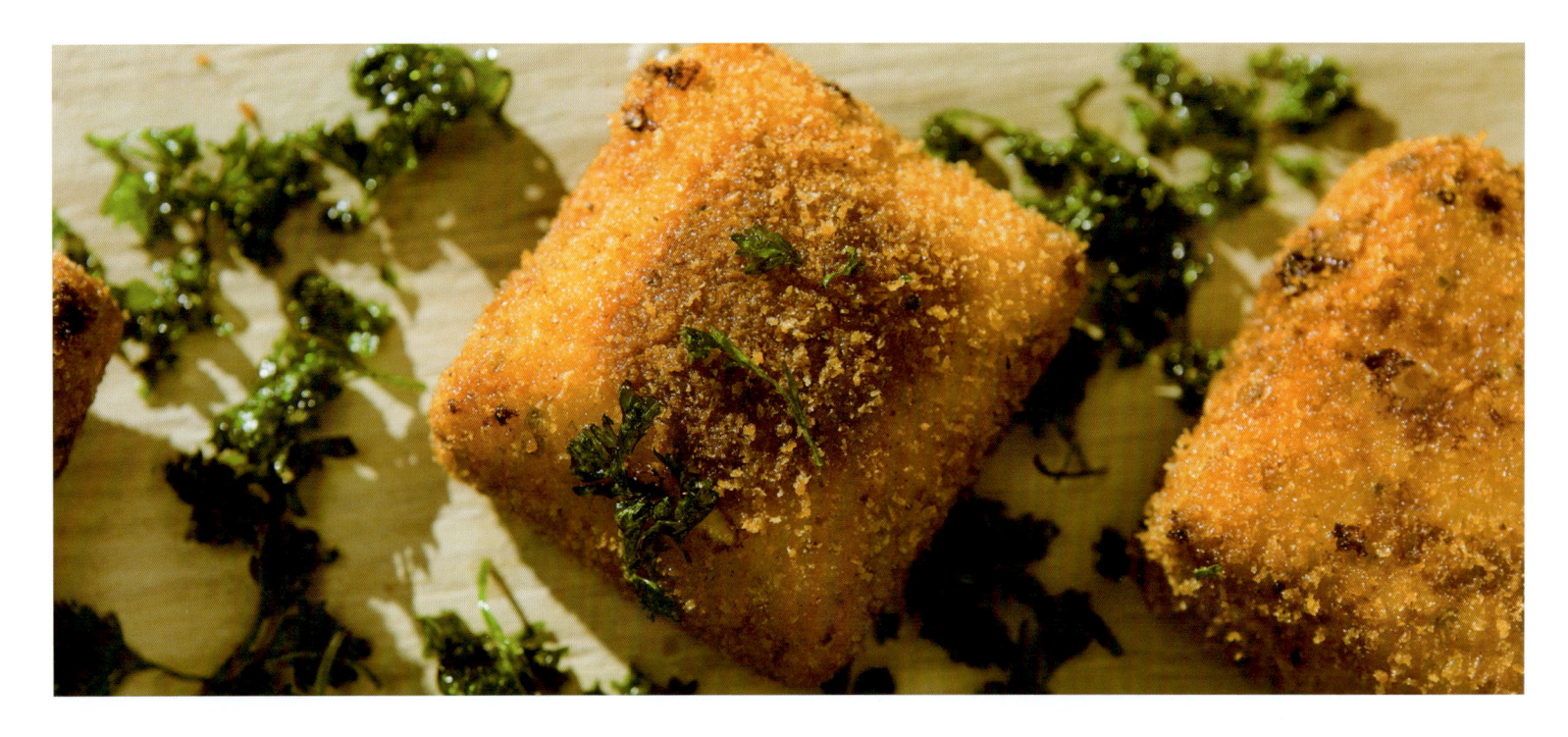

Ham and Cheese Croquettes

(Step By Step)

This is one of the first complex recipes I mastered when I was apprenticing at my father's shop. The chef taught me how to make a roux and why one is necessary when making béchamel. It really wasn't a big deal, but when you're 14 years old, it's impressive. One of the many uses of béchamel is as the base for these craveable croquettes. Packed with Gruyère, Grana Padano, and ham (Leoncini and Madrange produces some excellent options), the golden squares are decadent and delicious. If they're too rich for your taste, squeeze on fresh lemon juice. You really need a countertop deep-fryer for this recipe. Waring, All-Clad, and Delonghi all make excellent models. Gelatin sheets are also required; they can be purchased online through retailers such as Modernist Pantry.

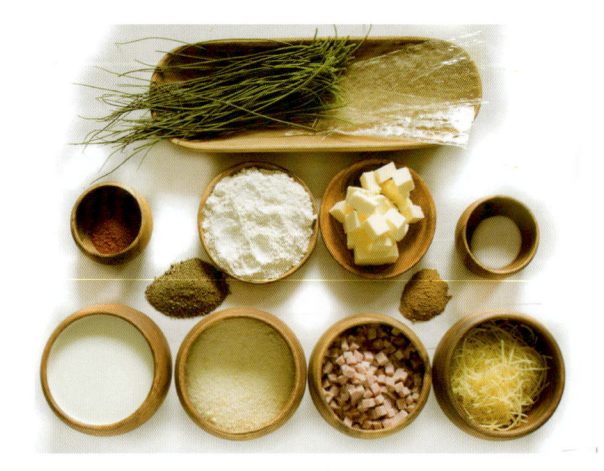

INGREDIENTS

1. 1 quart (1 liter) whole milk
2. 6 tablespoons (3/4 stick/90 grams) unsalted butter
3. 1 3/4 cups (210 grams) all-purpose flour, divided
4. 2 teaspoons (9 grams) kosher salt, divided
5. 1 3/4 teaspoons (4 grams) freshly ground black pepper
6. 1 teaspoon (2 grams) ground nutmeg
7. 1 teaspoon (2 grams) Espelette pepper
8. 10 sheets gelatin
9. 2 cups (200 grams) grated Grana Padano cheese
10. 1 cup (100 grams) grated Gruyère cheese
11. 1 1/2 cups (300 grams) diced deli ham
12. 1/4 cup + 3 tablespoons (20 grams) chopped fresh chives
13. Vegetable oil for frying
14. 3 large eggs (150 grams)
15. 1 teaspoon (5 grams) extra virgin olive oil
16. 5 cups (500 grams) dried breadcrumbs

DIRECTIONS

Spray a sheet pan with nonstick spray. Place parchment paper on the pan and then spray the paper. Set aside. [Image 6, 7 and 8]

In a medium saucepan over high heat, bring the milk to a boil. Immediately remove it from the heat and set aside.

Preheat the oven to 350°F (175°C). In a medium ovensafe saucepan over medium heat, melt the butter. Add 3/4 cup (90 grams) of the flour and whisk until the flour and butter are completely mixed. Place saucepan in the oven and bake for 5 minutes, until the mixture is brownish and smells like a freshly baked biscuit. [Image 1]

Place the butter-flour mixture back on the stove over medium heat. Add the milk and whisk until thoroughly combined.

Cook, constantly stirring gently, until it is smooth and thickened, about 20 minutes. Whisk in 1 teaspoon (5 grams) of the salt, the black pepper, nutmeg, and Espelette pepper. Remove from the heat.

In the meantime, put the gelatin sheets in a medium bowl and cover them with cold water. Let them soak until they have softened, then squeeze out the extra water. Whisk the gelatin sheets into the béchamel. Whisk in the Grana Padano and Gruyère until fully incorporated and the sauce is smooth. Use a wooden spoon to mix in the ham and chives until fully incorporated. [Image 2 through 5 and 9 through 11]

Cover the bottom and sides of a rimmed sheet pan with plastic wrap, pour in the mixture, cover with plastic wrap, and place in the refrigerator to set for 24 hours. (The mixture will keep for a week in the refrigerator if you don't want to fry the croquettes right away.) [Images 13 and 14]

When you are ready to cook, following the manufacturer's instructions, fill a deep-fryer with vegetable oil and heat it to 325°F (165°C). Fill one small bowl with the remaining 1 cup (120 grams) flour, a second small bowl with the eggs whisked with remaining 1/2 teaspoon (2 grams) salt and the olive oil, and a third bowl with breadcrumbs. Cut the ham and cheese mixture into 2-inch (5 cm) squares. [Images 15 and 16]

Bread the croquettes by dipping them first in the flour, then the egg wash, and then the breadcrumbs, making sure they get fully coated during each step. [Images 17 through 21]

As they are coated, place the croquettes on a clean sheet pan.

Place the croquettes in the deep-fryer in batches to ensure there's no overcrowding. Fry until golden brown. Place them on a sheet pan covered with paper towels to remove excess oil. Serve warm. [Image 22]

Stepwise Instructions

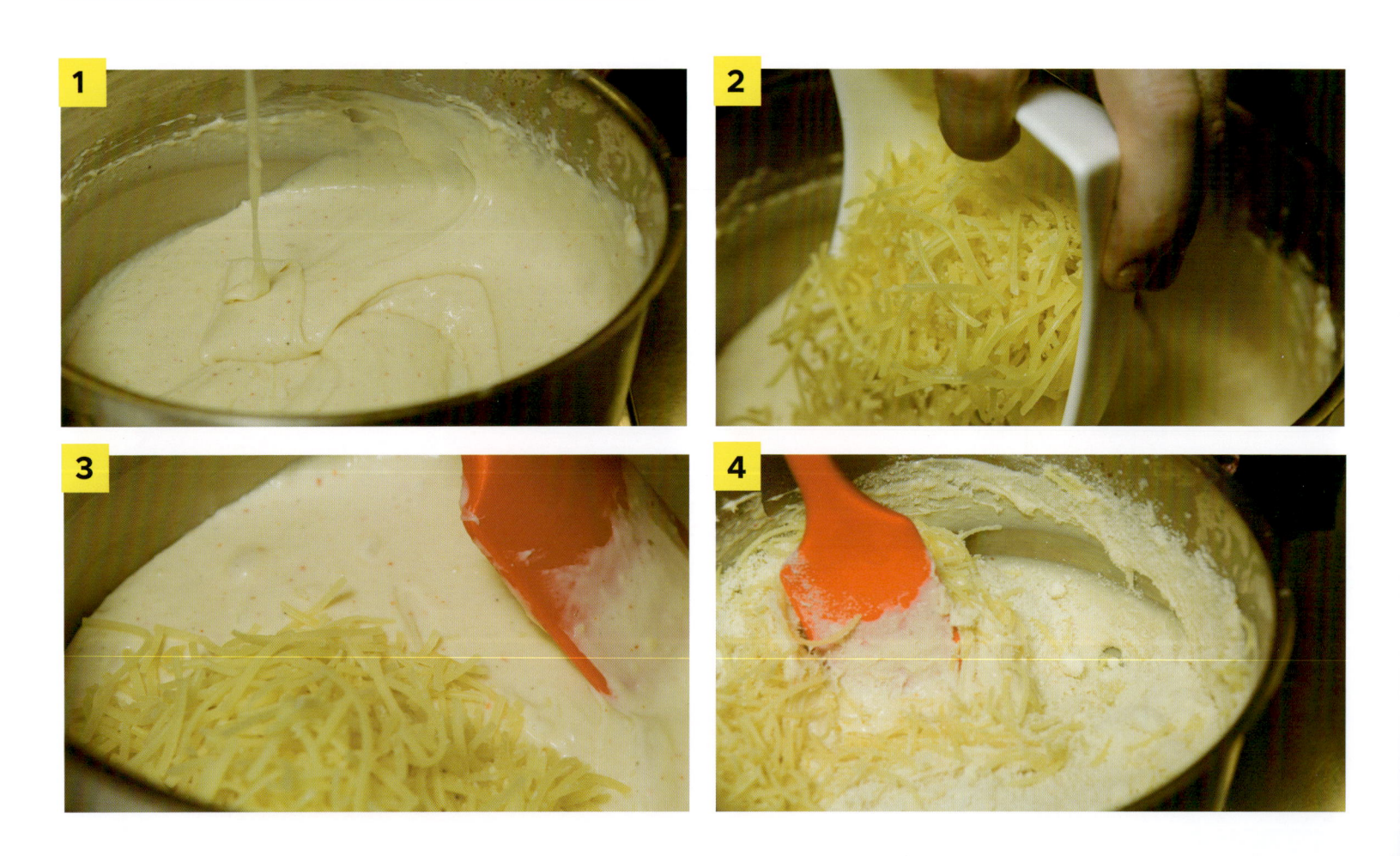

PAGE 137

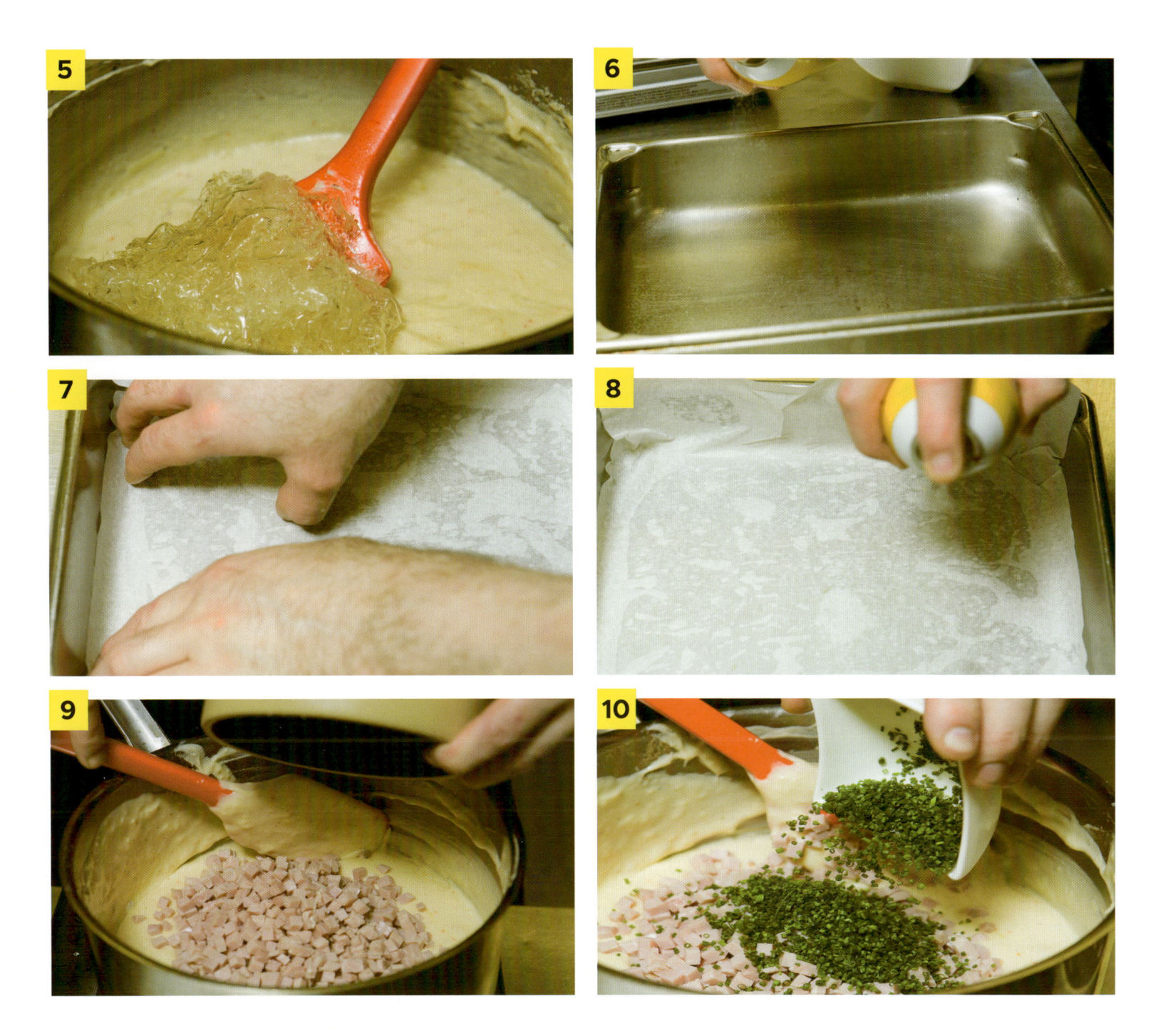

PAGE 138

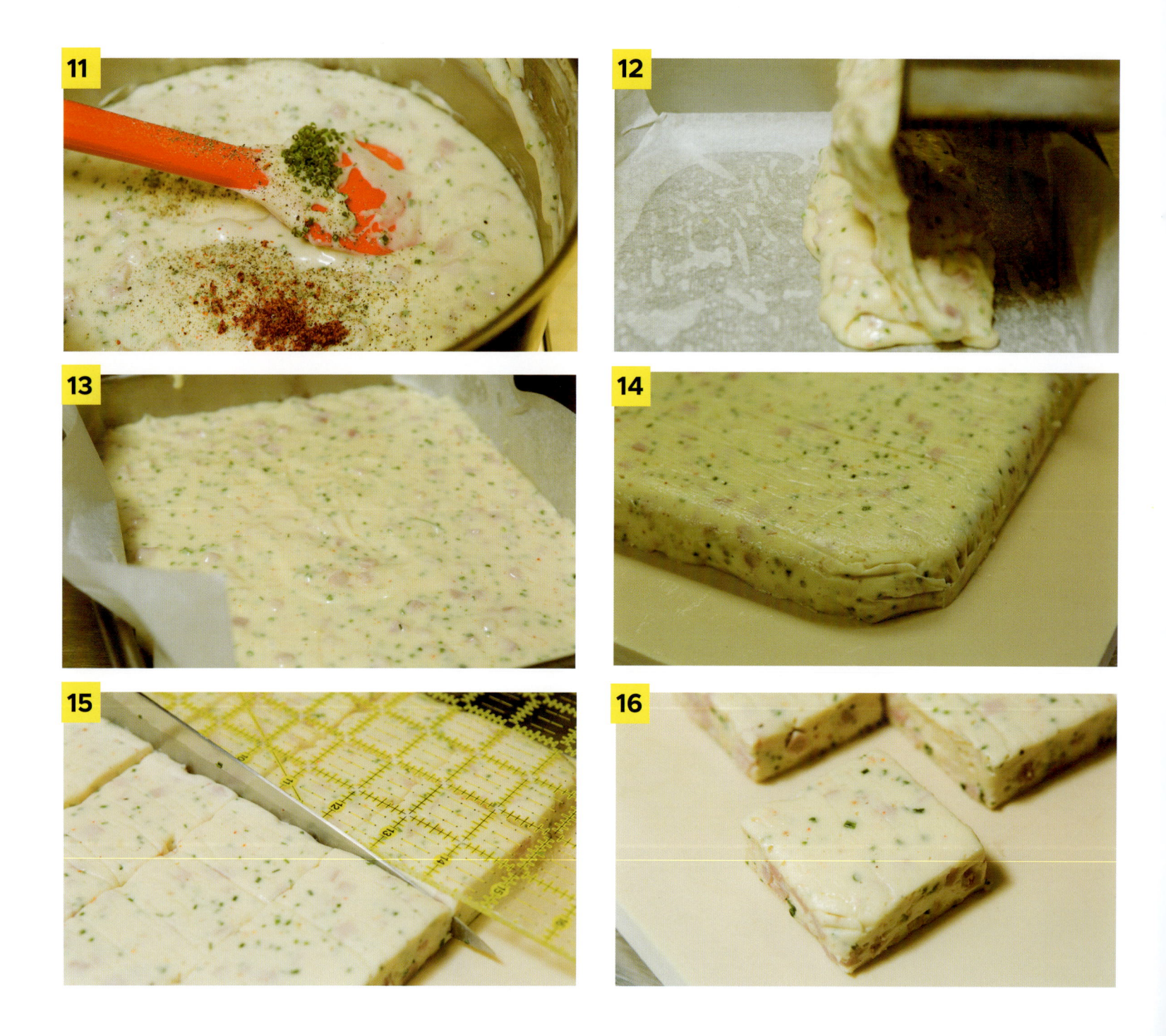

PAGE 139

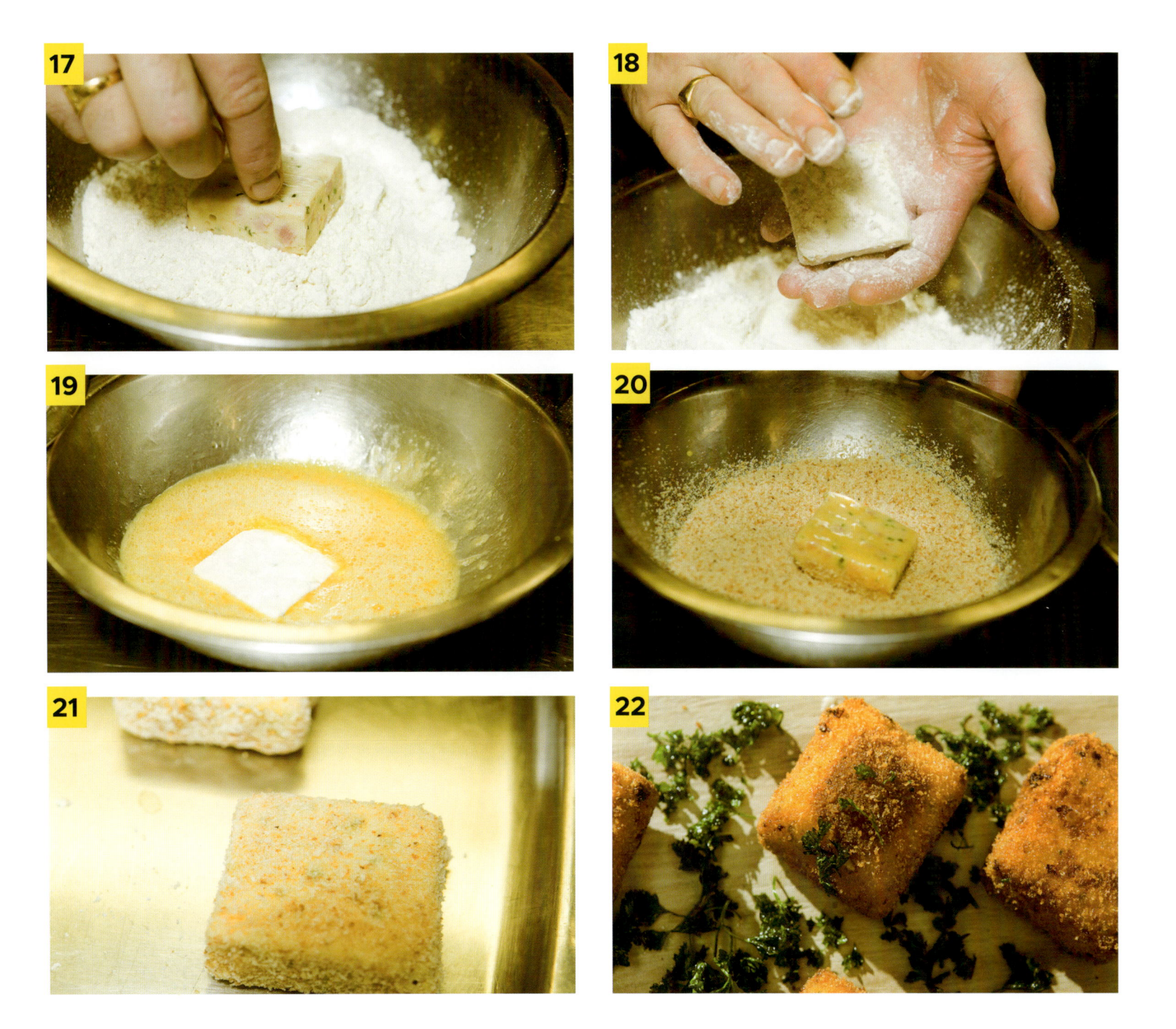

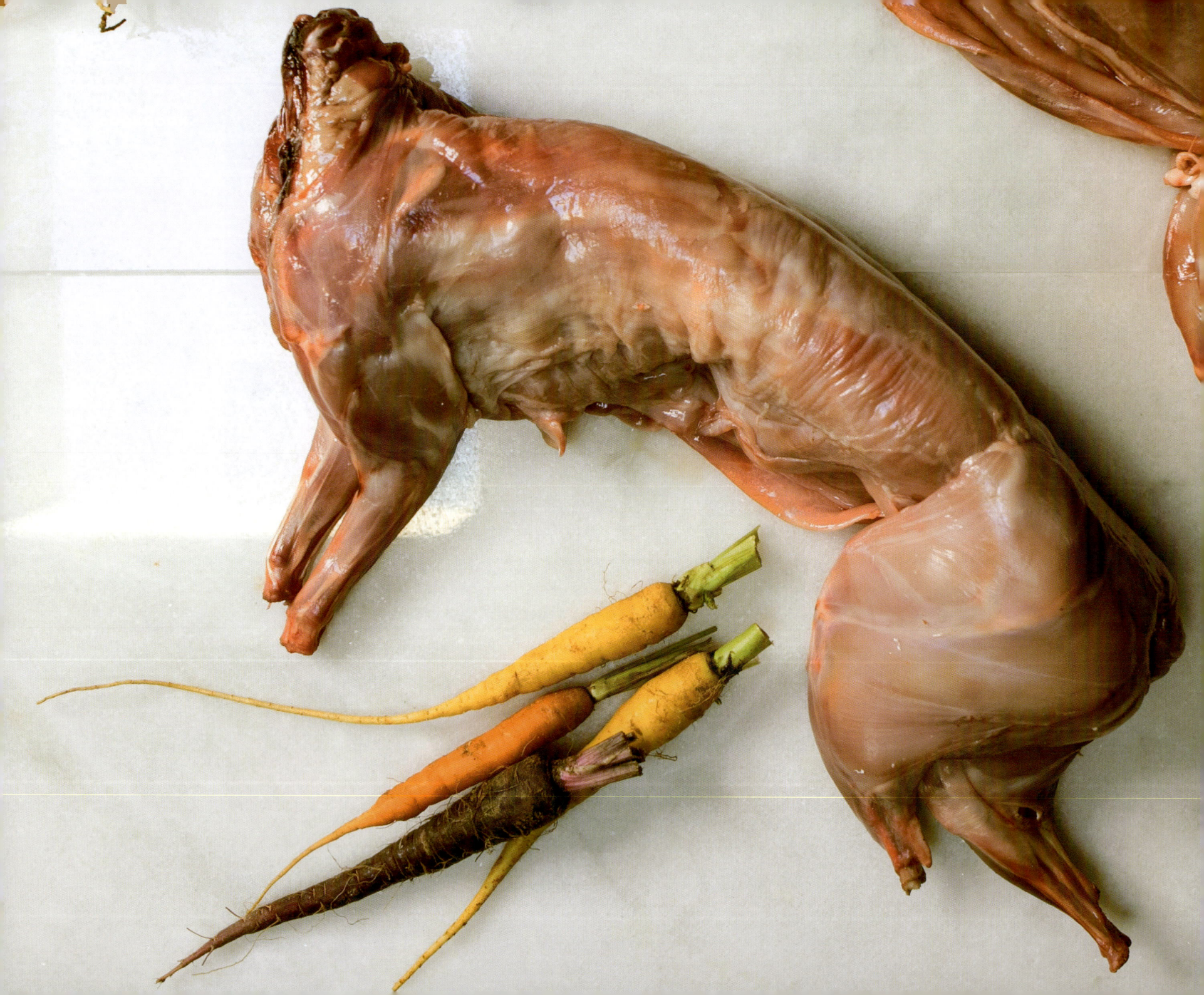

RABBIT

When I first started putting rabbit on the menu, my customers were hesitant to try it. But in the decade since we opened, diners have become more open to it—and many of them have fallen in love. For those that aren't familiar with this game meat, I compare it to a finer version of chicken, because it really soaks up whatever flavors you throw at it. Rabbit is available from specialty butchers, at many farmers markets, and online from gourmet purveyors such as D'Artagnan. Usually they are sold whole. Look for smooth, glossy flesh. Steer clear of those with dry or sticky flesh, or those with a metallic odor—they are past their proverbial use-by date.

37

SERVES 4

Rabbit Cannelloni

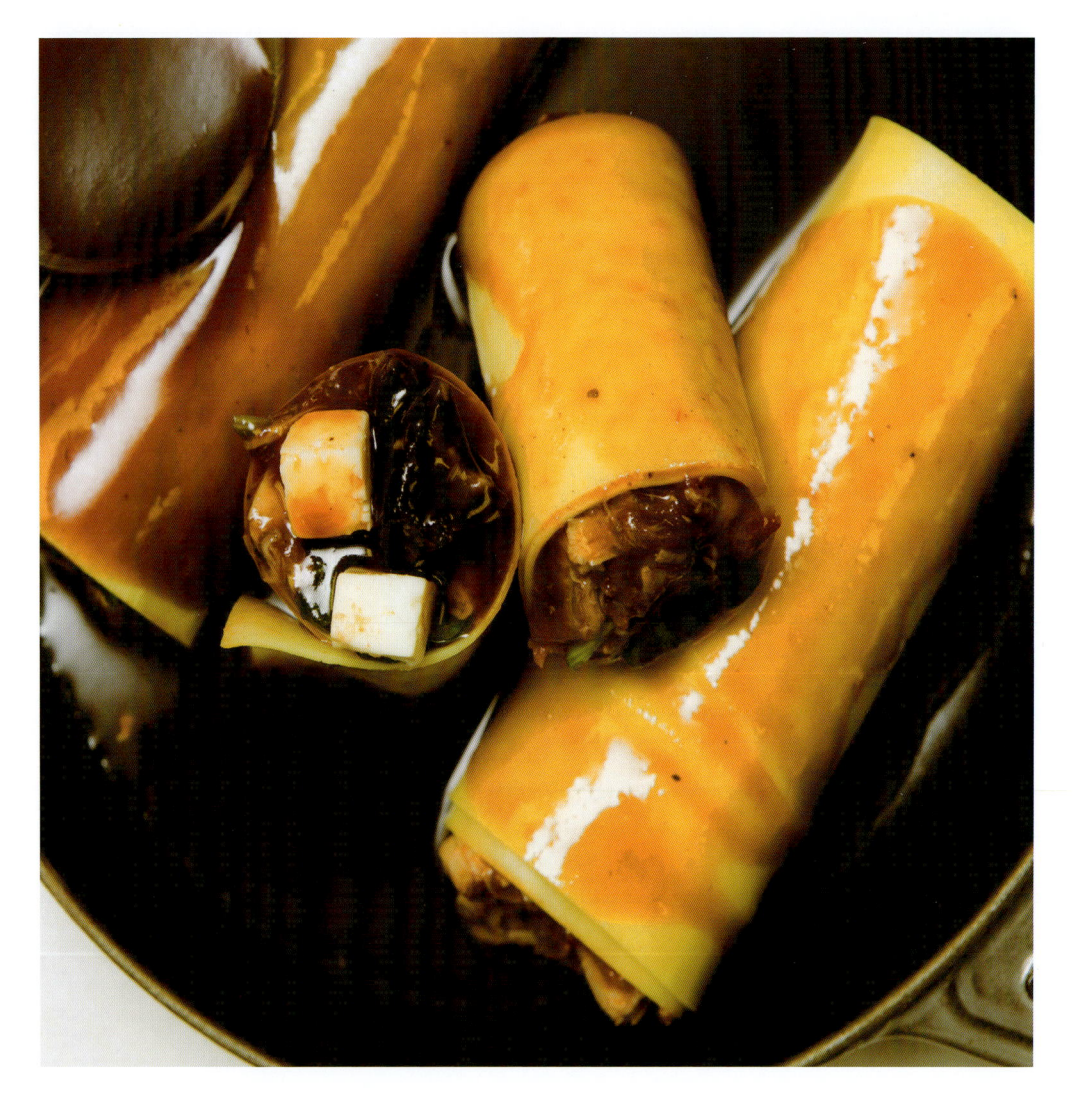

INGREDIENTS

1. 4 medium rear rabbit legs (about 2 1/4 pounds/1 kilogram total)
2. 3 tablespoons (42 grams) kosher salt, divided
3. 2 tablespoons (30 grams) vegetable oil, divided
4. 4 medium shallots, grated
5. 4 cloves garlic, grated
6. 2 stalks celery, grated
7. 1 large carrot, grated
8. 2 1/4 cups (500 milliliters) merlot or similar red wine
9. 1 sprig fresh thyme
10. 1 dried bay leaf
11. One 28-ounce (800 grams) can whole peeled San Marzano tomatoes
12. 3 sheets (12 by 6 inches/30 by 15 cm) fresh lasagna noodles (store-bought or page 216)
13. 3/4 cup + 2 tablespoons (200 grams) cooked spinach (page 213)
14. 6 prunes, pitted and diced
15. 1/2 cup (50 grams) diced Greek feta cheese
16. Grated zest from 2 medium oranges

Most people gravitate toward ground beef or veal when stuffing their cannelloni. I devised this recipe featuring braised rabbit mixed with spinach, prunes, and orange zest. The tubular pasta gets topped with feta and a reduction of the braising liquid. You will need a pasta machine for this recipe. Imperia makes affordable and reliable options. Rabbit can be purchased from good butchers and at some farmer's markets.

DIRECTIONS

Season both sides of the rabbit legs with 1 teaspoon (5 grams) of the salt. In medium sauté pan over medium heat, warm 1 tablespoon (15 milliliters) of the oil until smoking slightly, and then sear rabbit legs, two at a time, until both sides are golden brown. Remove from pan and set aside.

In a medium stew pot over medium heat, warm the remaining 1 tablespoon (15 milliliters) oil until shimmering, then add the shallots, garlic, celery, and carrots. Stirring continuously with a wooden spatula, cook the vegetables until they are softened, about 10 minutes. Add the wine, thyme, and bay leaf and cook until the liquid has reduced by half, 10 to 15 minutes. Add the tomatoes and their juices, 1 teaspoon (5 grams) of the salt, and the rabbit legs. Turn down heat to low, cover, and simmer until the meat is coming off the bones, about 1 1/2 hours.

While the rabbit is cooking, fill a large pot three-quarters full of water and add the remaining 2 tablespoons (28 grams) salt. Bring to a boil over high heat. Once the water has reached a rolling boil, add the lasagna noodles one sheet at a time and cook until al dente, about 5 minutes (or follow the manufacturer's instructions). Remove the noodle from the boiling water with a mesh skimmer, place in a strainer set in the sink, and run cold water over it. Lay a clean kitchen towel on a sheet pan and place the noodle on it. Repeat these steps until all 3 sheets of lasagna noodles are cooked.

Cut out 8 rectangles measuring 6 by 4 inches (15 by 10 cm) from the sheets of lasagna noodles. Set aside. Freeze the remaining lasagna noodle for another project.

Using a slotted spoon, remove the rabbit legs from the pot and set aside to cool. Pass the sauce through a fine-mesh strainer, pressing the mixture down with the back of a ladle. Discard the remaining solids. Divide the resulting liquid into two equal portions in two small bowls.

Remove all the rabbit meat from the bones and shred it. Place the meat and half of the sauce in a medium pot over low heat. Simmer until the sauce has reduced by half, about 20 minutes.

Preheat the oven to 350°F (175°C).

In a large bowl using a wooden spoon, gently mix together the spinach, prunes, rabbit mixture, feta, and orange zest. Place 2 tablespoons (28 grams) of the rabbit mixture lengthwise about 1 inch (2.5 cm) from the long edge of a pasta sheet. Roll up like a cigar. Place seam down in a 13 by 9-inch (33 by 23 cm) ovensafe glass baking pan, cover with the remaining sauce, and bake for 15 minutes.

To assemble, place two cannelloni on each plate and ladle on some of the sauce from the baking pan.

Cherry Beer–Braised Rabbit

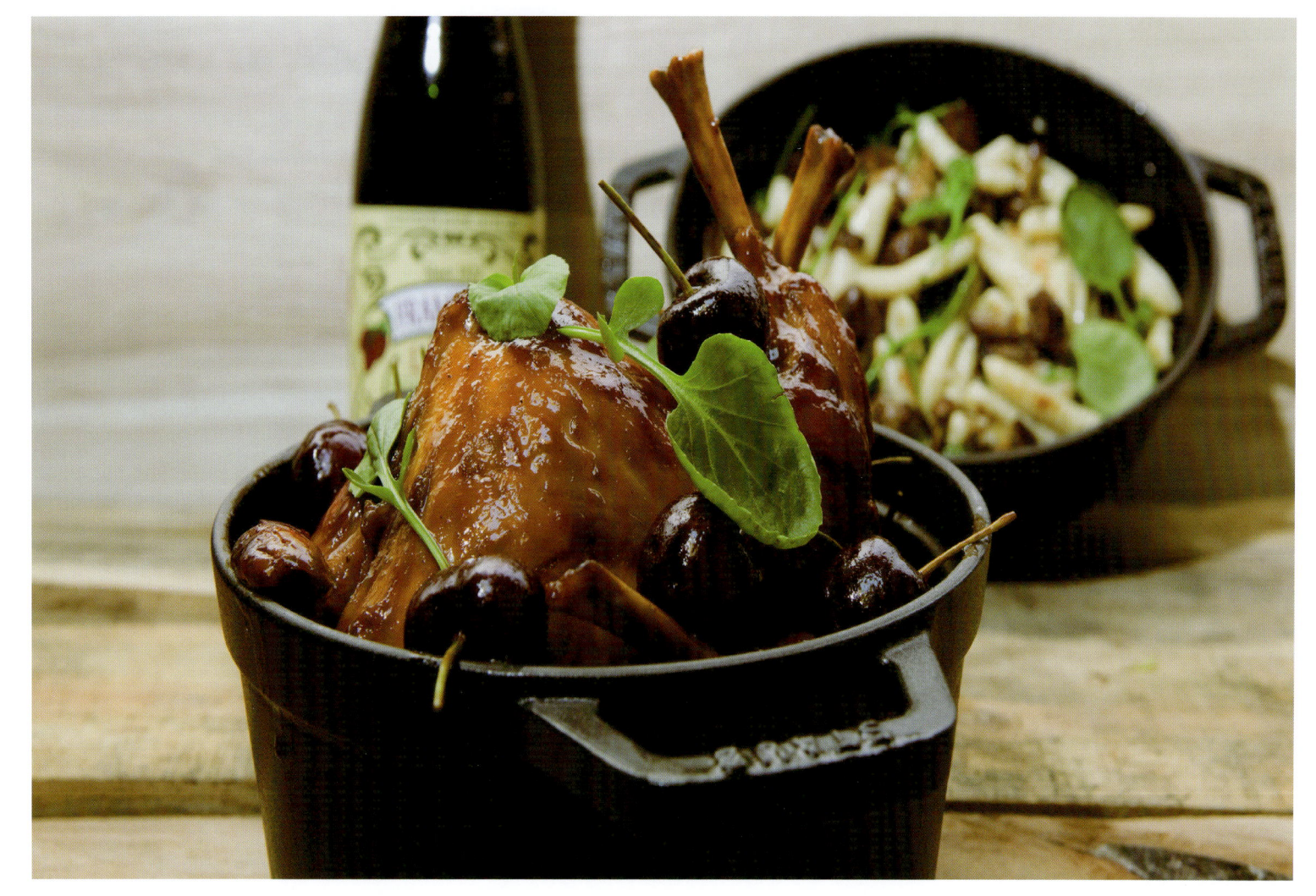

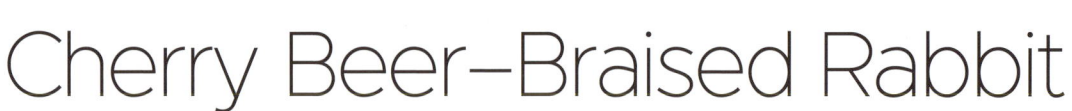

A beautiful photo of this dish sat atop Washington Post critic Tom Sietsema's lovely review of the restaurant in his 2014 Fall Dining Guide. I'm very proud of the recipe, which is much easier to execute than you probably think. Serve it at a winter dinner party and your guests won't be able to stop singing your praises. Accompany it with a Kriek beer to emphasize the cherry flavor. I like Lindemans Kriek, which can often be found at craft beer import shops or online at BelgianShop.com.

INGREDIENTS

1. 4 medium rear rabbit legs (about 2 1/4 pounds/1 kilogram total)
2. Kosher salt
3. 1/4 cup + 2 tablespoons (70 grams) canola oil, divided
4. 1/2 medium carrot, diced
5. 1/2 medium yellow onion, diced
6. 1 medium shallot, finely diced
7. 1/2 stalk celery, diced
8. 4 cloves garlic, finely chopped
9. 2 sprigs fresh thyme
10. 2 dried bay leaves
11. 1 teaspoon (5 grams) crushed black peppercorns
12. 1 bottle (26 ounces/750 milliliters) Kriek (cherry lambic) beer
13. 1 quart (1 liter) veal stock (store-bought, or page 207)
14. 2 cups (500 milliliters) chicken stock (store-bought, or page 208)
15. 3/4 cup (180 grams) fresh tart cherries, pitted
16. 1 1/4 cups (260 grams) Ricotta Cavatelli (store-bought, or page 51)
17. 2 tablespoons (30 grams) unsalted butter
18. 6 ounces (180 grams) nameko or brown beech mushrooms, separated and cleaned
19. 1 tablespoon (10 grams) chopped shallots
20. 1 tablespoon (10 grams) finely diced garlic
21. 1 cup (240 milliliters) chicken stock (store-bought, or page 208)
22. Watercress sprigs for garnish

DIRECTIONS

Preheat the oven to 350°F (175°C).

Season both sides of the rabbit legs with salt. Warm 2 tablespoons (30 milliliters) of the oil in a large sauté over medium heat and sear rabbit legs two at a time until both sides are golden brown color. Remove from the pan and set aside.

In a large ovensafe stew pot over medium heat, warm the remaining 2 tablespoons (30 milliliters) oil until shimmering, then add the carrots, onions, finely diced shallot, celery, and finely chopped garlic. Cook until softened and the onions are translucent, about 10 minutes. Add the thyme, bay leaves, peppercorns, and beer and cook until the liquid is reduced by half, 10 to 15 minutes. Add the veal and chicken stocks and bring to a boil. Add the rabbit, cover the pot, and place in the oven. Cook until rabbit is cooked through, about 1 1/2 hours. To check if the rabbit is cooked, press your finger against the meat. If it comes off the bone easily, it's ready.

Remove the rabbit from the sauce and set aside to keep warm. Pass the sauce through a fine-mesh strainer into a medium bowl, discard the solids, then transfer the sauce back into the stew pot. Spoon off all excess fat. Place the pot over medium heat and let the liquid reduce until the sauce coats the back of a wooden spoon, 20 to 25 minutes.

In a small sauté pan over medium heat, place the cherries and 3 tablespoons (45 milliliters) of the sauce. Simmer until the cherries have softened and are beginning to release their juices, about 5 minutes. Remove from heat.

Cook the cavatelli according to the instructions on page 51 (or the manufacturer's instructions) until al dente. Drain and set aside.

In a medium skillet over medium heat, melt the butter. Add the mushrooms, chopped shallots, and finely diced garlic and sauté until the mushrooms are golden brown, about 6 to 8 minutes. Add the cavatelli and chicken stock and sauté until the chicken stock has evaporated.

To assemble the dish, place a rabbit leg on each plate, ladle cherry sauce on top (rewarming first if necessary), and garnish with watercress. Serve the cavatelli and mushrooms on the side.

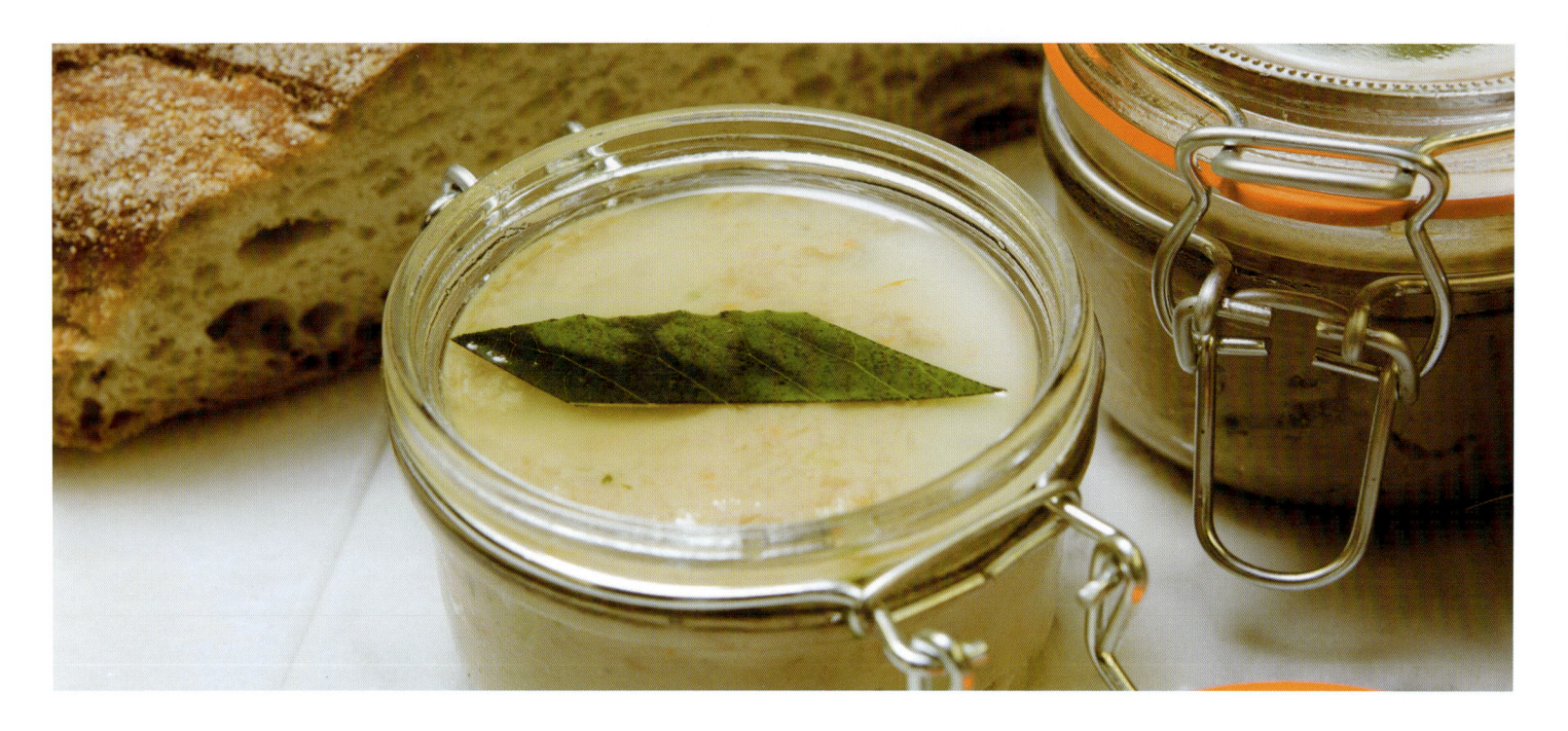

39

SERVES 8

Rabbit Rillettes

(Step By Step)

The chunky country-style pâté adds wow factor to a charcuterie board. Full of shredded rabbit, chunks of pork belly, and creamy sweet potato, it's best smeared on a round of crusty baguette and complemented by whatever pickled produce you have on hand. To make the rillettes' presentation daintier, I serve it in small swing top jars, which are available in the canning section of some hardware stores or online. You will need a stand mixer with the paddle attachment to best execute the recipe. Duck fat is available in many gourmet grocery stores or online from D'Artagnan; gray sea salt (sel gris) is available at some import stores and online at Yummy Bazaar and elsewhere; and Mason jars can be found in the canning section of most grocery stores and hardware stores.

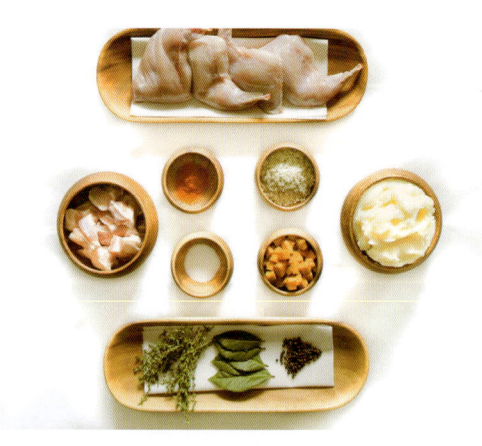

INGREDIENTS

1. 4 medium rear rabbit legs (about 2 1/4 pounds/1 kilogram total)
2. 1/4 cup + 3 tablespoons (100 grams) gray sea salt
3. 9 3/4 cups (2 kilograms) rendered duck fat
4. 2 sprigs fresh thyme
5. 1 dried bay leaf
6. 1 teaspoon (4 grams) whole black peppercorns
7. 1 pound (450 grams) pork belly with rind, diced into 1-inch (2.5 cm) pieces
8. 11 ounces (300 grams) sweet potato, peeled and diced into 3-inch (7.5 cm) pieces (about 1 1/2 cups)
9. 1 1/4 teaspoons (6 grams) kosher salt
10. 1/4 cup (25 grams) diced green onion (white and green parts)

DIRECTIONS

Place the rabbit legs on a rimmed sheet pan and sprinkle with sea salt on all sides. Let sit for 30 minutes, then wash off all the salt with cold water. Pat the legs dry with a kitchen towel. [Images 1, 2 and 3]]

In a large saucepan over medium heat, melt the duck fat. Add the rabbit legs, thyme, bay leaf, black peppercorns, and pork belly. Turn down the heat to low and cover. Cook until the rabbit and pork are tender, about 1 1/2 hours. [Images 4 and 5]

While the rabbit is cooking, place a medium pot over medium-high heat. Add the sweet potato and cover with cold water. Add the kosher salt. Bring to boil and cook until a fork easily pierces a potato about 40 minutes. Pour the potatoes into a strainer set in the sink to drain. [Image 6]

When the rabbit and pork belly are finished cooking, remove them from the duck fat and place them in a fine-mesh strainer over a bowl to drain. Strain the duck fat into a medium bowl through another fine-mesh strainer and set aside. When the rabbit legs are cool enough to touch, remove all the bones as well as any thyme, bay leaf, or peppercorns that have stuck to the meat. [Image 7]

In the bowl of a stand mixer fitted with the paddle attachment, mash the rabbit meat and the pork belly on low speed until it is shredded. Slowly pour in 3/4 cup (180 milliliters) of the strained duck fat and mix until fully incorporated. Add the sweet potatoes and mix for 2 minutes more, until fully incorporated and smooth. Add the green onions and mix until just combined. [Image 8, 9 and 10]

Divide the mixture evenly between eight 5.4-ounce (160 milliliter) Mason jars. Pour approximately 1 tablespoon (15 milliliters) of the strained duck fat on top of the meat mixture until the top is completely covered. Let them cool completely, then seal the jars and refrigerate them until you're ready to serve. The rillettes will keep for up to 6 months in the refrigerator. Freeze the remaining duck fat for further projects.

PAGE 148

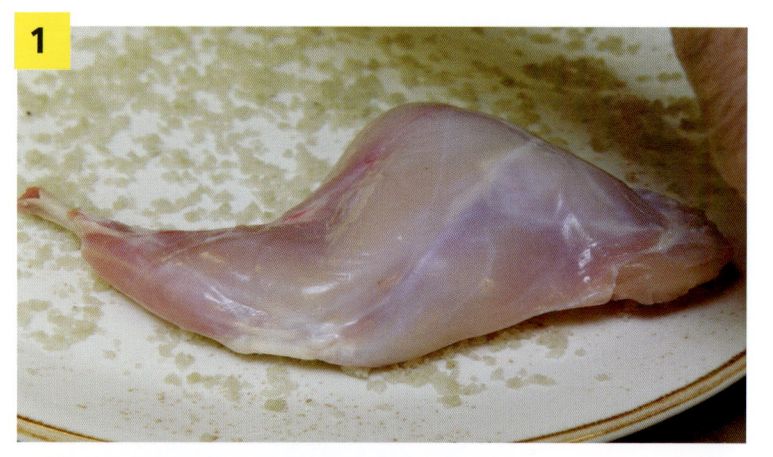

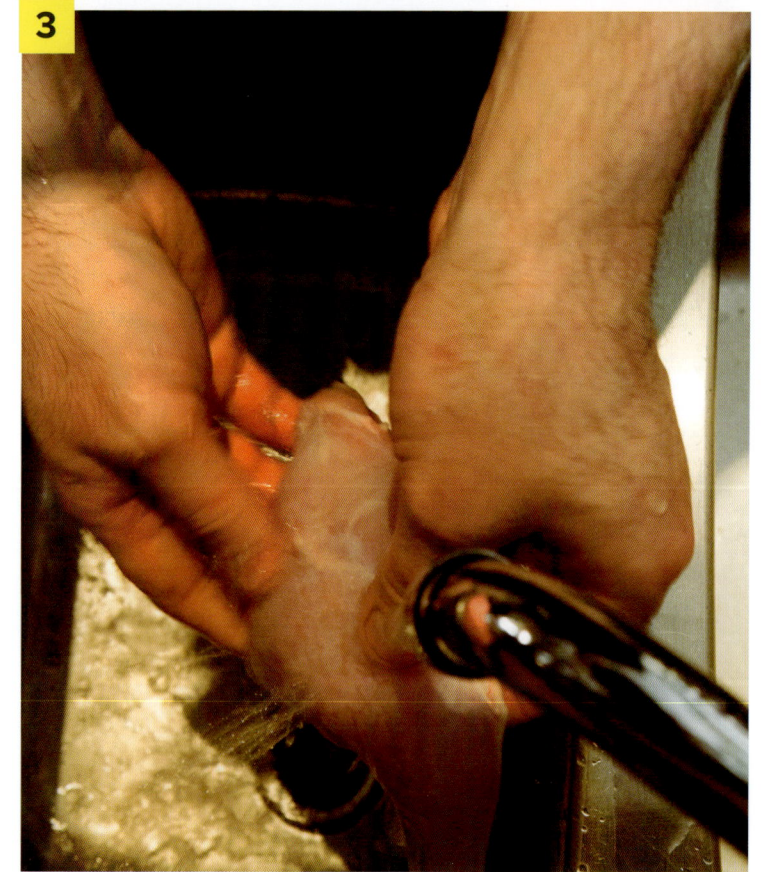

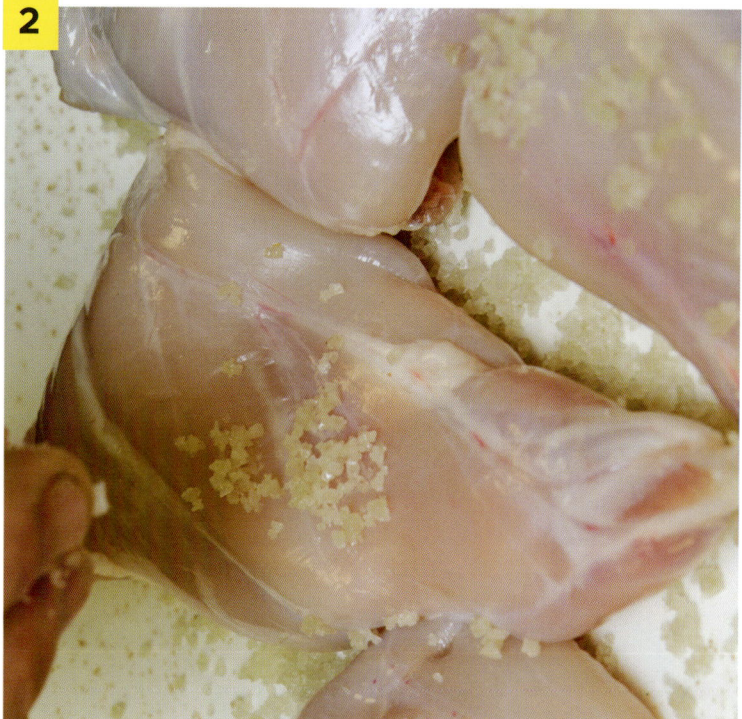

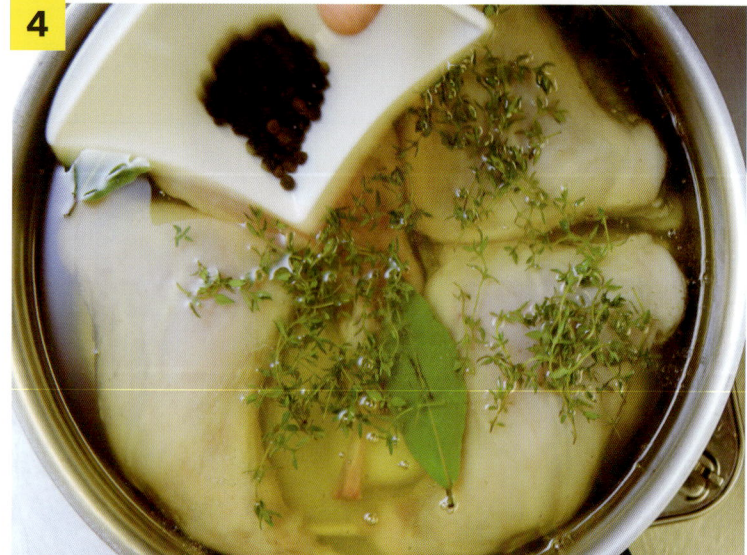

PAGE 149

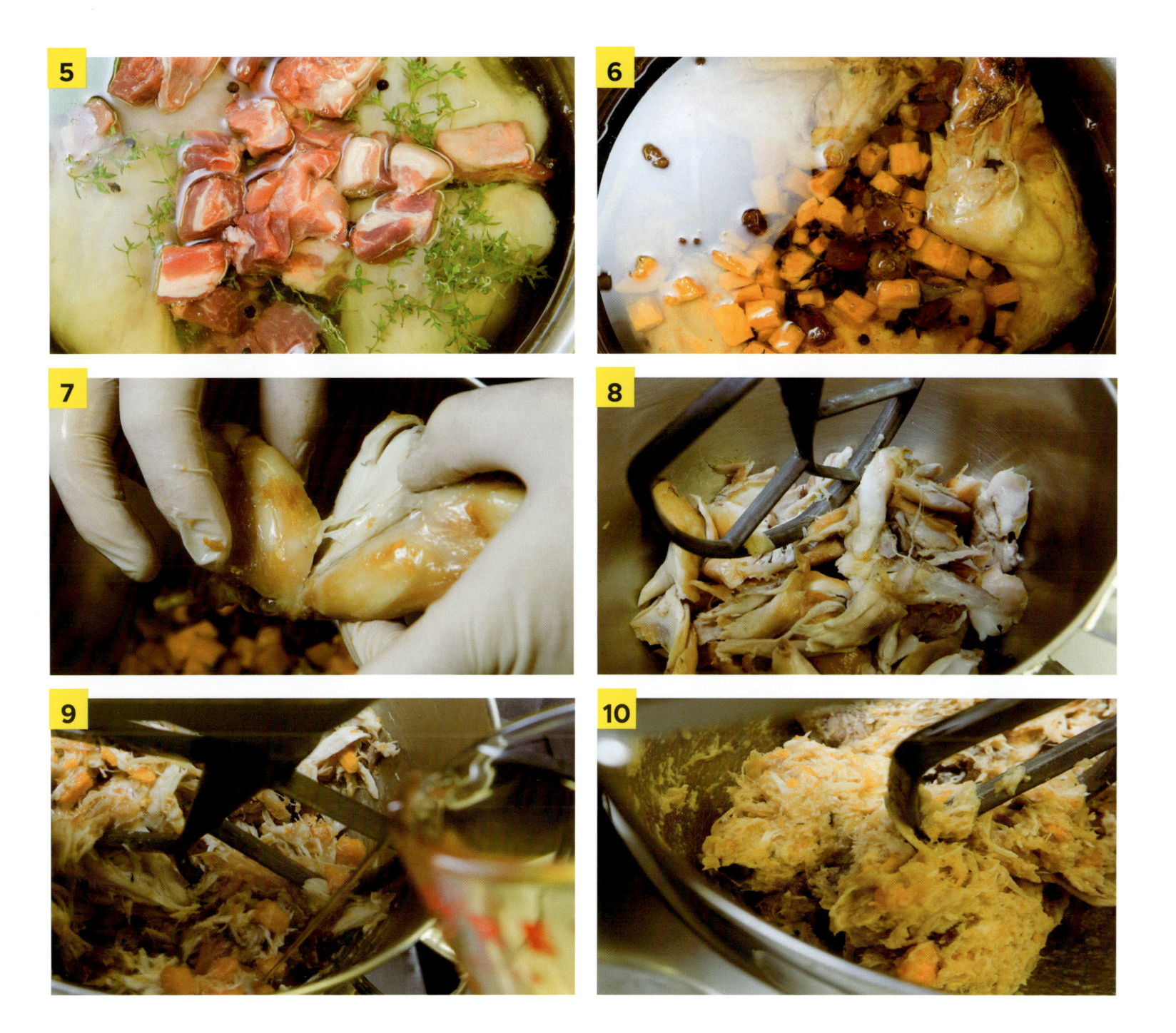

WORKING CLASS HEROES

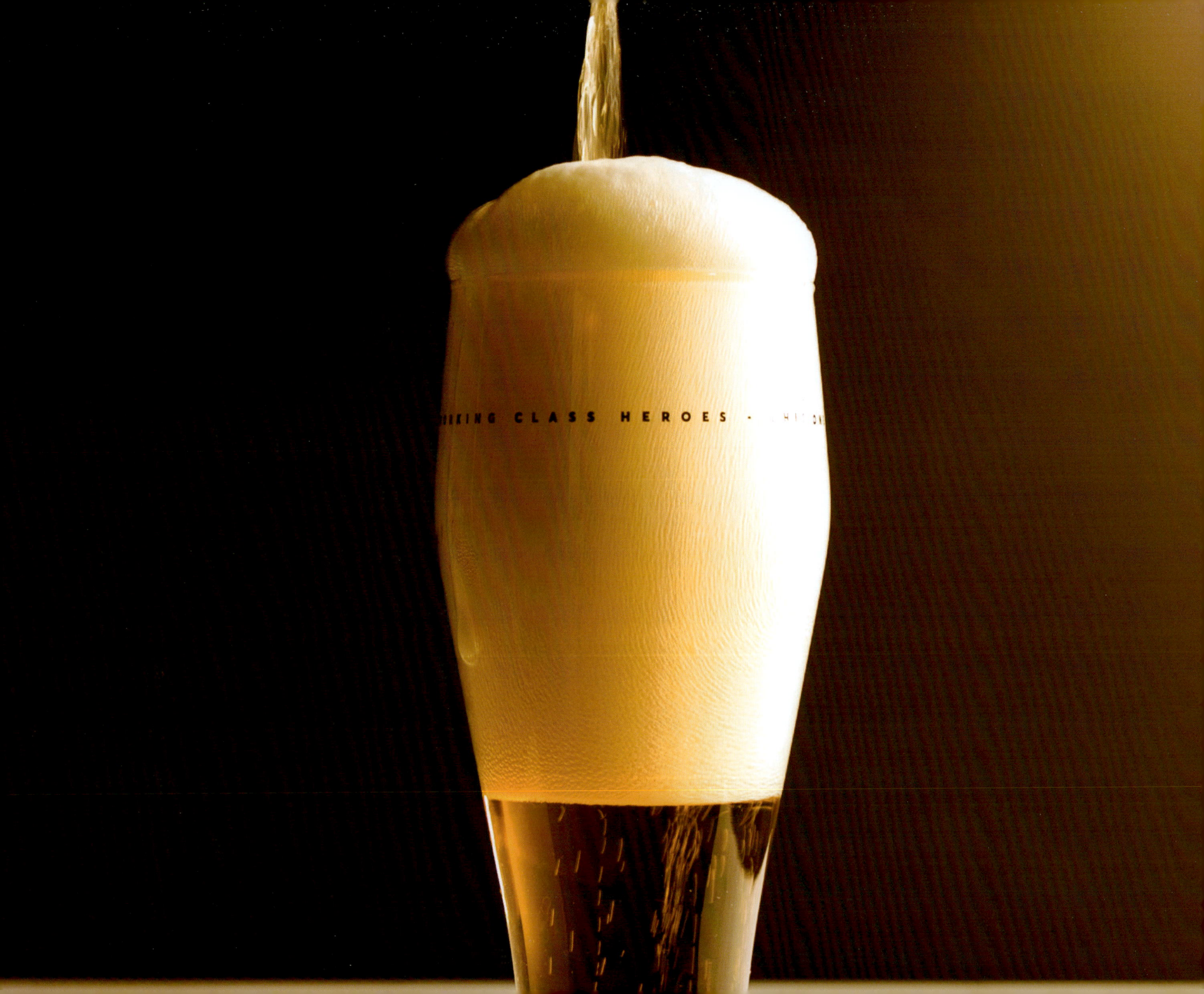

BEER

Beer bottles ring the shelf floating above our bar. We carry nearly 30 options, almost all of them Belgian, except for two French varietals and the occasional local craft brew. Though I cook with beer all the time, I rarely have the opportunity to sit down in my own restaurant to enjoy one myself. Maybe that will be my New Year's resolution next year. Let's hope it goes better than some of my previous resolutions! For those in the DC area, you can source a solid selection of Belgian beers at any Rodman's location, Calvert Woodley in Van Ness, or any Total Wine in Virginia, and readers anywhere can find purchase many options online at BelgianShop.com.

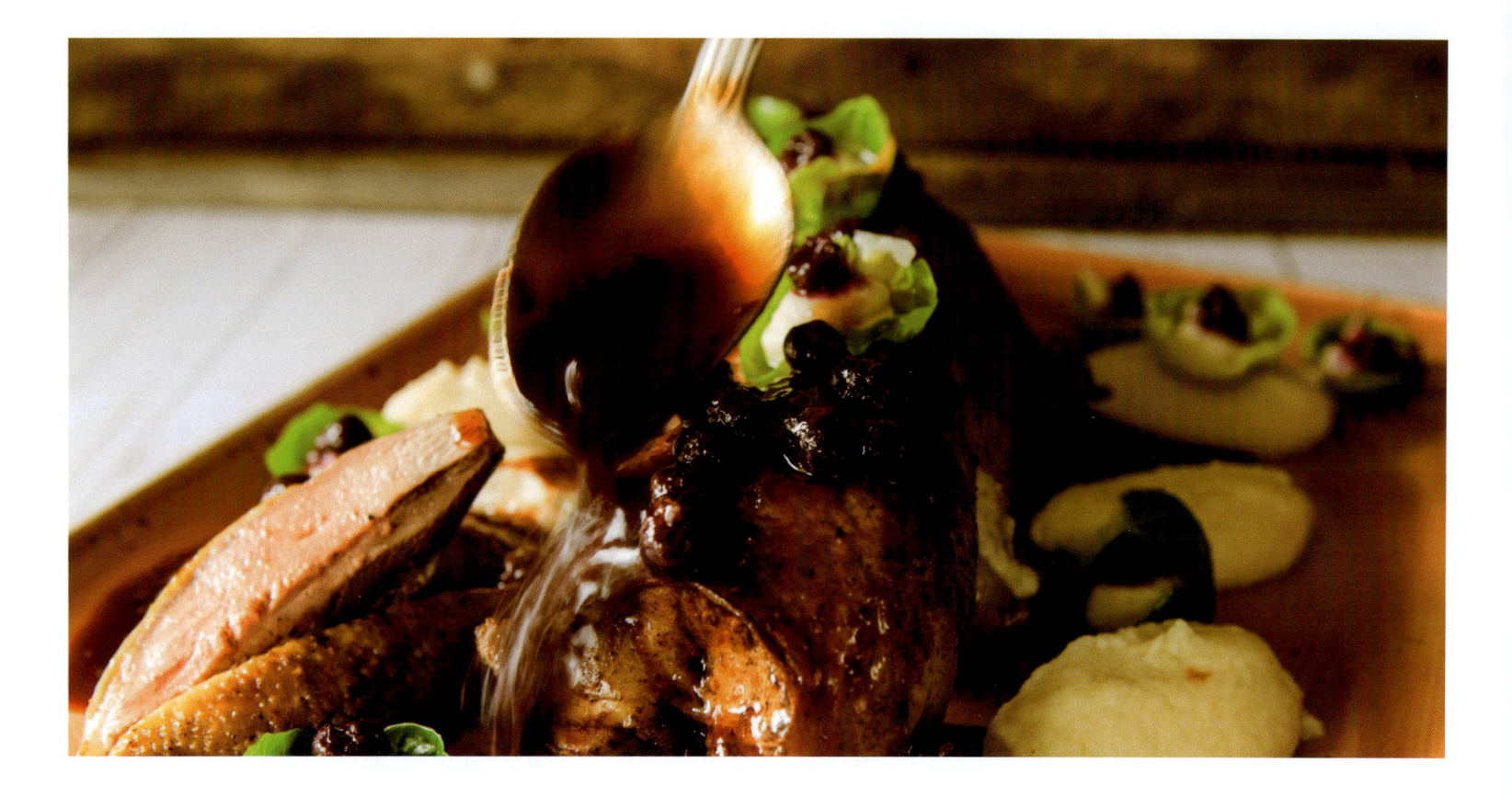

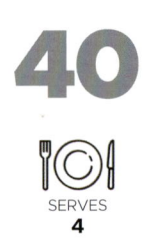

Roast Squab with Blackcurrant Beer Sauce and Celery Root Puree

Squab is a rarity on American menus. It's too bad, because the small bird packs big flavor. It tastes similar to foie gras, full of unctuous umami tones, but with a meatier texture. In this preparation, I cut through the meat's richness by pouring on an acidic, slightly sweet sauce made from blackcurrant beer. The celery root puree offsets squab's natural gaminess and adds a fresh undertone. Squab is available from some specialty butchers and online from gourmet purveyors such as D'Artagnan. Lindemans Cassis Lambic beer is an excellent choice to use in this recipe; it can often be found at craft beer import shops or online at BelgianShop.com.

INGREDIENTS

Celery root puree
1. 1 pound (450 grams) celery root, washed, peeled, and diced
2. 1 quart (1 liter) whole milk
3. Kosher salt
4. 3/4 teaspoon (2 grams) ground nutmeg
5. 4 tablespoons (1/2 stick/60 grams) unsalted butter,

Blackcurrant beer sauce
1. 4 tablespoons (1/2 stock/60 grams) unsalted butter, room temperature
2. 1 medium shallot, finely diced
3. 3 cloves garlic, roughly chopped
4. 1/2 cup (75 grams) diced celery
5. 1/4 cup (40 grams) diced carrot
6. Half a 12-ounce (355 ml) bottle blackcurrant beer
7. 1 cup (250 grams) veal stock (store-bought, or page 207)
8. 1/2 cup (125 grams) chicken stock (store-bought, or page 208)
9. 1 dried bay leaf
10. 1 sprig fresh thyme
11. 2 teaspoon (5 grams) crushed black peppercorns
12. 1/2 cup (50 grams) fresh

Squabs
1. 4 whole squabs (about 16 to 18 ounces/454 to 510 grams each), cleaned, internal organs removed
2. Kosher salt

DIRECTIONS

To make the celery root puree, in a medium stew pot over medium heat, add the milk, celery root, 1 teaspoon (5 grams) salt, and nutmeg. Cook at a low simmer until knife passes through the celery root with no resistance, about 1 hour. Drain the celery root through a strainer, discard the liquid, and place the solids in a food processor fitted with the stainless-steel blade. Puree until smooth. Add the butter and puree until it is incorporated. Season with more salt, if necessary. Set aside.

While the celery root is simmering, make the blackcurrant beer sauce. In a medium saucepan over medium heat, melt the butter. When it is bubbling, add the shallots, garlic, celery, and carrot, and cook until the vegetables are soft and mushy, about 10 minutes. Add the beer and reduce the liquid by half, 10 to 12 minutes. Reduce the heat to low and add the veal and chicken stocks, bay leaf, thyme sprig, and the peppercorns. Cook until the sauce has thickened and coats a spoon, about 30 minutes. Pass the liquid through a fine-mesh strainer into another medium saucepan; discard the solids.

Preheat the oven to 325°F (165°C).

To cook the squabs, season them all over with salt. In a large cast-iron skillet over medium-high heat, warm the oil until starting to smoke slightly. Place all the squabs in the skillet, turning them every 2 minutes or so to ensure every side is golden brown. Add the butter to the pan with the bay leaf, thyme, and garlic. When the butter begins to bubble, spoon it continually over the squab for about 2 minutes. Flip the squabs onto their breasts. Place the skillet in the oven and bake the squabs for 7 minutes, until golden brown. Remove the skillet from the oven and place the squabs on a cooling rack to cool for 7 minutes. Reduce the oven to 250°F (120°C).

After removing any yellowed or damaged leaves from the Brussels sprouts, peel the remaining leaves apart. Fill a medium bowl with ice and cold water. Set aside. In a medium stew pot over medium-high heat, bring well-salted water to a boil. Place the Brussels sprouts leaves in the boiling water for 2 minutes; their color will brighten slightly. Using a mesh skimmer or slotted spoon, immediately transfer them to the ice water. After 3 minutes, remove them from the water and let them drain for a few minutes on a paper towel–covered plate. In a small sauté pan over medium heat, melt the butter. Once the butter is bubbling slightly, add the Brussels sprout leaves and season to taste with salt and pepper. Set aside.

3. 2 tablespoons (30 grams) canola oil
4. 8 tablespoons (1 stick/125 grams) unsalted butter, room temperature
5. 1 dried bay leaf
6. 1 sprig fresh thyme
7. 1 clove garlic, smashed

To assemble
1. 10 Brussel sprouts
2. 1 tablespoon (15 grams) unsalted butter
3. Kosher salt and freshly ground black pepper

To assemble to dish, add the black currants to the sauce and reheat over medium-low heat. Slice the breast meat from the squabs, place them on a sheet pan and warm them in the oven for 5 to 8 minutes. Cut the legs off and place them in the sauce for 6 to 8 minutes to finish cooking them. Save the bones and wings for the stock pot. Reheat the celery root puree in the microwave. Place 2 squab breast halves on each plate, top them with the sauce and 8 to 10 Brussel sprout leaves, and put a dollop of celery root puree next to them

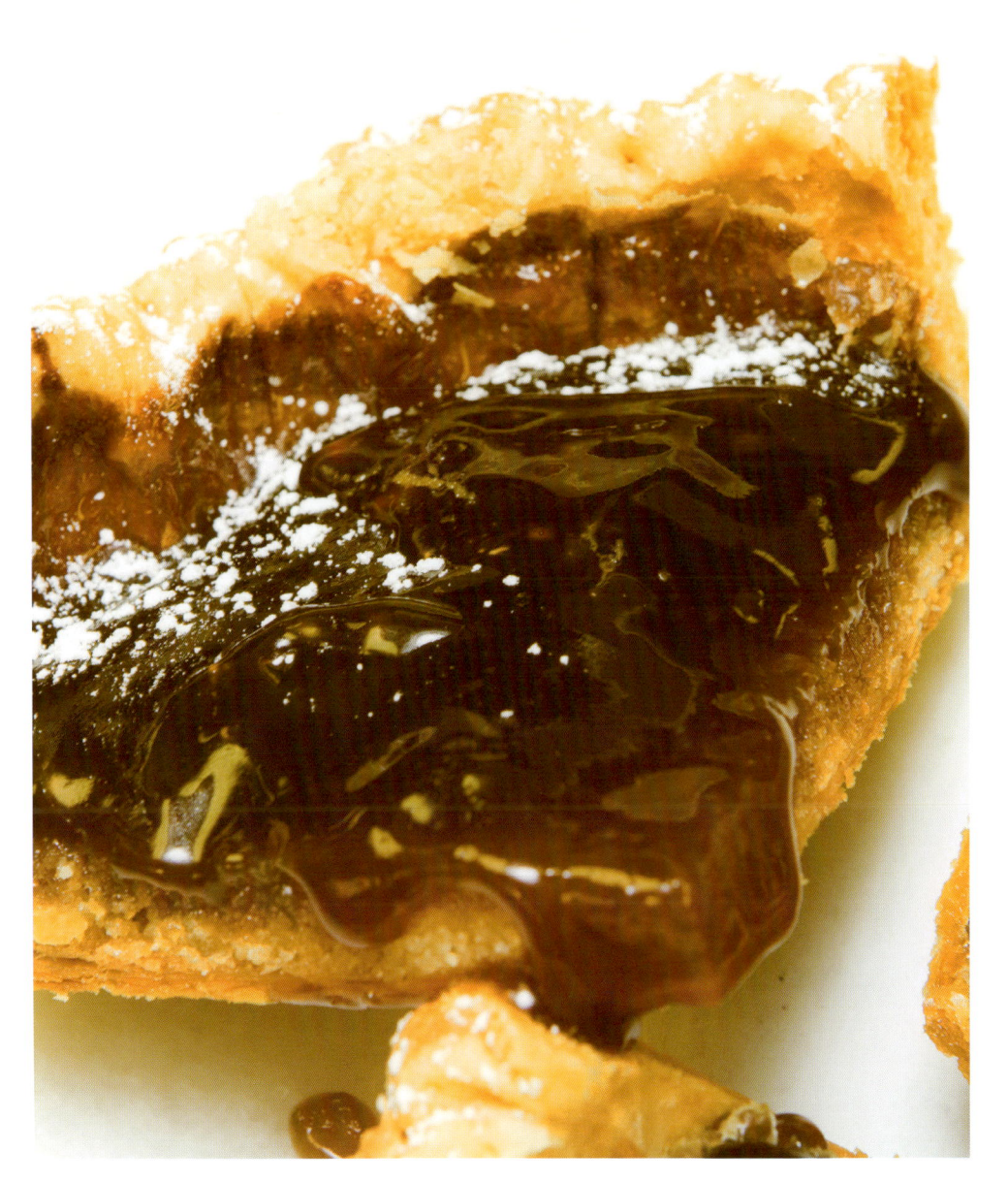

Raspberry Beer Tart

When Alex and I were working together in Switzerland, I was always visiting him in the pastry department to steal a leftover tarte au vin cuit or two. The little tarts feature Swiss cooked wine—a fruity syrup that's about as thick as molasses—and plenty of cream. I have such fond memories of them, so I always had it in the back of my mind to revive them at Et Voila!. After much pestering, Alex created them for a dinner a few years ago celebrating the Belgian National Day. His tarts aren't a carbon copy, since the raspberry beer takes on a beautiful caramel quality that goes above and beyond its inspiration. In fact, I think I like them even more than the original. Lindemans Framboise Lambic beer works well in this recipe; it can often be found at craft beer import shops or online at BelgianShop.com. You will need an 9-inch (23 cm) tart mold with 1-inch (2.5 cm) sides and a removable bottom, which can be purchased at any good cooking supply store. Serve the tart with Hoegaarden Ice Cream (page 155) or freshly whipped cream.

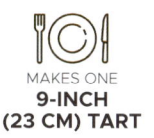

41

MAKES ONE
**9-INCH
(23 CM) TART**

PAGE 155

INGREDIENTS

1. 10 1/2 ounces (300 grams) puff pastry (store-bought, or page 214)
2. Half a 26.4-ounce (750 milliliter) bottle raspberry beer
3. 3/4 cup + 2 tablespoons (175 grams) granulated sugar
4. Pinch of ground cinnamon
5. 1/4 cup (28 grams) all-purpose flour, plus more for dusting
6. 1 tablespoon + 1 teaspoon (20 grams) unsalted butter

DIRECTIONS

1. Preheat the oven to 300°F (150°C).
2. Spray a 9-inch (23 cm) tart mold with nonstick spray, sprinkle the inside with flour, turn it over, and tap the bottom to shake off the excess flour. Set aside.
3. Sprinkle flour on a clean surface and roll out the puff pastry dough into a circle approximately 12 inches (30 cm) in diameter and 1/4 inch (6 mm) thick. Drape the dough over the inside of the mold and gently push it in, making sure to work it into the corners, then cut off any excess dough that rises above the sides. Using a fork, poke several sets of holes in the dough. Place a piece of parchment paper over the dough, making sure to cover it completely. Weigh the paper down with dried beans or pie weights. Bake until dry looking and light golden brown, about 20 minutes. Place on cooling rack to cool after removing dried beans and parchment paper.
4. Increase the oven to 325°F (165°C).
5. In a large bowl, whisk together the beer, sugar, cinnamon, and flour. In a medium saucepan over medium heat, bring the beer mixture to a boil, stirring constantly, until thickened and glossy, 5 to 8 minutes. Remove from the heat and whisk in the butter until fully melted.
6. Pour the mixture into the tart shell. Bake until filling is shiny and has a jammy consistency, about 30 minutes.
7. Let the tart cool completely on a cooling rack before removing it from the mold.

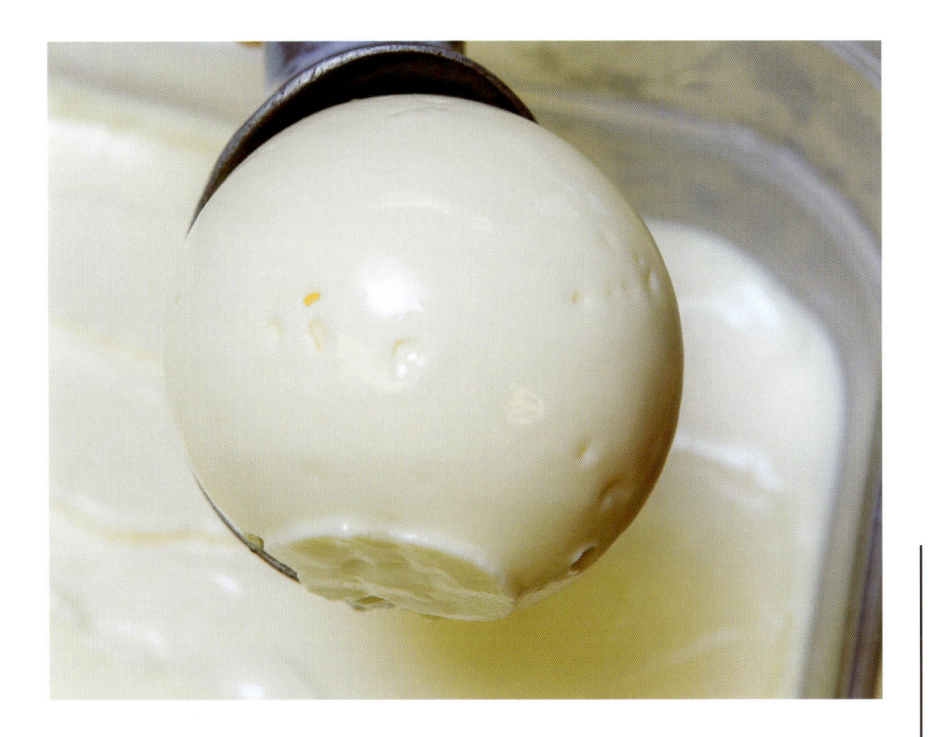

Hoegaarden Ice Cream

Rich with honey, coriander, and a hint of orange peel, Hoegaarden is one of the original craft beers. Its flavor translates well into ice cream, especially if you let the mixture rest in the refrigerator overnight before you put it in the ice cream maker so the intensity of its elements have a chance to build. It pairs well with an apple or pear tart, fruit crumble, or a generously cut slice of lemon pound cake. Sometimes I'll even put a couple of scoops in a tall glass of Hoegaarden to make the ultimate beer float. Hoegaarden can be found at many beer import stores and even at good grocery stores. Serve with the Raspberry Beer Tart (page 153) or with fresh raspberries.

INGREDIENTS

1. 1 quart (1 liter) whole milk
2. 3/4 cup (250 grams) honey
3. 16 large egg yolks (320 grams)
4. 1 1/2 cups (300 grams) granulated sugar
5. Three 11-ounce (330 milliliter) bottles Hoegaarden White beer

DIRECTIONS

1. In a medium pot over medium-high heat, bring the milk and honey to a boil. Remove from the heat and set aside to cool slightly. [Image 1, 2 and 3]
2. In a medium bowl whisk the egg yolks and sugar until fully combined and frothy. Add the milk mixture and whisk until fully incorporated. [Image 4]
3. Pour the mixture into a large pot over medium-low heat and whisk constantly until it reaches 185°F (85°C). [Image 5]
4. Remove from the heat and add the beer, whisking until it is fully incorporated. [Image 6]
5. Let the ice cream base cool down, then transfer it to a covered container and refrigerate until cold. [Image 7]
6. Following the manufacturer's instructions, place mixture in an ice cream maker and spin to create ice cream. Depending on the size of your machine, you may need to spin it in several batches. Place the ice cream in the freezer for 2 to 3 hours before serving it. [Image 8]

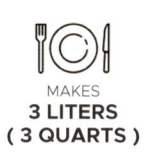

42

MAKES
3 LITERS
(3 QUARTS)

PAGE 158

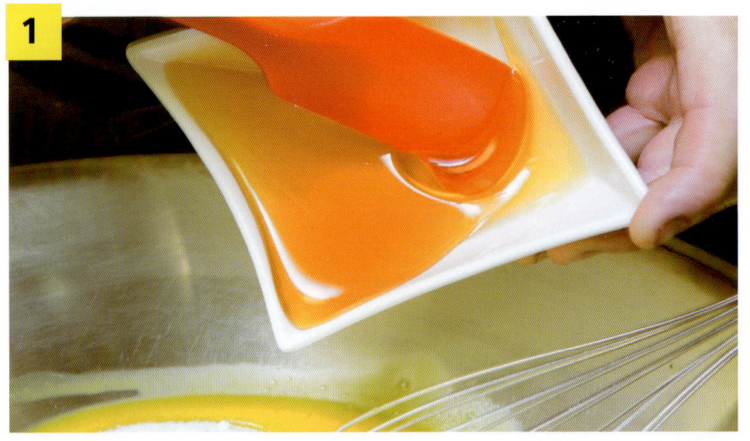

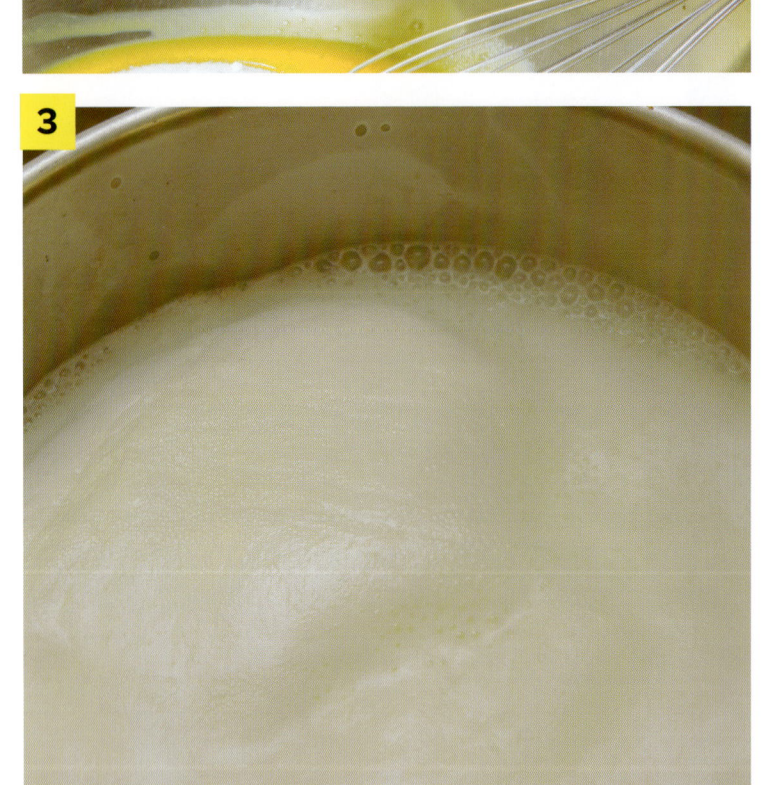

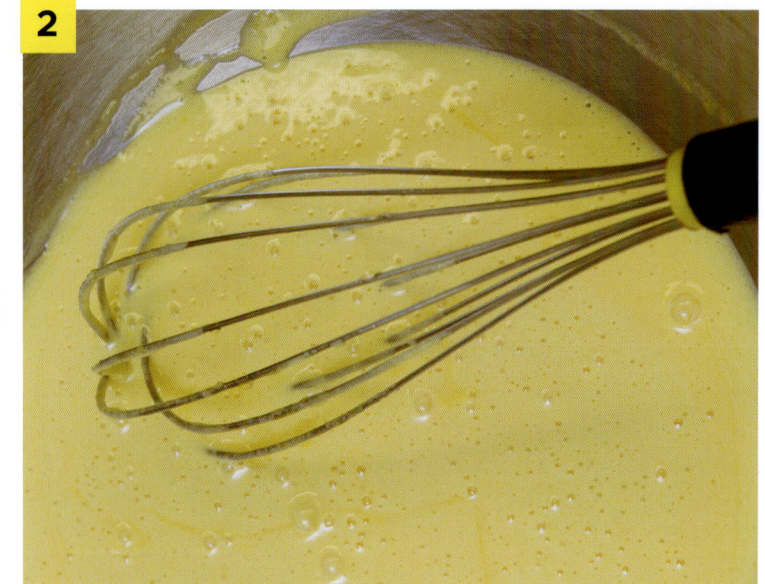

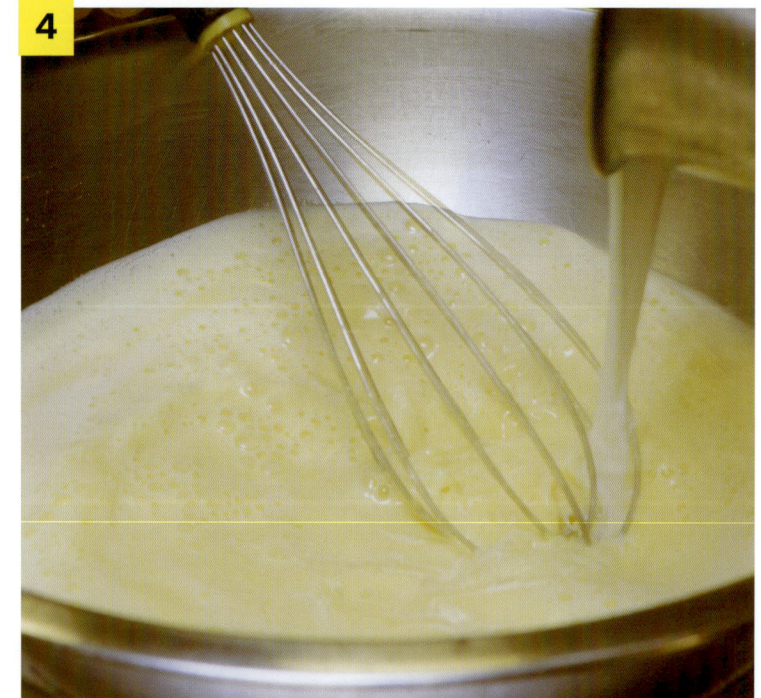

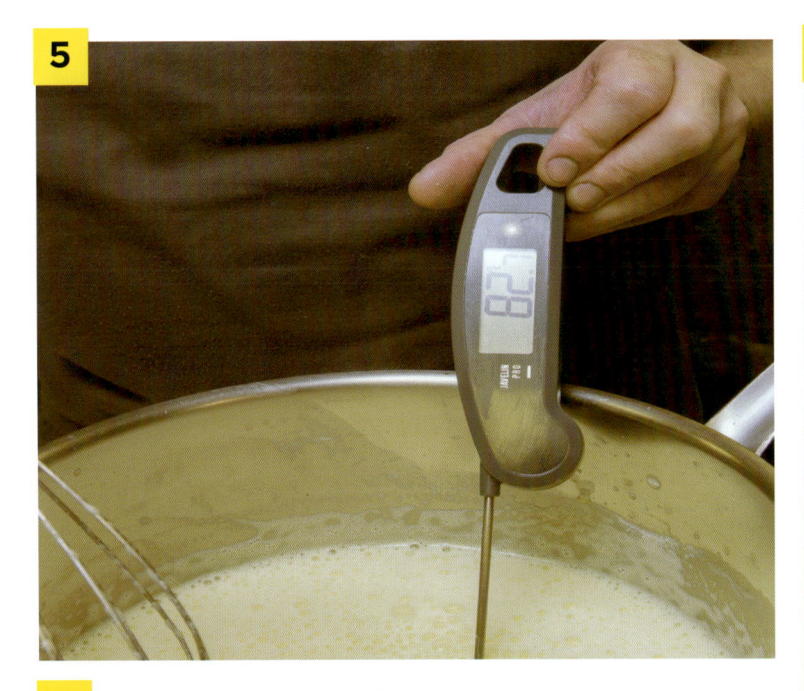

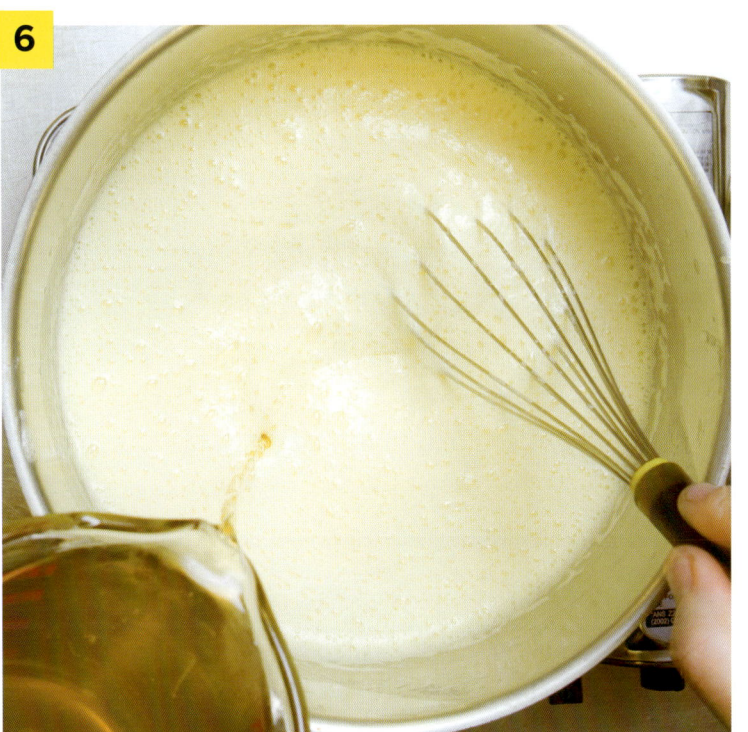

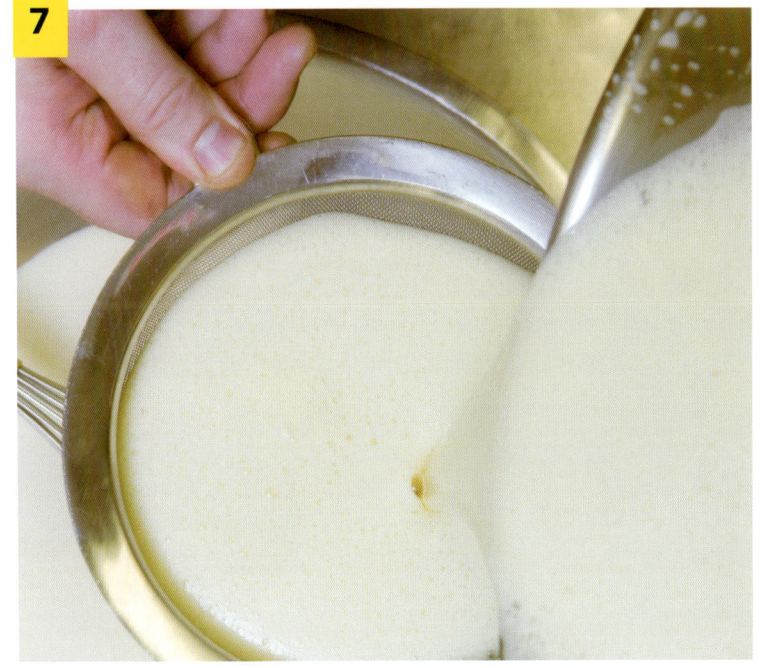

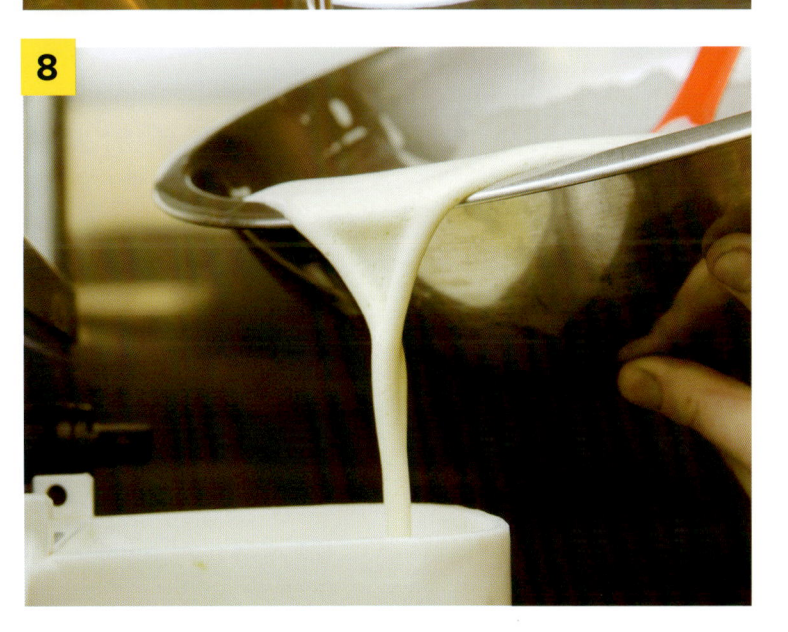

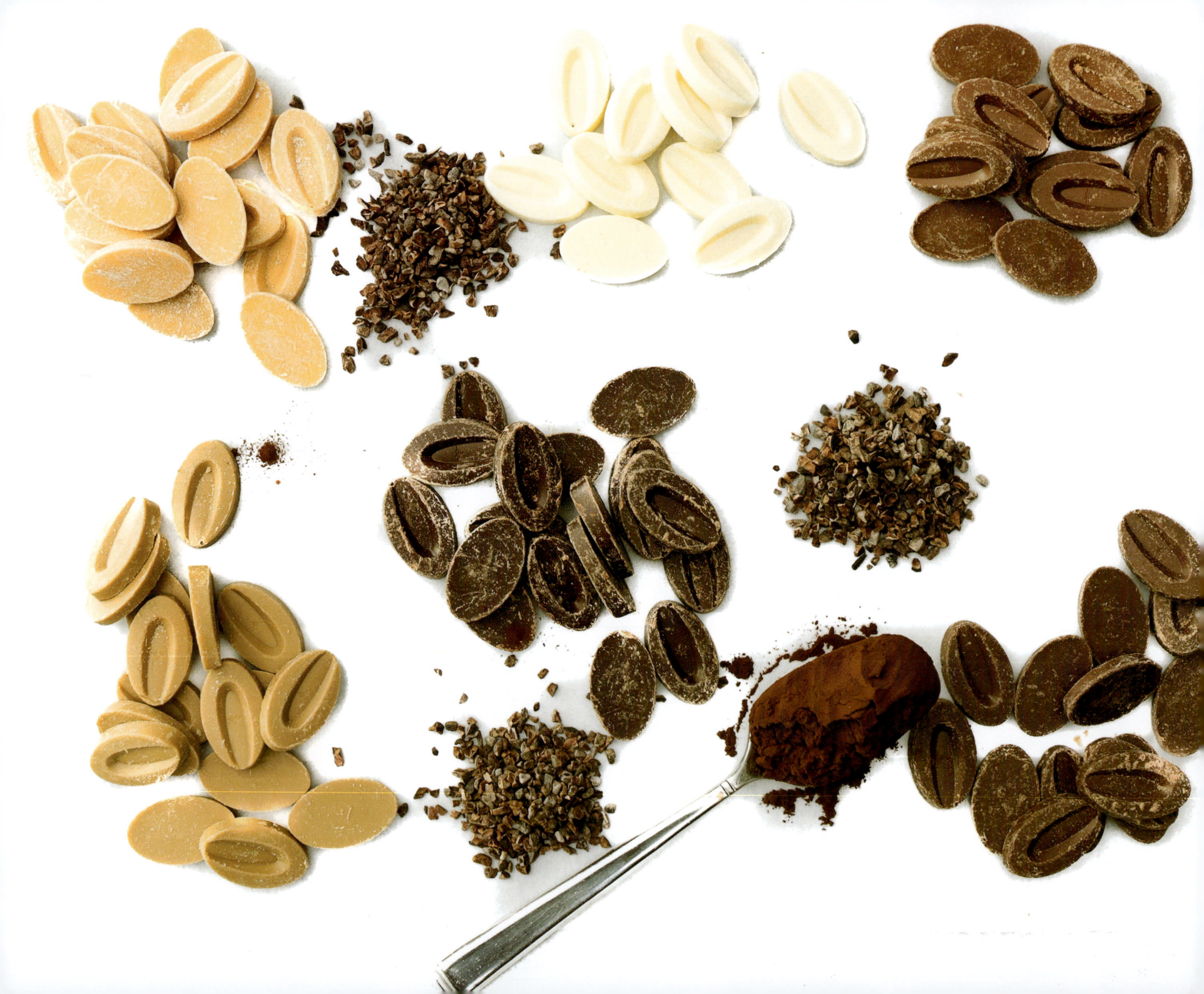

CHOCOLATE

I can devour a box of chocolates without thinking twice. Sometimes without thinking at all! Sweet milk chocolate is my favorite, especially when it's paired with a fruit element such as raspberries, blueberries, or oranges. That's why I'm so particular about the chocolatey desserts Alex puts on our menu. They might be the most debated dishes in the kitchen. Luckily, the taste testing is always a pleasure, even if we don't get it right the first time. Callebaut and Valrhona make the best chocolate for baking and confections; they're widely available in high-end grocery stores and online.

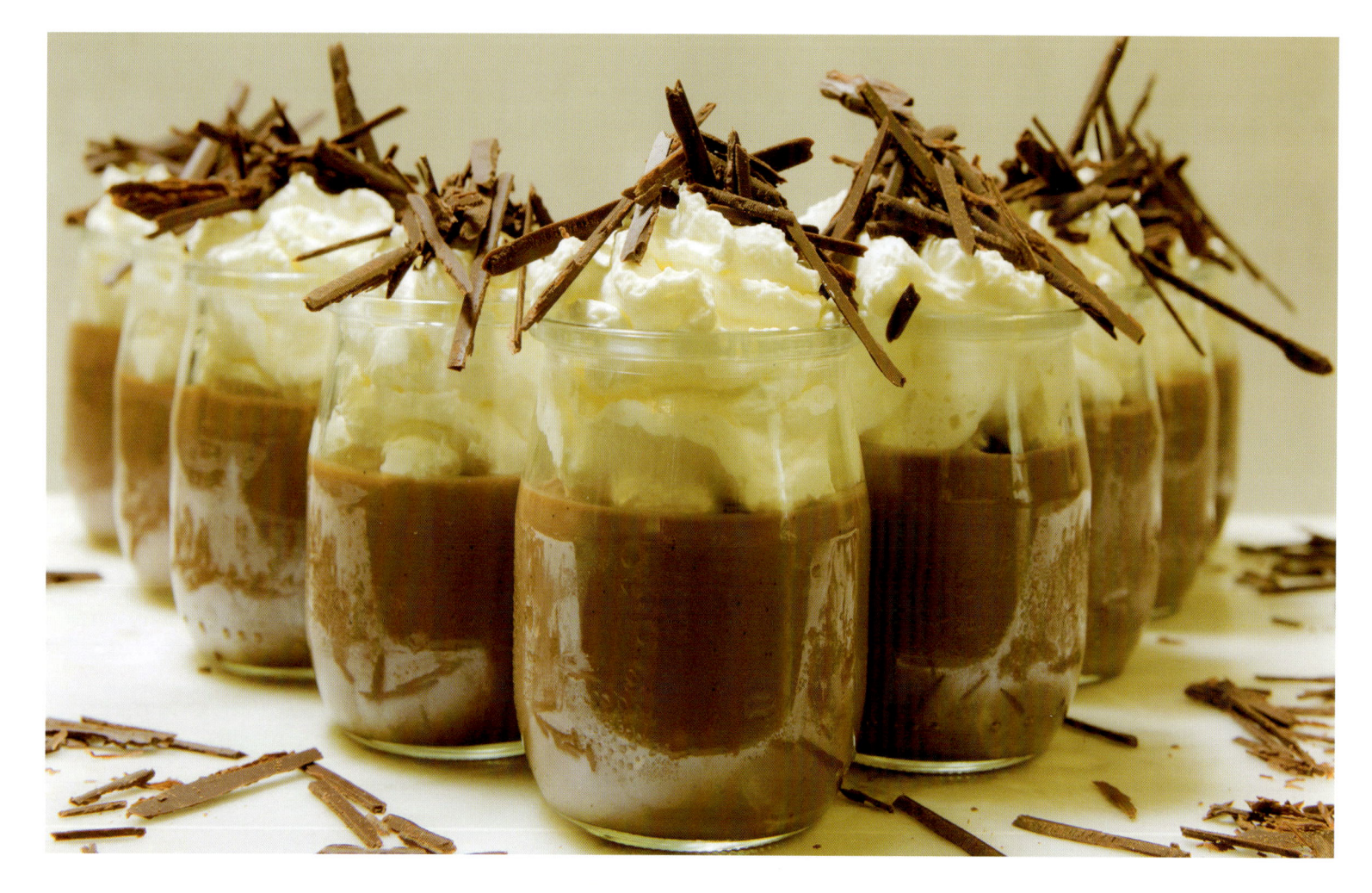

43

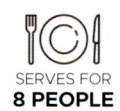

SERVES FOR
8 PEOPLE

Dark Chocolate Petits Pots

I have the fondest memories of Nestlé's La Laitière, my ultimate after-school snack. The dainty chocolate and vanilla pots de crème have a custardy, flan-like texture that always drove me to spoon out every last morsel from the charming little glass jars they come in. This dessert is a heartfelt homage to those afternoon treats. To add a textural component, we top ours with chocolate shavings and a pirouette of whipped cream. To complete the experience, they are served in 4-ounce (120 milliliter) clear glass jars, which you purchase online or in the canning section of many hardware stores, though ramekins work just as well. For this recipe, I prefer to use 64% bittersweet chocolate pistoles from Valrhona or Callebaut.

INGREDIENTS

Chocolate custard
1. 2 1/4 cups (500 grams) whole milk
2. 2 vanilla beans
3. 3/4 cup + 2 tablespoons (200 grams) heavy cream
4. 7 large egg yolks (140 grams)
5. 1/2 cup + 2 tablespoons (120 grams) granulated sugar
6. 1 1/4 cups (220 grams) 64% dark chocolate pistoles or chips

whipped cream
1. 1 1/4 cups (300 grams) heavy cream
2. 2 tablespoons + 1 teaspoon (30 grams) granulated sugar
3. 1 drop pure vanilla extract
4. 2 teaspoon (5 grams) crushed black peppercorns
5. 1/2 cup (50 grams) fresh black-currants

To assemble
1. 3 tablespoons (20 grams) shaved chocolate

DIRECTIONS

To make the chocolate custard, in a bowl of a stand mixer fitted with the whisk attachment on medium speed, whisk together the egg yolks and sugar until the mixture becomes very pale yellow, about 6 to 8 minutes. Set aside.

Pour the milk into a medium saucepan over medium heat. Cut the vanilla beans in half lengthwise and scrape the seeds into the milk. Add the vanilla bean pods and cream. Bring to a boil, then remove from the heat. Pass the liquid through a fine-mesh strainer into a medium bowl. Discard any solids.

Pour the hot milk mixture over the egg mixture and mix the together with a whisk. Return this to the saucepan over medium heat. Cook, stirring constantly with a wooden spoon, until the temperature reaches 181°F (83°C). If you don't have a thermometer, cook until the mixture coats the spoon. Add the chocolate and mix with a whisk until it has completely melted. Pour the chocolate mixture into eight 4-ounce (120 milliliter) glass jars, about three-quarters full, cover them with plastic wrap, and place them in the refrigerator to chill for at least for 2 hours or up to overnight.

When you are ready to serve the dessert, make the whipped cream. In the bowl of a stand mixer fitted with the whisk attachment, place the cream, sugar, and vanilla extract. Whisk at medium speed until strong peaks form.

To assemble, top each jar with whipped cream and finish it off with a sprinkling of shaved chocolate.

44

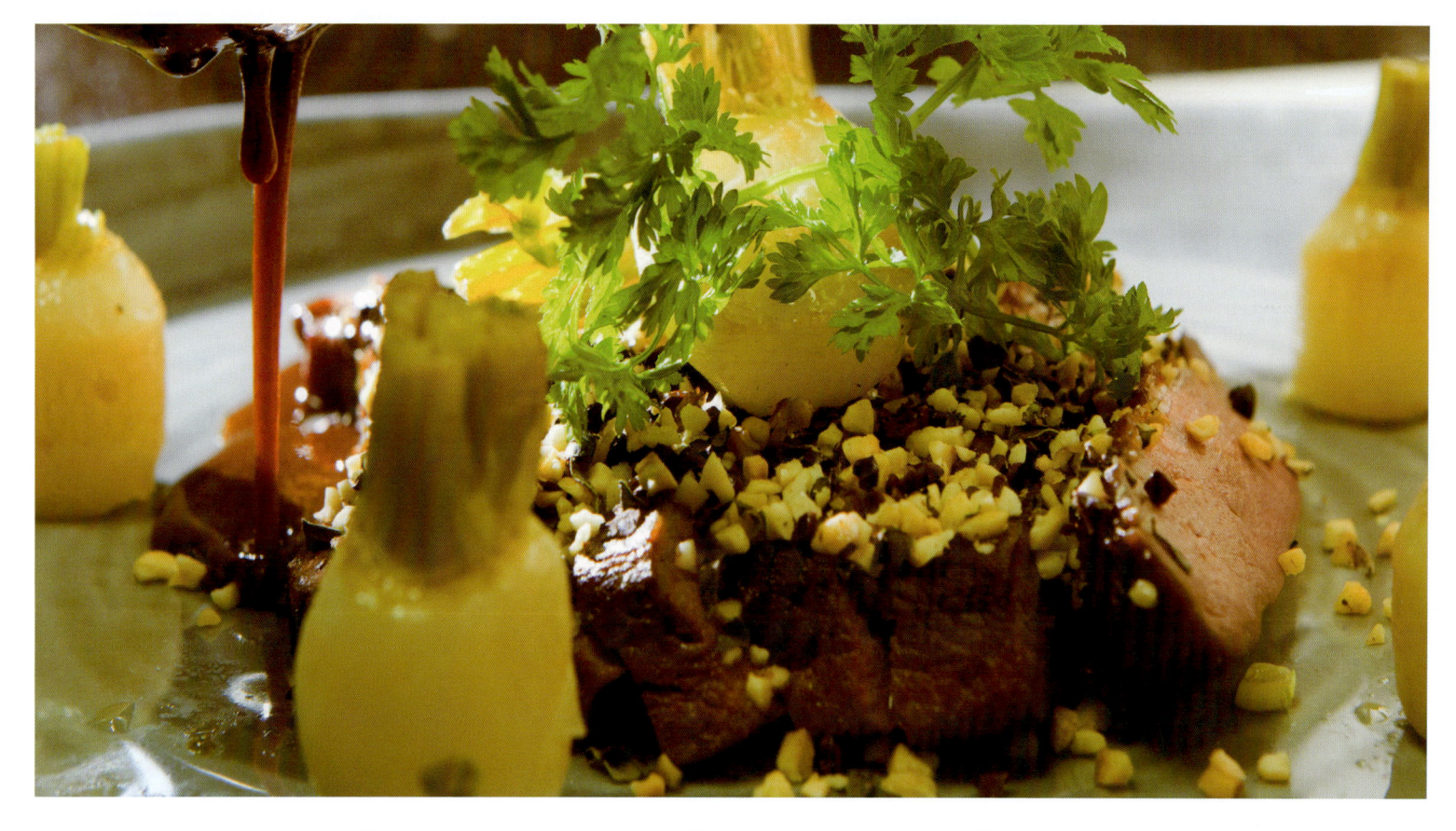

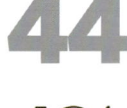

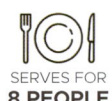

SERVES FOR
8 PEOPLE

"Ferrero Rocher" Crusted Duck Breast

with Chocolate-Balsamic Sauce and Cauliflower Puree

Gold-wrapped Ferrero Rocher bonbons, equally rich with hazelnuts and chocolate, are one of Italy's greatest exports. We mimic them with more savory results in the coating for this roasted duck by mixing Piedmont hazelnuts (the best in the world and worth seeking out) and cacao nibs with a few Italian herbs. There's still a pleasant smack of sweetness from chocolate-balsamic sauce and cauliflower puree enhanced with a touch of white chocolate, but it's not overwhelming. Duck can be purchased from any good butcher, some farmers' markets, and online from gourmet purveyors such as D'Artagnan. For the chocolate, I recommend the 64% dark chocolate Valrhona or Callebaut pistoles, though dark chocolate chips also work. Savory is a fresh herb that can be found at some farmers markets; rosemary is an acceptable substitute.

INGREDIENTS

Cauliflower puree

1. 12 tablespoons (1 1/2 sticks/180 grams) unsalted butter
2. 2 pounds (900 grams) cauliflower, cut into florets
3. 1/2 cup + 2 tablespoons (100 grams) chopped shallots
4. 1 dried bay leaf
5. 1 sprig fresh thyme
6. 2 cups (474 grams) chicken stock (store-bought, or page 208)
7. 2 cups (474 grams) heavy cream
8. 1/2 teaspoon (2 grams) kosher salt
9. 1/4 cup (45 grams) white chocolate chips

Chocolate-balsamic sauce

1. 1 1/2 cups + 2 tablespoon (400 milliliters) balsamic vinegar
2. 1 tablespoon + 1 teaspoon (18 grams) vegetable oil
3. 2 medium shallots, finely diced
4. 2 cloves garlic, smashed
5. 1/2 medium yellow onion, diced
6. 1/2 stalk celery, diced
7. 1/2 medium carrot, diced
8. 1 quart (1 liter) merlot or similar red wine
9. 1 quart (1 liter) veal stock (store-bought, or page 207)
10. 1/4 cup (40 grams) 64% dark chocolate pistoles

DIRECTIONS

To make the cauliflower puree, in a medium stew pot over medium heat, melt the butter. Add the cauliflower, shallots, bay leaf, and thyme and cook, stirring occasionally, until the shallots are translucent but not golden, about 10 minutes. Add the chicken stock, cream, and salt and cook until the cauliflower is completely softened, about 30 minutes. Transfer the cauliflower mixture to a strainer set in the sink and let drain for 30 minutes. Remove the thyme stem and bay leaf. Place the cauliflower mixture in a food processor fitted with the stainless-steel blade and blend until completely smooth. Transfer the cauliflower puree to a medium saucepan over medium heat. Add the white chocolate and whisk until the chocolate has melted completely and is fully incorporated. Remove from the heat and set aside.

To make the chocolate-balsamic sauce, in a small saucepan over medium heat, cook the balsamic vinegar until it has reduced by half, about 10 minutes. Heat the oil in a medium saucepan over medium heat until starting to smoke slightly. Add the shallots, garlic, onions, celery, and carrots, and cook until the vegetables have started to soften and are light golden brown, 8 to 10 minutes. Add the wine and cook until the liquid has reduced by half, about 10 minutes. Add the veal stock and cook until the sauce thickens and coats a spoon, about 20 minutes.

Pass the sauce through a fine-mesh strainer into a medium bowl. Return the sauce to the medium saucepan over medium heat; discard the solids. Add the balsamic reduction, whisking it in until fully incorporated and bring it to a boil. Remove from the heat, add the chocolate, and whisk until the chocolate has melted completely and is fully incorporated. Set aside.

To make the chocolate-balsamic sauce, in a small saucepan over medium heat, cook the balsamic vinegar until it has reduced by half, about 10 minutes. Heat the oil in a medium saucepan over medium heat until starting to smoke slightly. Add the shallots, garlic, onions, celery, and carrots, and cook until the vegetables have started to soften and are light golden brown, 8 to 10 minutes. Add the wine and cook until the liquid has reduced by half, about 10 minutes. Add the veal stock and cook until the sauce thickens and coats a spoon, about 20 minutes.

Turnips
1. 4 tablespoons (1/2 stick/60 grams) unsalted butter
2. 24 baby turnips, trimmed and washed
3. 2 tablespoons + 1 teaspoon (30 grams) granulated sugar
4. 1 dried bay leaf
5. 1 sprig fresh thyme
6. 2 cups (475 milliliters) chicken stock (store-bought, or page 208)

Duck
1. 1/4 cup (30 grams) cacao nibs
2. 1/4 cup + 1 tablespoon (15 grams) chopped fresh savory
3. 1/2 cup (60 grams) crushed blanched and roasted hazelnuts
4. 4 duck breasts (each about 8 ounces/225 grams)
5. Kosher salt

Pass the sauce through a fine-mesh strainer into a medium bowl. Return the sauce to the medium saucepan over medium heat; discard the solids. Add the balsamic reduction, whisking it in until fully incorporated and bring it to a boil. Remove from the heat, add the chocolate, and whisk until the chocolate has melted completely and is fully incorporated. Set aside.

To make the turnips, in a small stew pot over medium heat, melt the butter. Add the turnips and cook for 8 to 10 minutes, until you can slip a knife into them without any resistance. Raise the heat to medium-high, add the sugar, bay leaf, thyme, and chicken stock, and bring to boil. Reduce the heat to medium and simmer until a knife passes easily through the center of the turnips, about 25 minutes. Remove from the heat and set aside

To make the duck, in a food processor fitted with the stainless-steel blade, place the cacao nibs, savory, and hazelnuts, and pulse them a few times until roughly chopped and lightly combined. Set aside.

Preheat the oven to 450°F (230°C).

Season both sides of the duck breasts with salt. Heat a large ovensafe sauté pan over high heat. Once it has warmed, place all the duck breasts skin side down. Cook until the fat is a light golden brown, about 4 minutes, then turn and cook the other side for 4 minutes. Place the sauté pan in the oven to cook for 5 minutes, until medium rare. Remove the duck from the oven and let rest for 5 to 10 minutes. Slice the duck breasts into 1/2-inch-wide (1 cm) strips. Place them on a sheet pan and sprinkle with the cacao nib mixture.

Turn on the broiler.

Broil the duck breast slices until the cacao nib mixture is light golden brown, 4 to 5 minutes.

Gently reheat the cauliflower puree, sauce, and turnips if necessary. To assemble, put a large spoonful of the cauliflower puree in the middle of a plate, place the duck on top, and pour on some chocolate-balsamic sauce. Arrange the turnips around the plate.

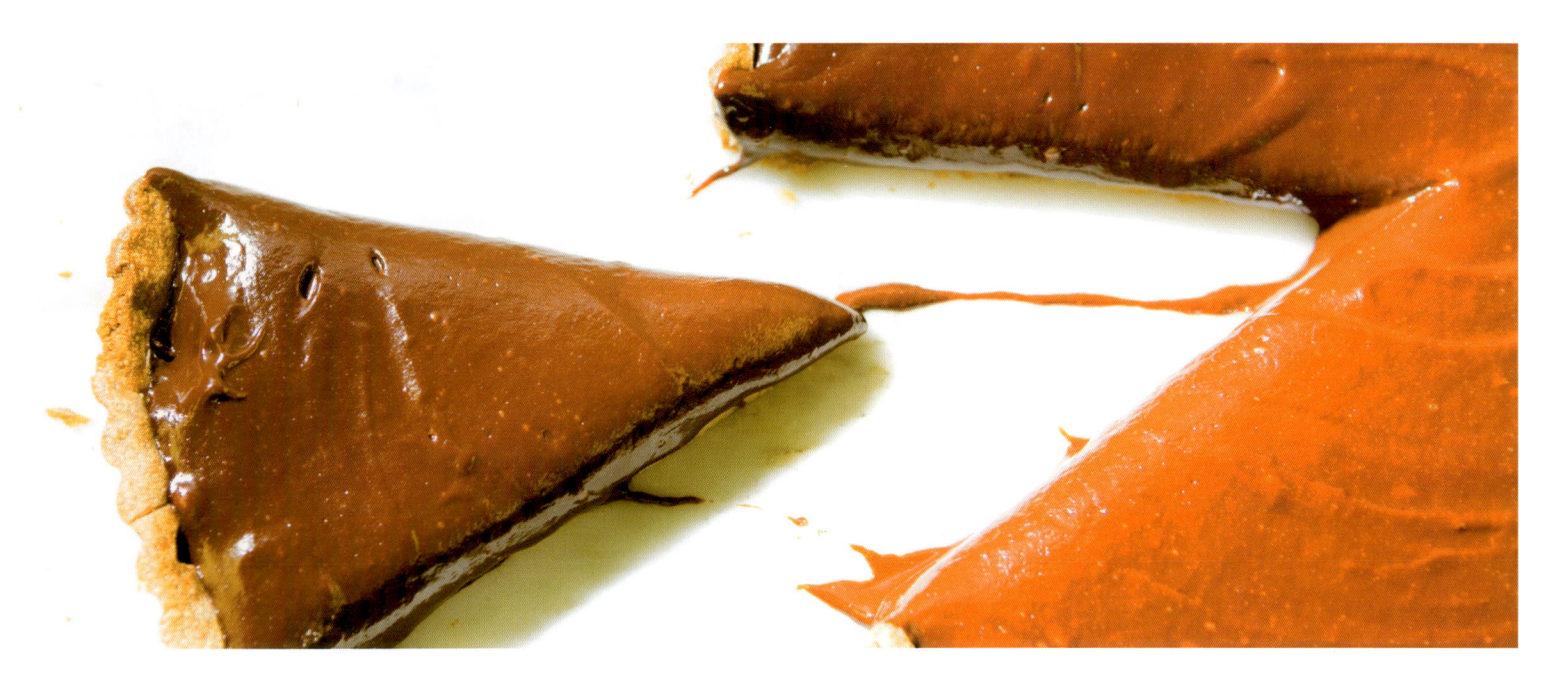

Chocolate Raspberry Hazelnut Tart

(Step By Step)

The tang of the raspberry intertwines harmoniously with the chocolate in the fudgy topping of this hazelnut cream tart. Make sure you serve it at room temperature, so the flavors really sing. For this recipe, I prefer to use 66% bittersweet chocolate pistoles or chips from Valrhona or Callebaut. Almond flour and hazelnut flour can be purchased online or at some grocery stores; Anthony's Goods make great nut flours. You will also need a pair of 9-inch (23 cm) tart molds with 1-inch (2.5 cm) sides and removable bottoms, which can be purchased at any good cooking supply store. Frozen raspberry puree is available at some gourmet grocers and online at GourmetFoodStore.com and elsewhere. Serve with vanilla ice cream, whipped cream, and/or fresh raspberries.

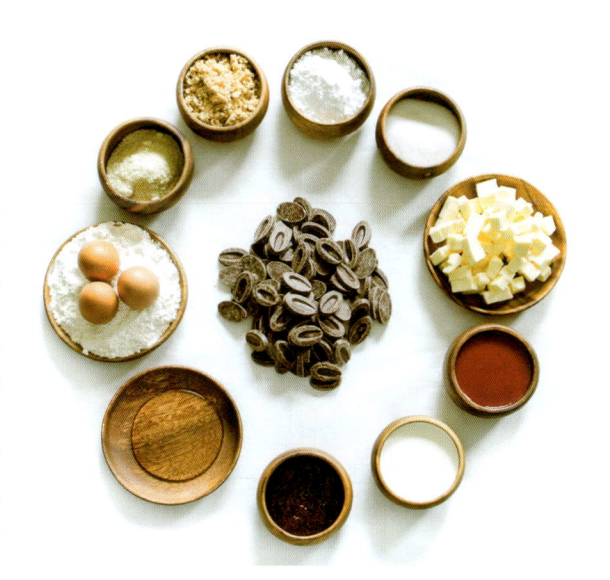

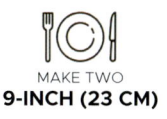

45

MAKE TWO
9-INCH (23 CM)

PAGE **167**

INGREDIENTS

Dough

1. 2 cups (250 grams) all-purpose flour, plus more for rolling
2. 3/4 teaspoon (3 grams) kosher salt
3. 3/4 cup (95 grams) confectioners' sugar
4. 1/4 cup (30 grams) almond flour
5. 10 tablespoons (1 1/4 sticks/150 grams) unsalted butter, cut into small pieces
6. 1 large egg (50 grams)

Hazelnut cream

1. 3/4 cup (75 grams) hazelnut flour
2. 3 tablespoons (40 grams) granulated sugar
3. 5 tablespoons (75 grams) unsalted butter, room temperature
4. 1 large egg (50 grams)

Chocolate ganache

1. 2 1/4 cups + 2 tablespoons (375 grams) 66% dark chocolate pistoles or chips
2. 3/4 cup (175 grams) heavy cream
3. 1 1/2 cups (200 grams) frozen raspberry puree, thawed
4. 3 tablespoons (60 grams) light corn syrup

To assemble

1. 1/2 cup (165 grams) raspberry jam

DIRECTIONS

To make the dough, in the bowl of a stand mixer fitted with the dough hook attachment, on medium speed combine the all-purpose flour, salt, sugar, almond flour, and butter and mix until combined. Add the egg and mix until thoroughly combined. [Images 1 through 4]

Gather the dough into a ball, wrap it in a plastic wrap, and place in the refrigerator to chill for 8 hours or overnight. [Images 5 through 8]

To make the hazelnut cream, in a small bowl mix together the hazelnut flour, sugar, and butter until creamy. Add the egg and mix thoroughly. Place the cream in a pastry bag and refrigerate until ready to use. [Image 31 through 36]

Take the dough out of the refrigerator and separate it into equal halves. On well-floured surface, roll each half of the dough out into a 12-inch (30 cm) wide circle about 1/4 inch (6 mm) thick. [Image 9 through 16]

Using a fork or dough docker, prick the dough all over. [Image 17]

Place the dough in the molds, letting the edges drape over the side, and then press it gently into place. Use a rolling pin to remove the excess dough by rolling it over the top of the rim of the mold. [Image 18 through 25]

Cover the dough with parchment paper and weight it down with dried beans or pie weights. Place it in the refrigerator to chill for 1 hour. [Image 26 through 30]

To make the chocolate ganache, place a medium pot filled with water over medium heat and bring a simmer. Place the chocolate in a heatproof mixing bowl wider than the pot. Place the bowl on top of the pot and melt the chocolate, stirring occasionally until the chocolate is smooth. Remove the bowl from over the water. [Image 44]

In another medium pot over medium heat, bring the cream, raspberry puree, and corn syrup to a boil. Take the pot off the heat. [Image 37 through 43]

Pour in the melted chocolate, whisking until it is well incorporated and the mixture is glossy. [Image 45 though 59]

Preheat the oven to 300°F (150°C).

Remove the tart shells from the refrigerator and bake until light golden brown, about 20 minutes. Place them on a cooling rack. Gently remove the beans and parchment paper. Using the pastry bag, pipe the hazelnut cream on the bottom of both shells.

Return the tarts to the oven to bake until the hazelnut cream is golden brown and a toothpick inserted into its center comes out clean, about 15 minutes. Remove the tarts from the oven and let them cool on the rack for 10 minutes. Gently remove the molds and place the tarts back on the rack to cool completely.

To assemble, stir the raspberry jam to loosen it up. Using a spatula, spread the half of the jam evenly surface of the hazelnut cream of each tart. Pour the chocolate ganache into the shells to cover completely. Let the tarts sit at room temperature until the chocolate firms up, about 2 hours. [Image 60 though 71]

Tarts may be refrigerated. After removing them from the refrigerator, let them sit for an hour at room temperature before serving. [Image 72]

Stepwise Instructions

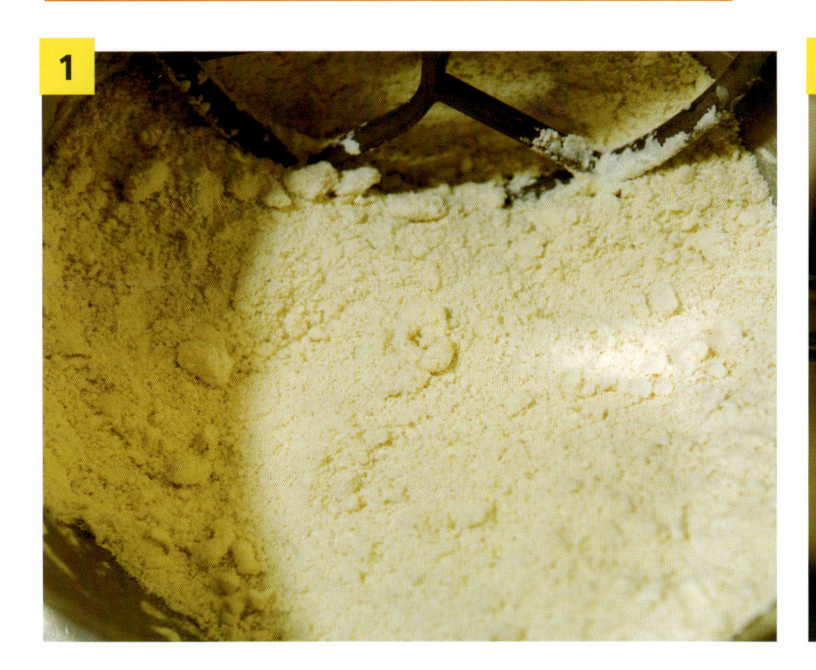

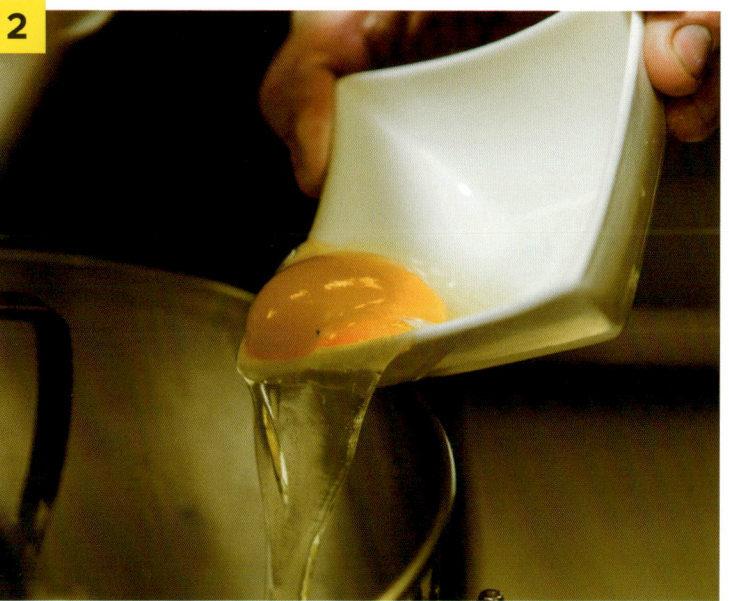

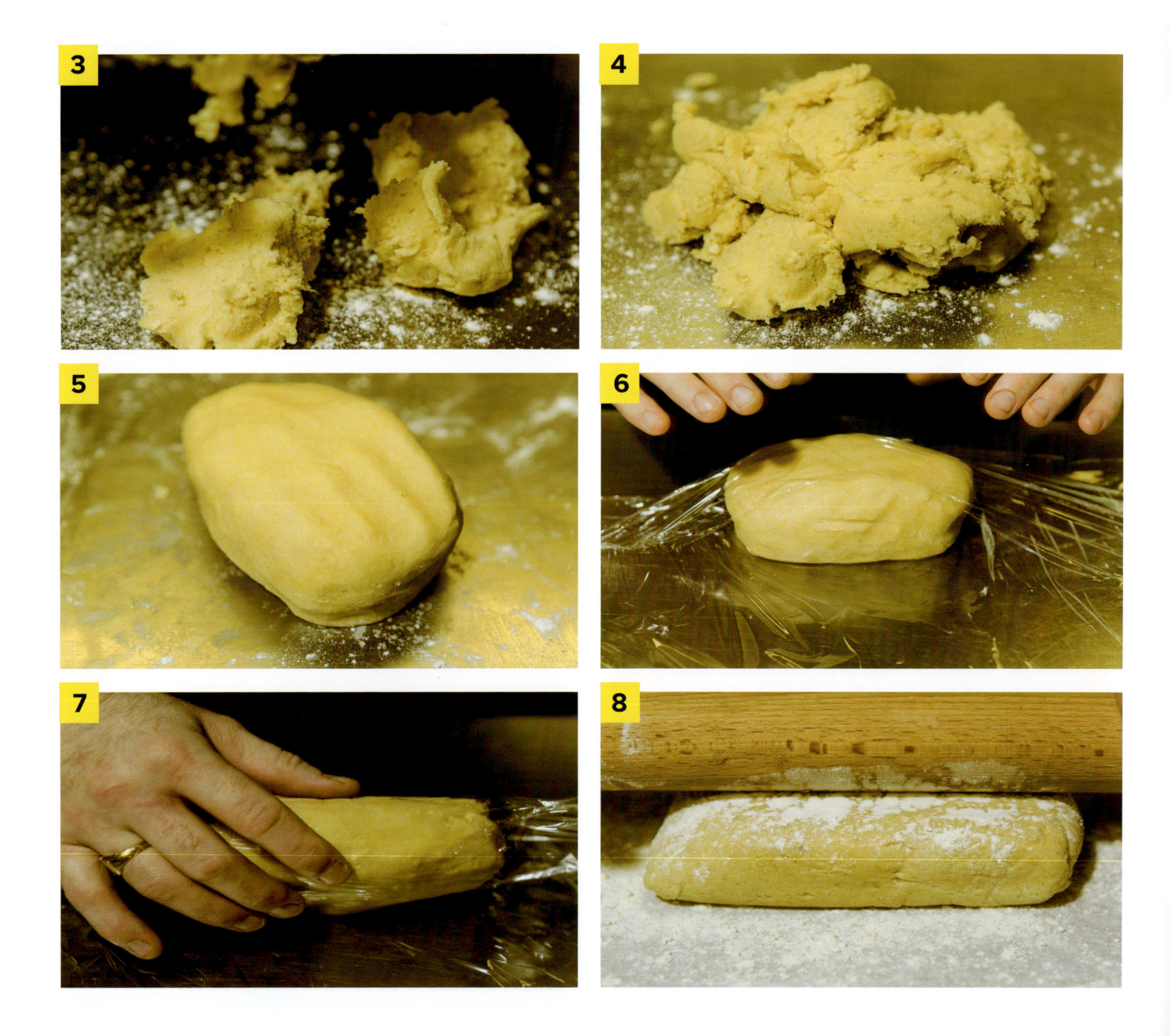

PAGE 171

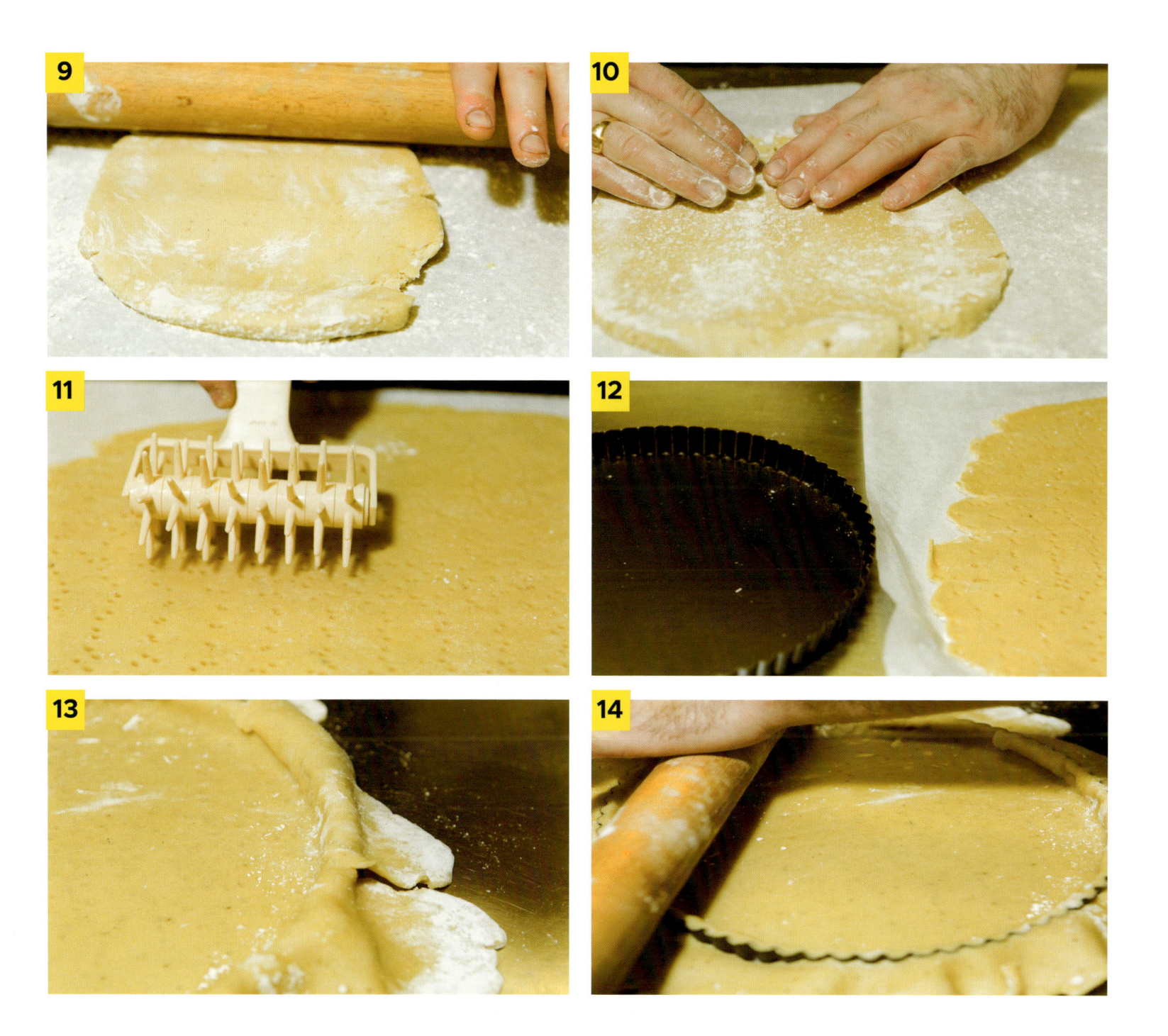

PAGE 172

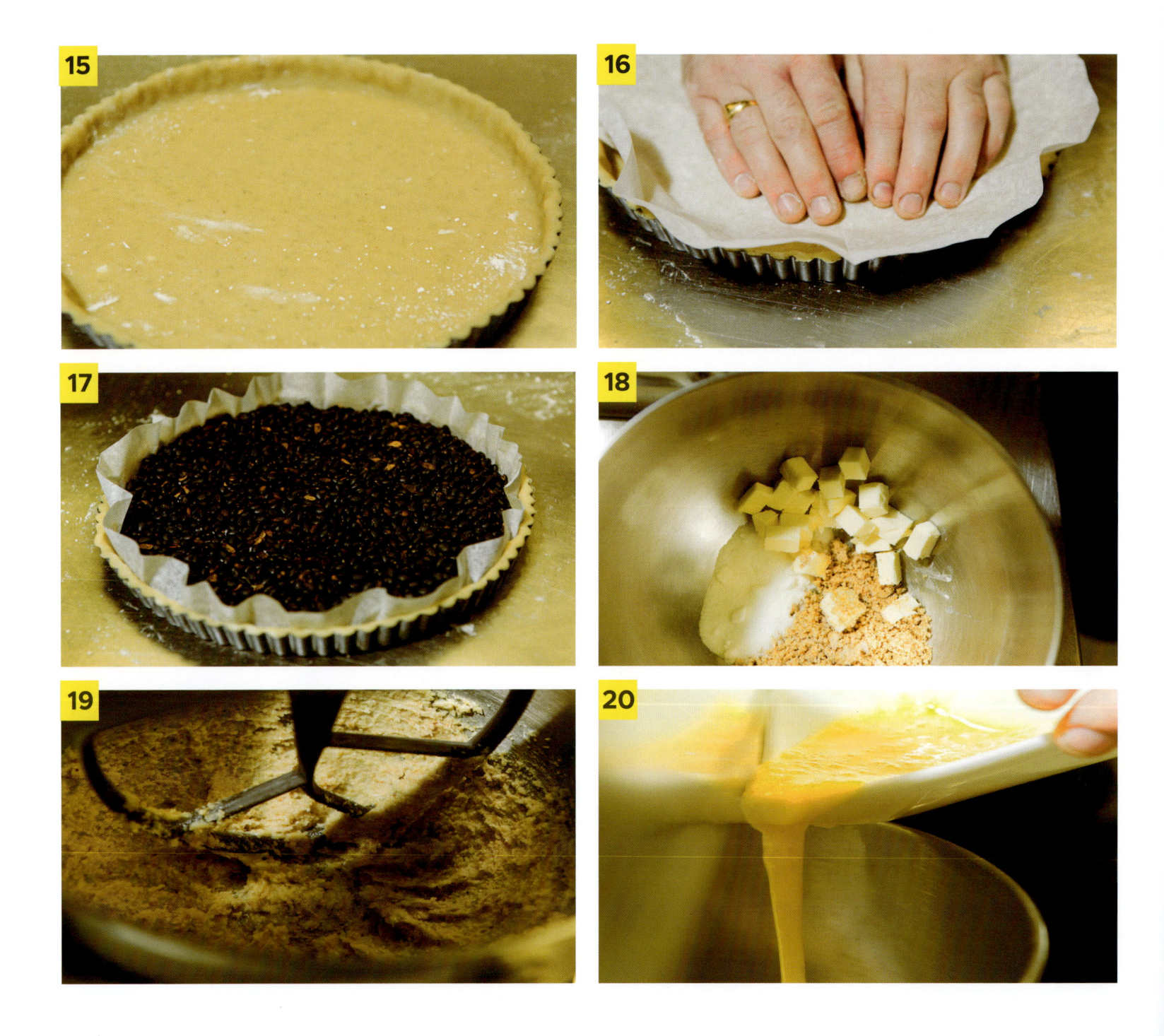

PAGE 173

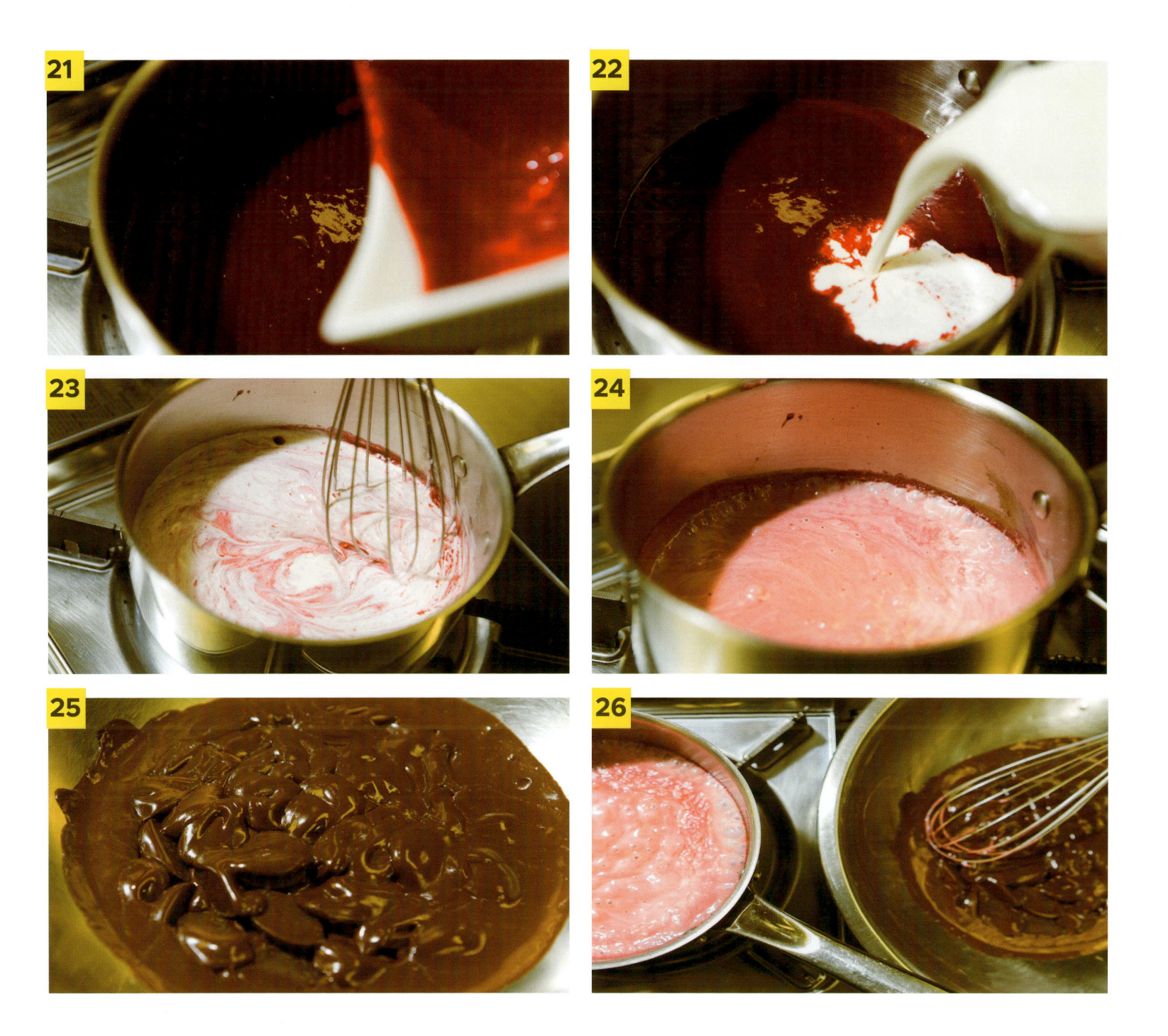

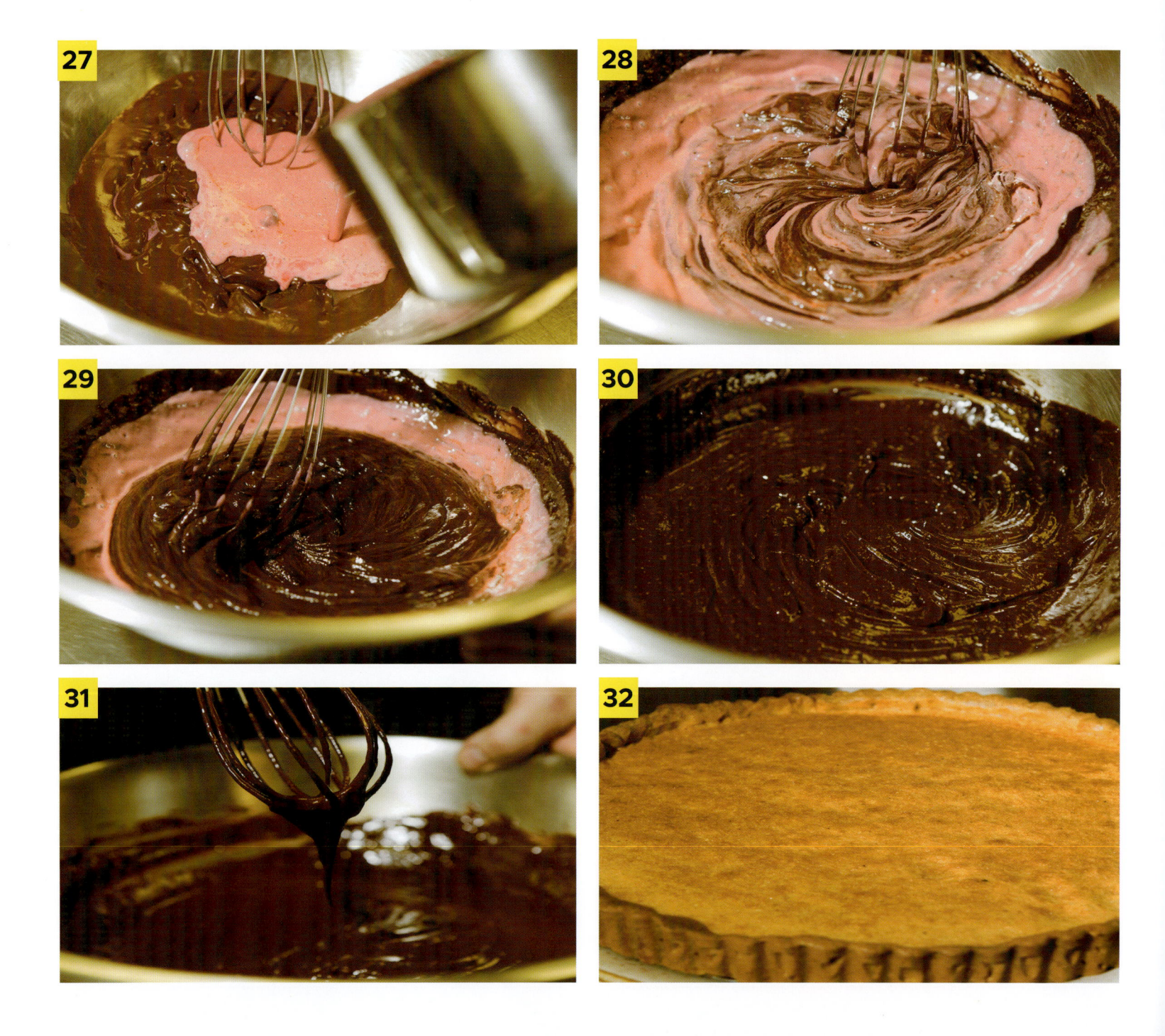

PAGE 175

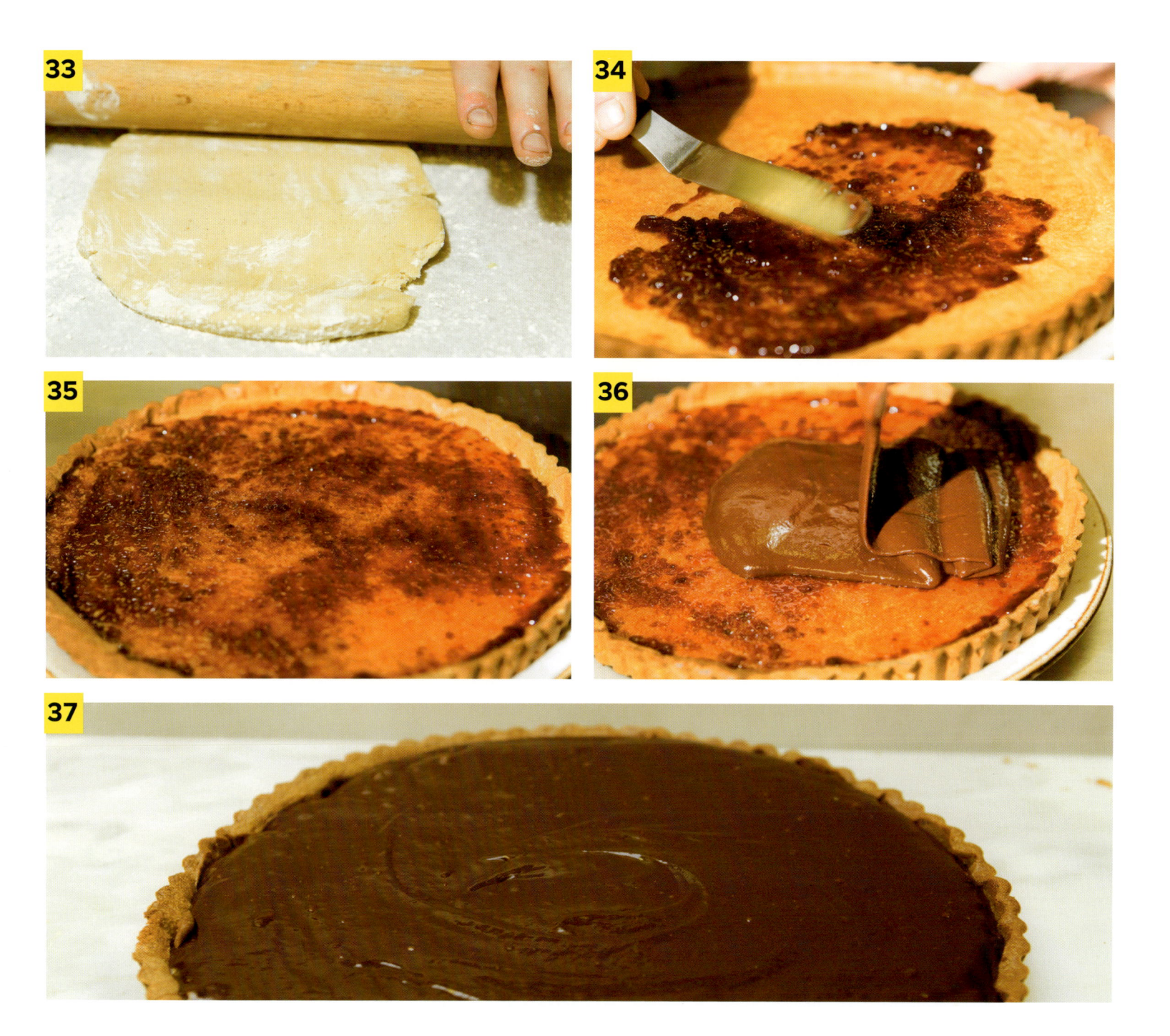

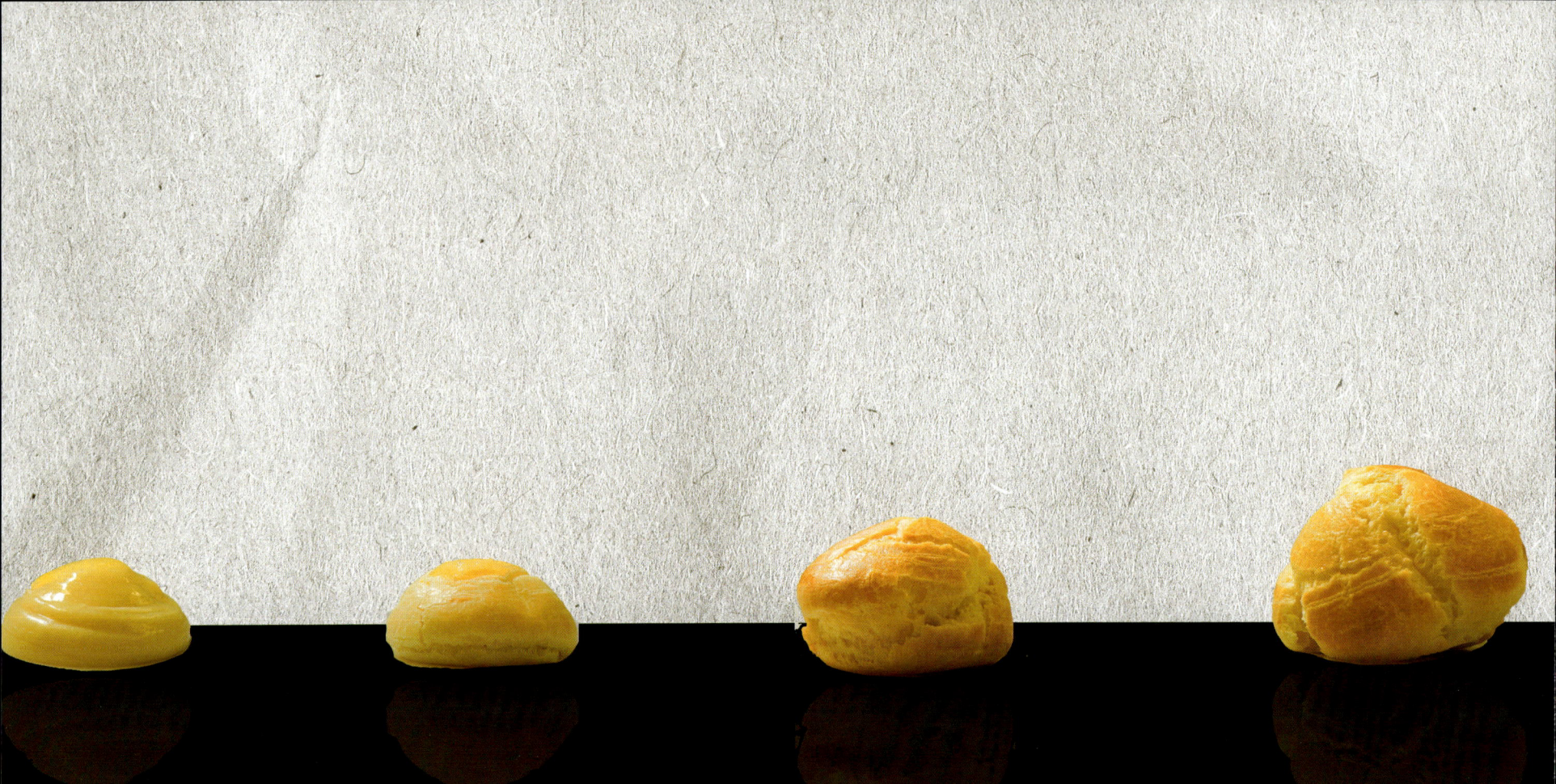

PÂTE À CHOUX

This dough is the basis for some of the greatest pastries on the planet. Along with the recipes that follow, pâte à choux can also be used to make cream puffs, éclairs, gougères, profiteroles, Paris-Brest, and St. Honoré. With a crispy golden exterior that gives way to a cloud-like core, it can be formed into balls, bars, or rings; packed with a sweet or savory filling; frosted or left bare. Its possibilities are nearly endless.

46

SERVES FOR 8-10 PEOPLE

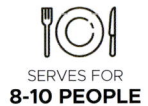

Dauphine Potatoes

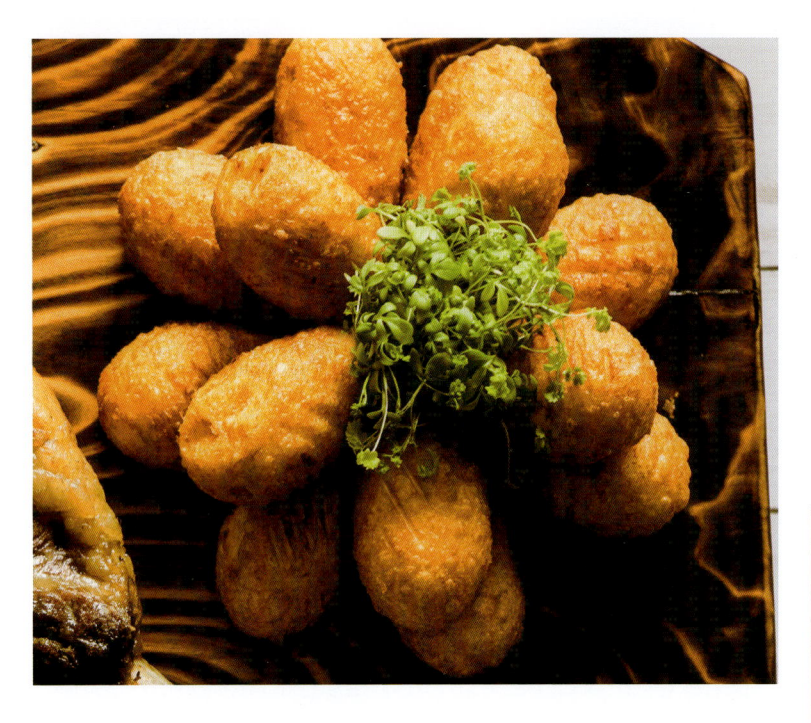

Once you've made the pâte à choux, this recipe is a breeze. All you need to do mix dough and mashed potatoes in equal amounts. Dollops are deep-fried until they're crispy golden brown on the outside but still fluffy and creamy white on the inside. Dauphine potatoes make a fantastic appetizer for any party; they go well with Flemish Beef Stew (Carbonnade à la Flamande) (page 122), Pork Chops with Blackwell Sauce (page 130), and Cherry Beer–Braised Rabbit (page 142); and they're a wonderful addition to a Thanksgiving or Christmas dinner. You will need a countertop deep-fryer, or a deep thick-bottomed pot and a deep-frying thermometer.

To make this recipe, you will first need to make a batch of pâte à choux dough, but don't bake it (page 179).

INGREDIENTS

1. 1/2 batch (1 3/4 pounds/800 grams) Pâte à Choux (page 179), unbaked
2. 3 pounds (1.4 kilograms) Yukon gold potatoes, washed
3. 2 teaspoons (10 grams) kosher salt, plus more for finishing
4. 3/4 teaspoon (2 grams) freshly ground black pepper
5. Canola oil for frying

DIRECTIONS

1. Prepare the pâte à choux dough and set it aside at room temperature.
2. Place the potatoes and salt in a large pot and fill to cover with cold water. Cook over high heat until a knife passes through a potato without resistance, about 45 minutes to 1 hour. Drain them in a colander set in the sink and let cool slightly for 5 minutes. To peel the hot potatoes, one at a time hold each in a folded kitchen towel and use a sharp paring knife to take off the skin. While they are still hot, place the potatoes in bowl of a stand mixer fitted with the paddle attachment and mix on medium speed until smooth. Add the salt, pepper, and pâté à choux dough, and mix until smooth and well combined.
3. Cover a plate with paper towels and set it aside.
4. Following the manufacturer's instructions, fill a deep-fryer with oil and heat it to 375°F (190°C). Scoop 1 tablespoon (15 milliliters) of the batter at a time into oil, being sure to not overcrowd the fryer. Using a mesh skimmer, rotate the balls so both sides are fried to golden brown, about 2 minutes a side.
5. Remove the balls from the fryer and place them on the prepared plate. Salt them to taste and serve warm.

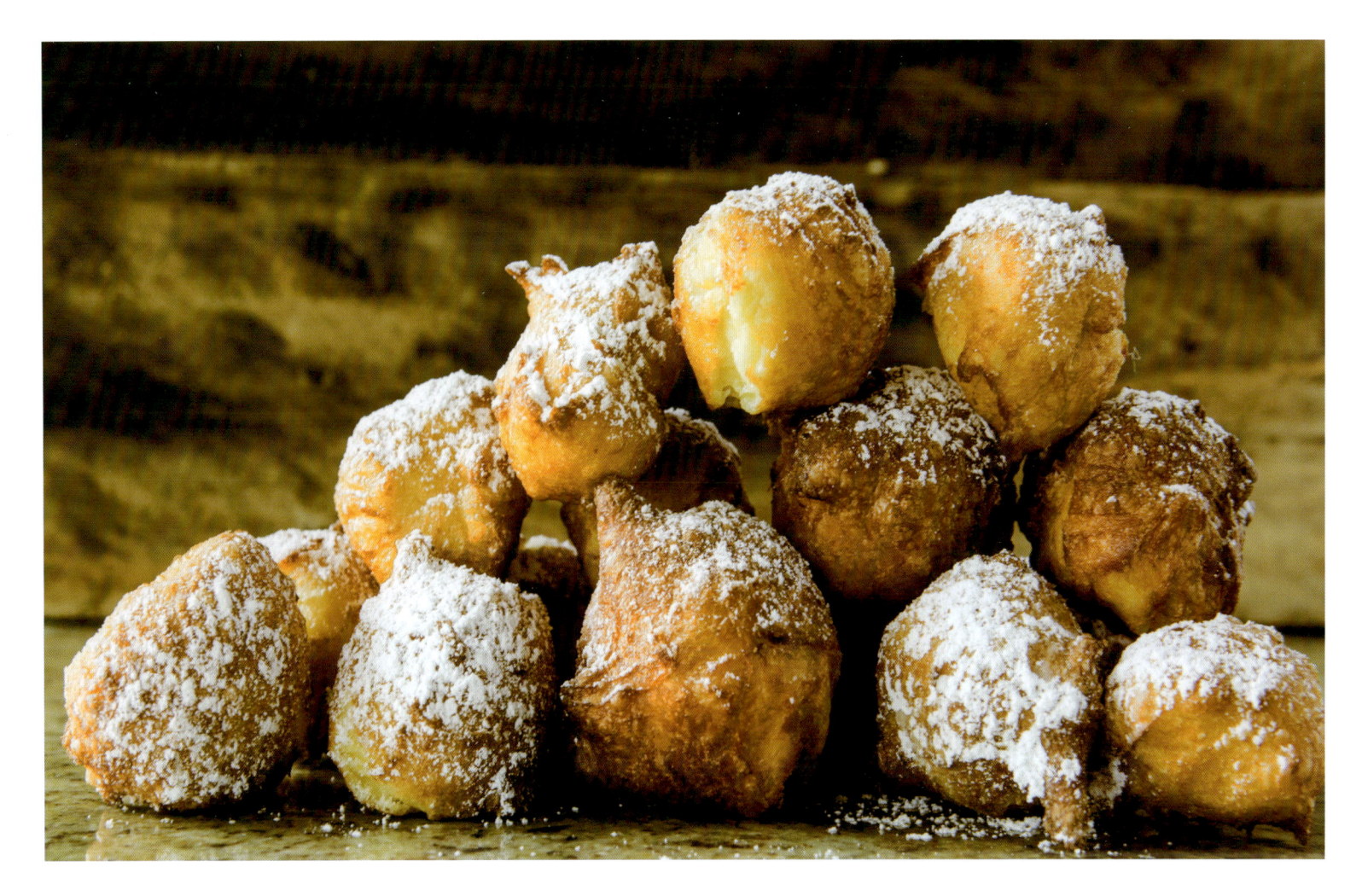

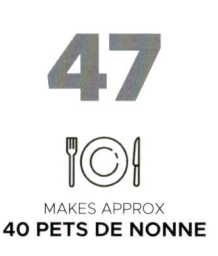

Pets de Nonne with Vanilla Custard

MAKES APPROX
40 PETS DE NONNE

The French name for these delightful desserts is more elegant than the English translation: nun's farts. They're essentially stuffed beignets. Deep-friend puffs of pâte à choux are sprinkled with a snowfall of confectioners' sugar and piped full of vanilla custard. As if that weren't enough, I like serving them with raspberry coulis or chocolate cream sauce to dunk them in.

To make this recipe, you will first need to make a batch of Pâte à Choux batter, but don't bake it (page 179).

INGREDIENTS

1. 5 large egg yolks (100 grams)
2. 1/2 cup (100 grams) granulated sugar
3. 1/4 cup + 2 teaspoons (35 grams) cornstarch
4. 2 cups (500 grams) whole milk
5. 4 vanilla beans, halved lengthwise, seeds scraped out
6. 3 tablespoons + 1 teaspoon (50 grams) heavy cream
7. 1/2 teaspoon (2.5 grams) dark rum
8. Canola oil for frying
9. 1 batch Pâte à Choux dough (page 179), unbaked
10. Confectioners' sugar for sprinkling

DIRECTIONS

To make the vanilla custard, in a medium bowl, whisk together the egg yolks, granulated sugar, and cornstarch until well incorporated. Set aside.

In a medium pot over high heat, whisk together the milk, vanilla bean pods, and seeds. As soon as it boils, remove from the heat and whisk in the egg mixture until smooth. Return the pot to the stove over medium heat, whisking continuously until the mixture becomes thick and smooth, 5 to 8 minutes.

Remove the pot from the stove. Mix in the cream and rum until fully incorporated. Strain out and discard the solids. Cover and place the custard in the refrigerator to chill for at least 2 hours or up to overnight.

When you're ready to assemble the pets de nonne, cover a plate with paper towels and set it aside. Following the manufacturer's instructions, fill a deep-fryer with oil and heat it to 350°F (175°C). Scoop generous 1 tablespoon (15 milliliters) of the pâte à choux dough at a time into oil, being sure to not overcrowd the fryer. Using a mesh skimmer, rotate the balls so both sides are fried golden brown, about 2 minutes a side. Remove the balls from the fryer with the skimmer and place them on the prepared plate. Let them cool for 5 to 10 minutes.

While they are still warm, fill a pastry bag fitted with an 8 mm plain tip with the vanilla custard. Insert the tip of the pastry bag into the bottom center of each pet de nonne and fill the pastry with cream. Sprinkle them with confectioners' sugar, making sure to cover all the sides. Serve immediately.

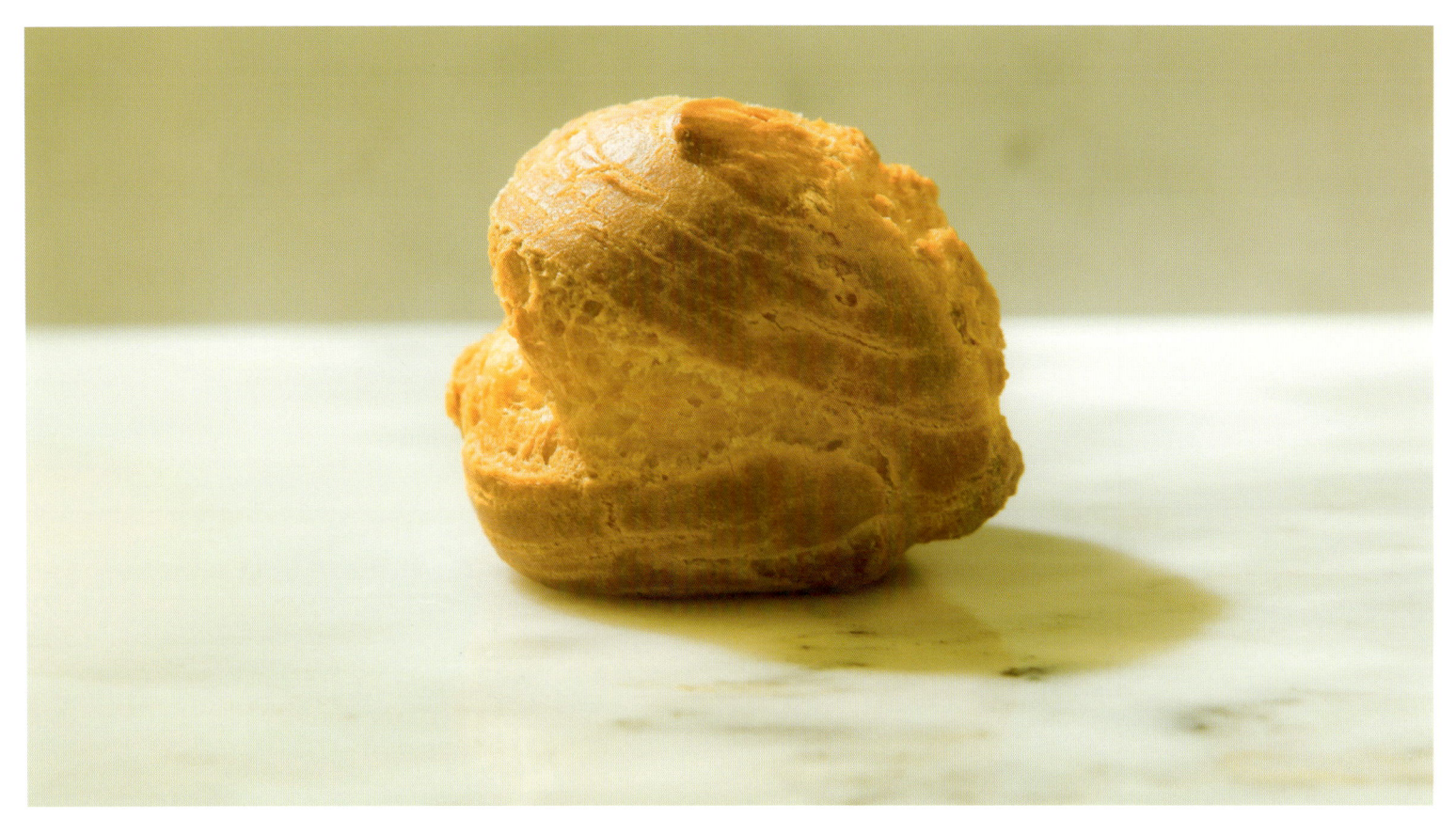

Pâte à Choux

(Step By Step)

48

MAKES APPROX
50 PUFFS

Once you master this recipe—don't worry, it's easy—this versatile dough will be a workhorse in your culinary repertoire. My one tip for perfect pâte à choux is to make sure the dough hangs like pointy icicles off the paddle. That's when you know it's ready to go. To make this recipe, you need a stand mixer with a paddle attachment and a pastry bag with a plain tip. Both are available at kitchenware stores.

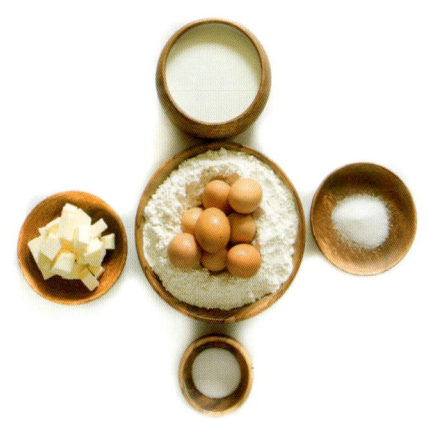

INGREDIENTS

1. 2 cups (500 grams) whole milk
2. 3 tablespoons + 1 teaspoon (40 grams) granulated sugar
3. Pinch of kosher salt
4. 1/2 pound (2 sticks/250 grams) unsalted butter
5. 2 3/4 cups (300 grams) pastry flour
6. 10 large eggs (500 grams), divided

DIRECTIONS

In a medium pot over high heat, whisk together the milk, sugar, and salt, and bring to a boil. Add the butter. When the butter has melted completely, take the pot off the stove.

Add the flour all at once and mix with wood spoon until fully combined. Put the pot back on the stove over medium heat and mix constantly until the mixture forms a big ball, about 10 minutes.

Transfer the mixture to the bowl of a stand mixer fitted with a paddle attachment. With the mixer on low speed, add the eggs one by one, mixing until each egg is fully incorporated before adding the next.

After adding the sixth egg, lift the paddle from the bowl. If the dough hangs off of the paddle in a triangular icicle shape, it's ready. If not, add 3 more eggs, one at a time, checking after each addition, until the desired consistency is achieved.

Spray 2 rimmed sheet pans with nonstick cooking spray and cover with parchment paper. Preheat the oven to 350°F (175°C).

Using a spatula, put the dough in a pastry bag fitted with a 12 mm plain tip attachment. Squeeze out 1 1/2-inch-wide (4 cm) spheres of dough onto the prepared sheet pans, leaving 2 inches (5 cm) between them.

Using a whisk and a small bowl, mix the remaining egg with 1 1/2 teaspoons (7.5 mL) water to create an egg wash. Brush it on the top of each sphere of dough.

Reduce the oven temperature to 325°F (165°C). Bake the puffs for 25 minutes. Open the oven door for 1 minute, while still baking, then close the door and bake for another 10 minutes, until they are golden brown and puffy.

Transfer the pâte à choux to a cooling rack and let cool before filling and serving, or wrap them in cling-wrap, place in a freezer-safe container, and freeze them for 2 months or longer.

Stepwise Instructions

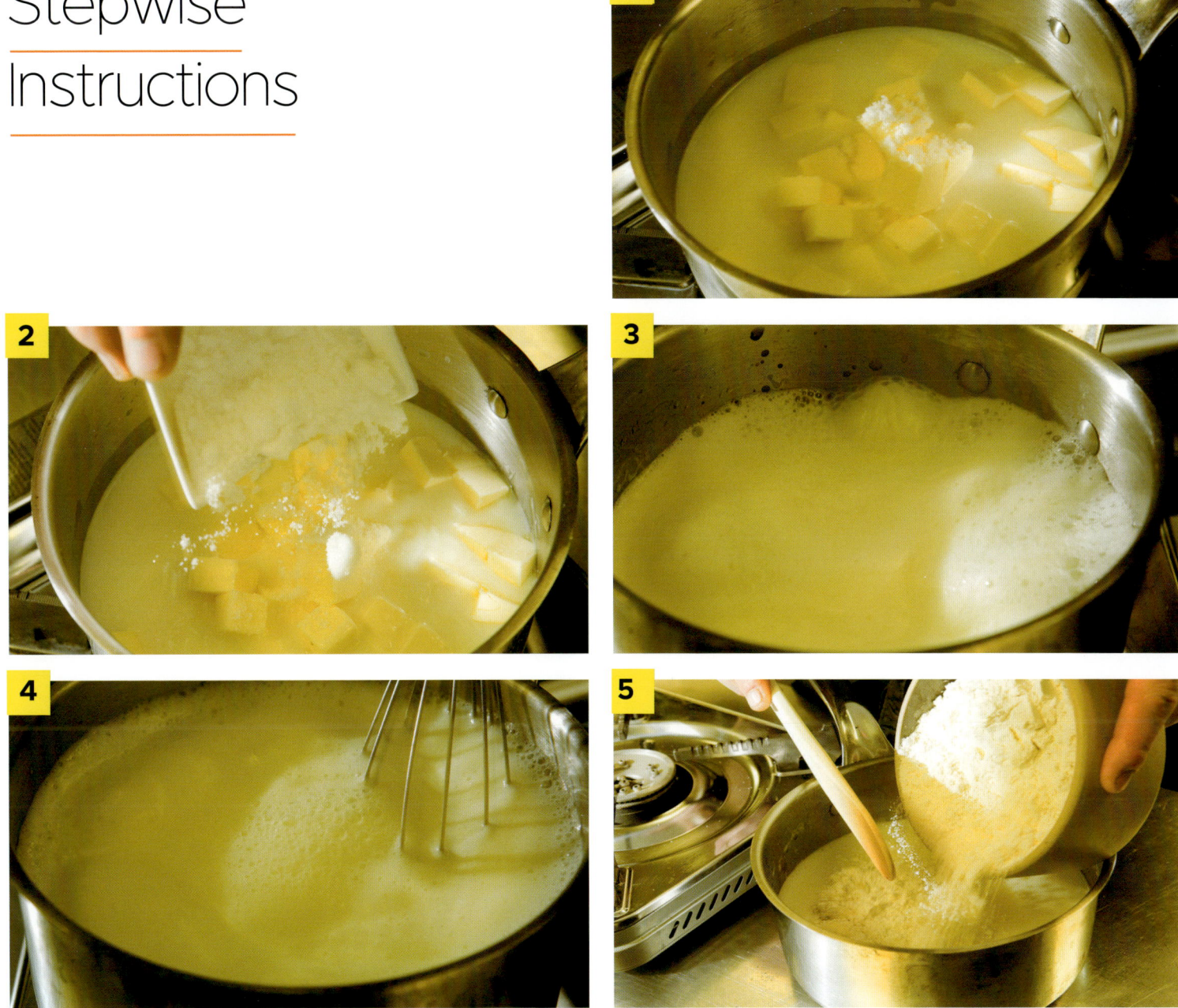

PAGE 183

PAGE 184

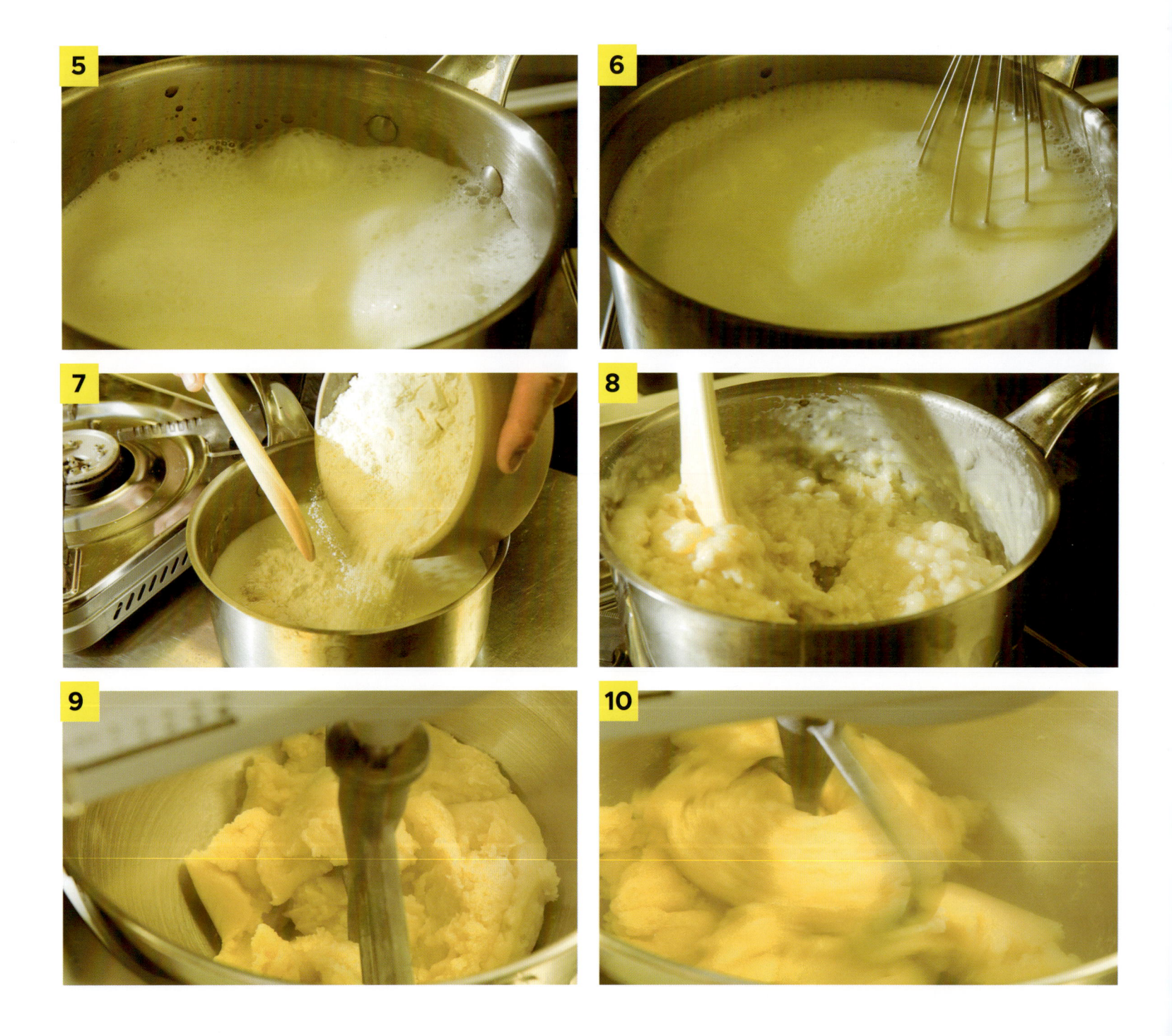

PAGE 185

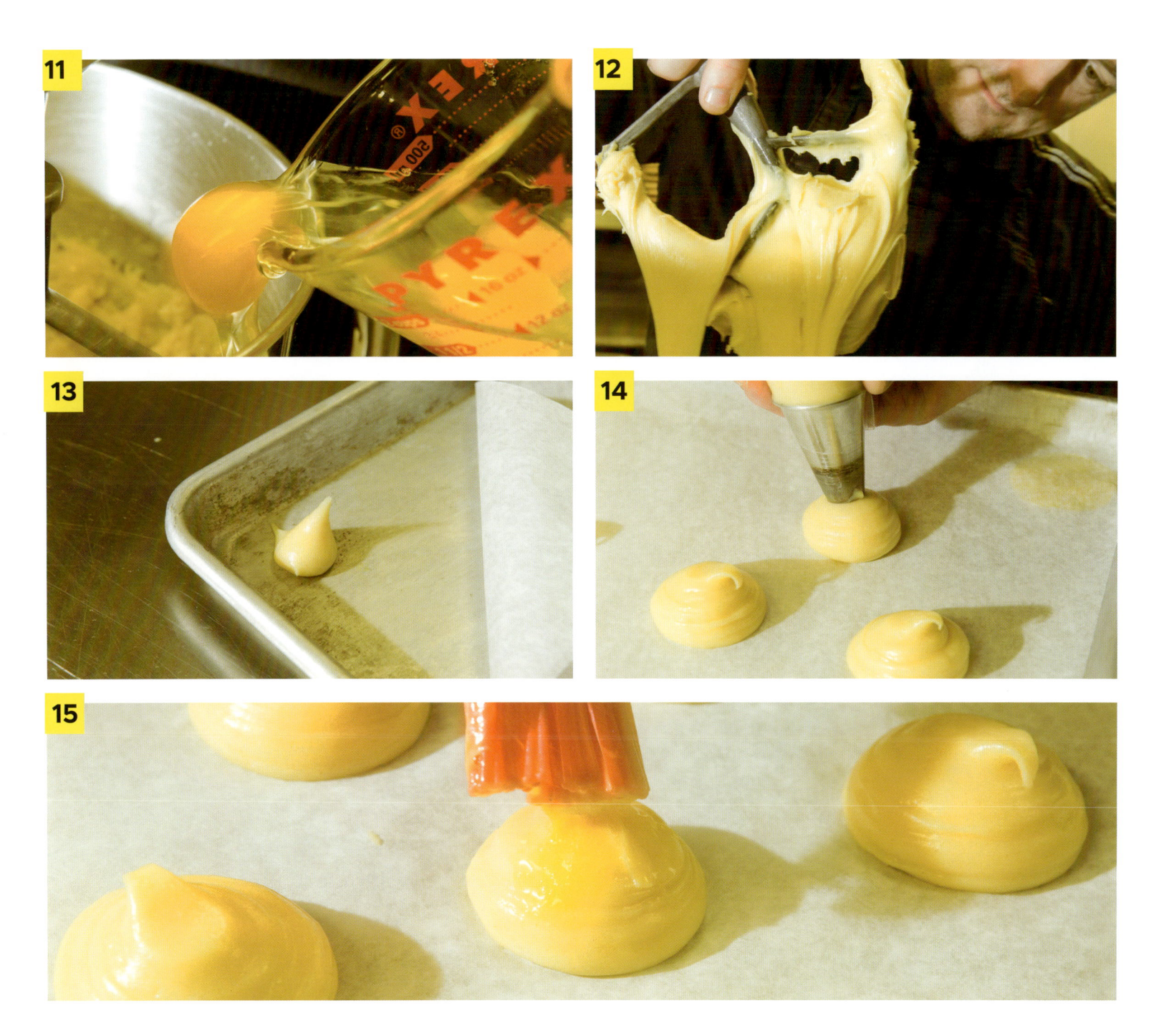

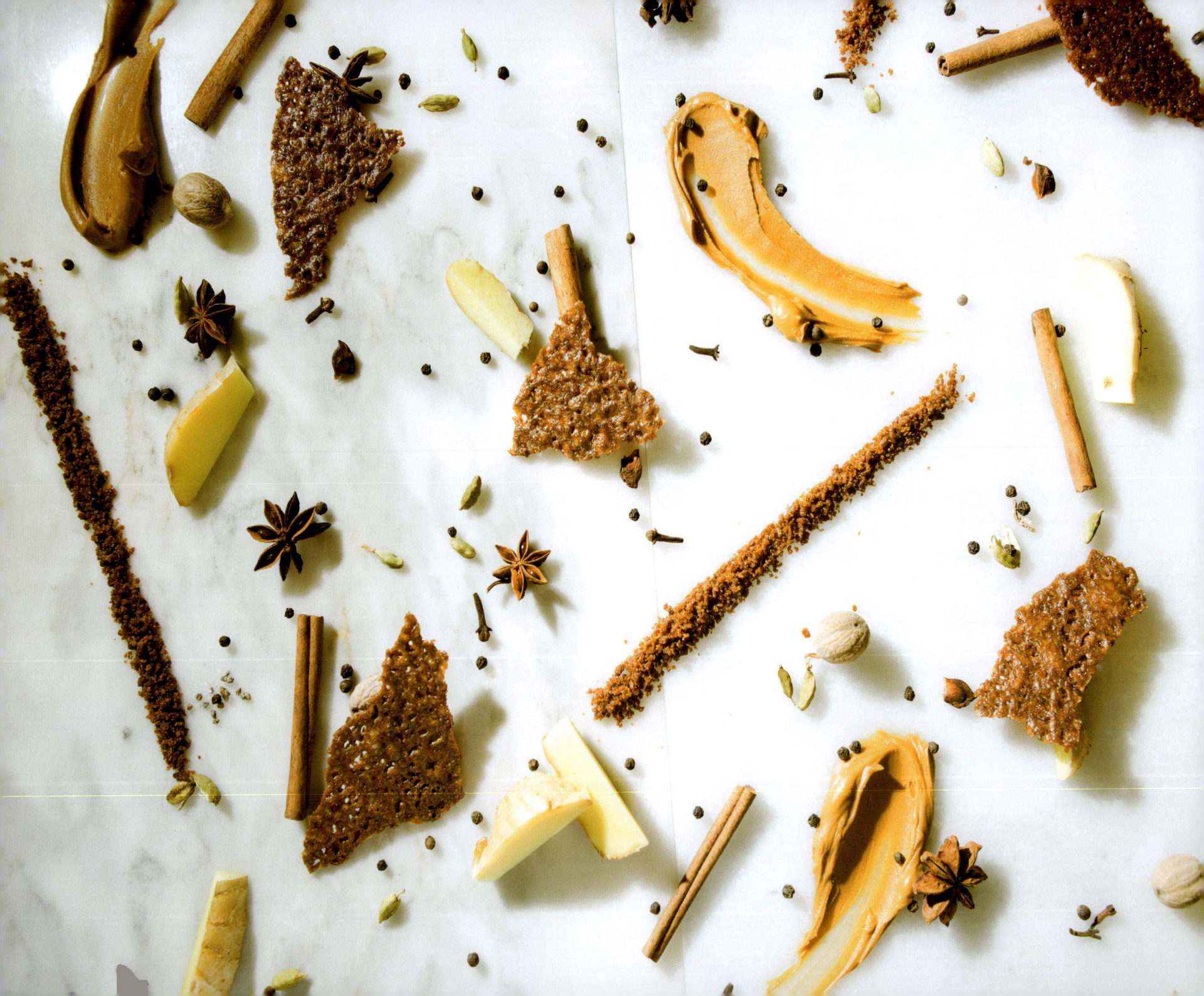

SPECULOOS

In Belgium, December 6 is Saint Nicholas Day. When I was a child, I would put a shoe out the night before and wake up to find that Sinterklaas (St. Nick) had left me a clementine orange, a small gift, and a speculoos cookie in the shape of himself. Snappy and full of buttery, the crunchy cookies are packed with wintry, warming spices: ginger, nutmeg, cinnamon, and cloves. It's a versatile flavor that lends itself to both savory and sweet preparations. You can buy speculoos (they are sometimes labeled as Biscoff cookies) in many grocery stores, including Trader Joe's, and online; my favorite brands are Vermeiren and Lotus.

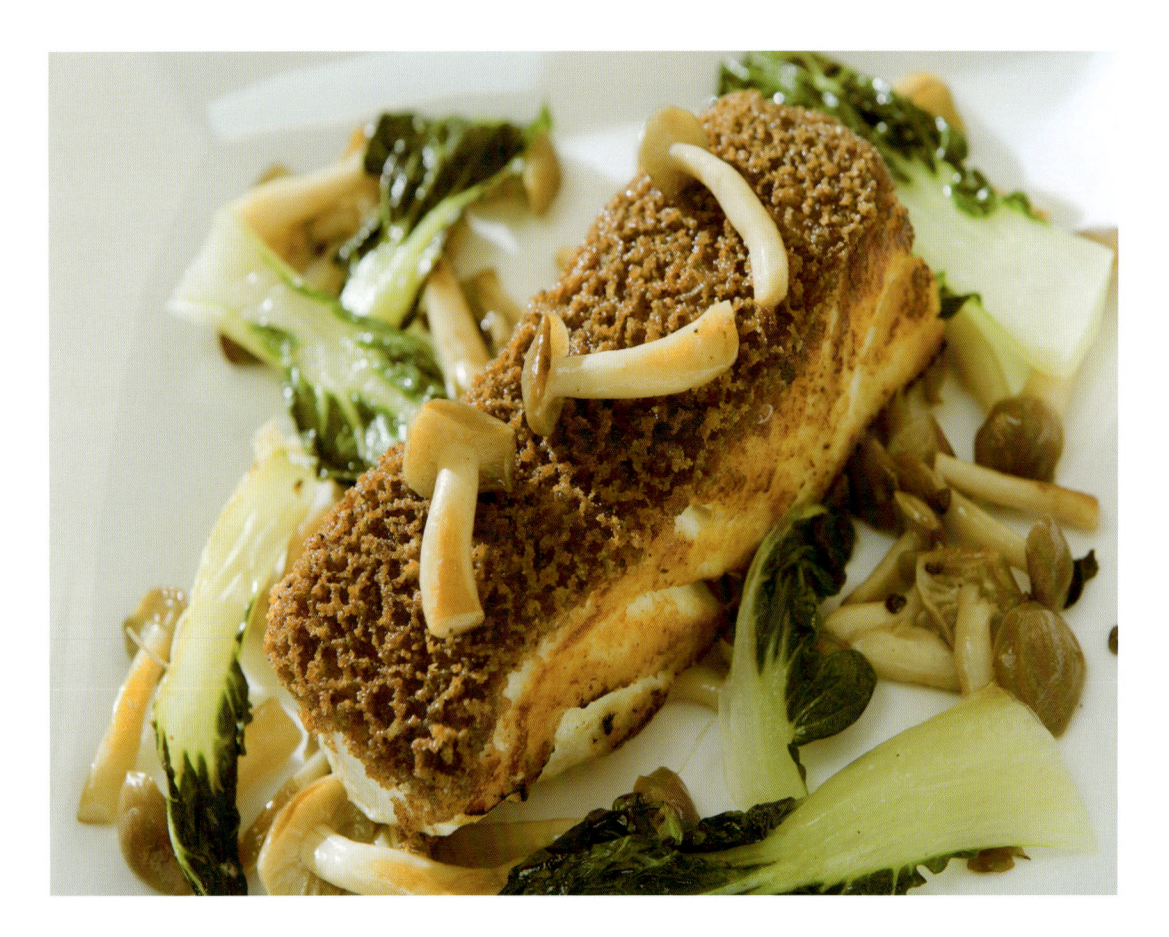

Speculoos-Crusted Halibut with Mushroom Emulsion

49

SERVES FOR **4 PEOPLE**

INGREDIENTS

Crust

1. 8 tablespoons (1 stick/125 grams) unsalted butter, room temperature
2. 1 tablespoon + 1 teaspoon (10 grams) speculoos spice mix (store-bought, or page 211)
3. 1/2 teaspoon (2 grams) kosher salt
4. 1/4 teaspoon (1 gram) freshly ground black pepper
5. 1/2 cup (90 grams) plain dried breadcrumbs
6. 1 tablespoon (20 grams) all-purpose flour

To start this recipe, I create a "dough" with speculoos spice mix (if you don't feel like making it, I like the one King Arthur Flour makes), breadcrumbs, flour, butter, salt, and pepper. After rolling it out, I place squares of it on halibut fillets and let the broiler drape it over the fish. I complement it with an emulsion that showcases the land and the sea thanks to the use of mushrooms and mussels, and serve it with sautéed shiitake mushrooms and seared bok choy. An artful dish with sophisticated flavors, it will surprise dinner party guests as much as it will satisfy them.

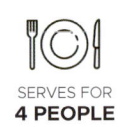

Mushroom sauce

1. 2 cups white mushroom consommé (page 209)
2. 1 cup + 1 tablespoon (250 grams) heavy cream

To assemble

1. 2 tablespoons (30 grams) vegetable oil, divided
2. 7 ounces (200 grams) nameko or brown beech mushrooms, separated and cleaned
3. Kosher salt and freshly ground black pepper
4. 1 medium shallot, finely diced
5. 2 sprigs fresh thyme, divided
6. 2 cloves garlic, finely diced
7. 8 tablespoons (1 stick/125 grams) unsalted butter, room temperature
8. 4 heads bok choy
9. Four 6-ounce (170 gram) halibut fillets (Alaskan preferred)

DIRECTIONS

To make the crust, place 8 tablespoons (125 grams) of the butter and the speculoos spice mix in a food processor fitted with the stainless-steel blade and process for 1 minute, until fully incorporated and creamy. Add the salt and pepper and process for 1 minute, until fully incorporated and smooth. Add the breadcrumbs and flour and process until everything is well combined and looks like a soft dough, about 2 minutes. Remove the dough from the food processor and shape it into a ball. Wrap in plastic wrap and chill in the refrigerator for 1 hour, until firm.

Remove the dough from the refrigerator and use a rolling pin to roll it into a large rectangle about 1/4 inch (6 mm) thick. Cut the dough into four smaller rectangles, each the size of one of the halibut fillets. Place the dough rectangles on a sheet pan covered with parchment paper, cover with plastic wrap, and refrigerate.

To make the sauce, place the white mushroom consommé in a medium saucepan over medium heat. Bring to a simmer and cook until reduced by half, about 20 minutes. Stir in the cream, reduce the heat to low, and cook until the sauce has reduced again by half, about 20 minutes. Remove from the heat and set aside.

In a large sauté pan over high heat, heat 1 tablespoon (15 grams) of the oil until starting to smoke slightly. Add the mushrooms, 1/4 teaspoon (1 gram) salt, 1/4 teaspoon (1 gram) pepper, shallots, 1 thyme sprig, the garlic, and 2 tablespoons (30 grams) of the butter. Cook until the mushrooms have softened, about 2 minutes. Remove from the heat and set aside.

Fill a large bowl with ice cubes and cold water and set aside. Remove the first layer of leaves and any leaves that have yellowed from the bok choy. Bring a large pot of well-salted water to a boil over high heat. Place the bok choy into the boiling water and cook until al dente, about 5 minutes. Place the bok choy into the ice water bath to stop the cooking. When the bok choy has fully cooled, remove it from the water and place on a paper towel–lined plate to drain. Set aside.

In a medium sauté pan, melt 4 tablespoons (60 grams) of the butter. Add the remaining thyme sprig. Add the bok choy and stir to coat. Season with salt and black pepper to taste, and cook until soft, about 4 minutes. Remove from pan and let cool on a cooling rack set in a sheet pan.

Preheat the broiler.

Season the fish with salt on both sides. In a large nonstick sauté pan over medium heat, warm the remaining 1 tablespoon (15 grams) oil and the remaining 2 tablespoons (30 grams) butter. When the butter is completely melted and begins to bubble, place the fish in the pan and sear until light golden brown, 3 to 5 minutes. Place the fish with the seared side up on a sheet pan. Spoon approximately 1 tablespoon (15 milliliters) of the butter and oil mixture over each fillet. Place a rectangle of the dough on each fillet and broil until the crust is crispy and golden brown, 6 to 8 minutes.

Meanwhile, rewarm the mushroom sauce over medium heat until boiling. Using a hand blender, blend the sauce frothy. Reheat the bok choy and sautéed mushrooms.

To serve, divide the mushrooms between four plates, then place fillet on top and spoon on 2 tablespoons (30 milliliters) of the froth from the mushroom sauce (save the sauce itself for another project). Divide the bok choy between the plates. Serve immediately.

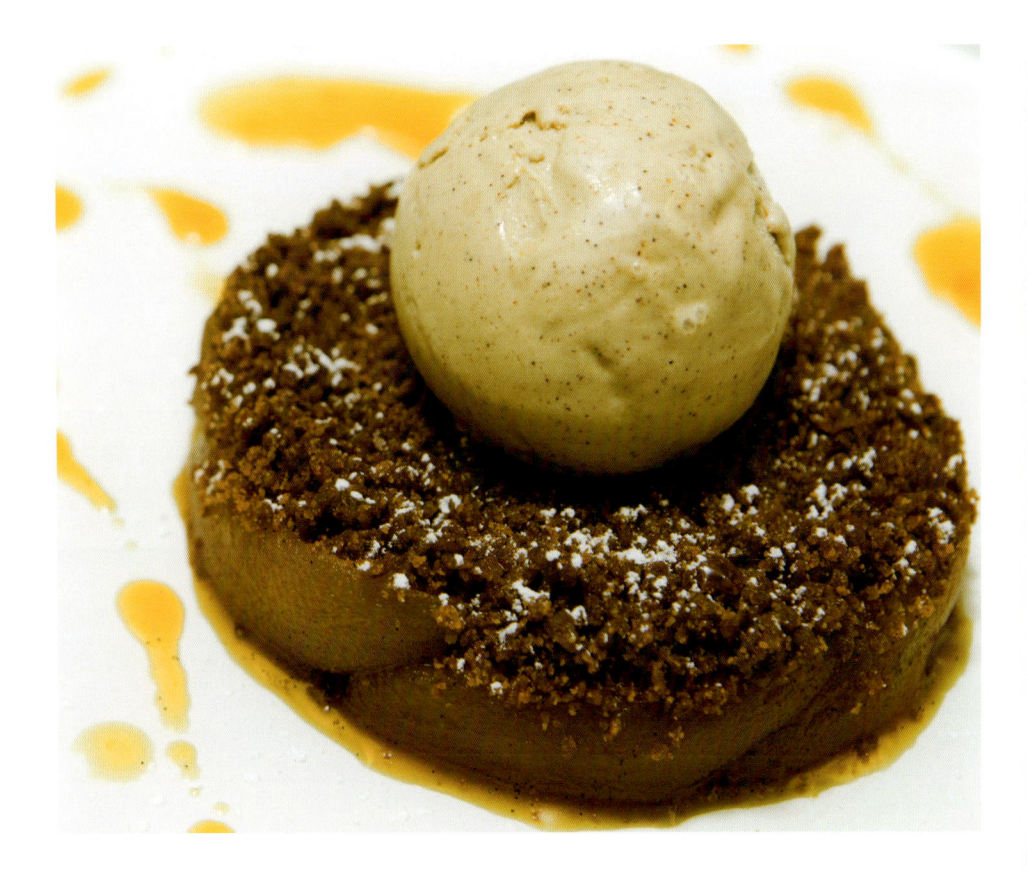

Apple Crumble
with Speculoos Ice Cream

This is not your grandma's apple crumble. I elevate the humble dessert to a more elegant plane by cooking apples (Gala or Red Delicious work best) in blond caramel before covering them with the brown sugar topping and baking them. If you're not in the mood to make speculoos spice mix, it can be purchased online; I like the one King Arthur Flour makes. Almond flour can be purchased online or at some grocery stores; Anthony's Goods makes a good option. The ice cream needs to be made a day beforehand and requires an ice cream maker; Cuisinart makes reasonably priced, efficient models that work well.

INGREDIENTS

Speculoos ice cream

1. 2 cups (500 grams) whole milk
2. 1/2 teaspoon (1 gram) freshly grated orange zest
3. 2 cinnamon sticks
4. 1 vanilla bean, halved lengthwise, seeds scraped out
5. 8 large egg yolks (160 grams)
6. 3/4 cup (100 grams) confectioners' sugar
7. 2 tablespoons + 1 teaspoon (50 grams) honey
8. 1 tablespoon + 1 teaspoon (10 grams) speculoos spice mix (store-bought, or page 211)
9. 1 cup (250 grams) heavy cream

Crumble topping

1. 2 tablespoons (25 grams) light brown sugar
2. 3 tablespoons (25 grams) confectioners' sugar
3. 4 tablespoons (1/2 stick/60 grams) unsalted butter, room temperature
4. 1/2 cup (50 grams) almond flour
5. 1/4 cup + 3 tablespoons (50 grams) all-purpose flour

Apple filling

1. 1 1/2 cups + 1 tablespoon (200 grams) confectioners' sugar
2. Scant 3 tablespoons (40 grams) water
3. 3 tablespoons (45 grams) unsalted butter
4. 3 large Gala apples or similar, peeled, cored, and each cut into 8 pieces
5. 2 vanilla beans, halved lengthwise, seeds scraped out

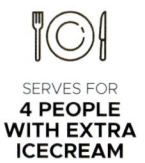

50

SERVES FOR
4 PEOPLE WITH EXTRA ICECREAM

PAGE 191

DIRECTIONS

To make the ice cream, in a medium pot over medium heat, place the milk, orange zest, cinnamon sticks, and vanilla bean pod and seeds. Bring to boil, then remove the pot from the heat and cover it with aluminum foil. Let the flavors infuse for 10 minutes. Pass the milk mixture through a fine-mesh strainer and return it to the pot; discard the solids.

In a large bowl, whisk together the egg yolks, sugar, and honey until the mixture is pale and smooth. Set aside.

Return the pot to the stove over medium heat and bring the milk mixture to a boil. When boiling, add the egg mixture and gently whisk until thoroughly combined. Add the speculoos spice and whisk steadily until the mixture reaches 180°F (83°C). Remove the pot from the heat, add the heavy cream, and whisk until fully incorporated. Fill a large bowl halfway with ice and cold water. Place a medium bowl on top of the ice water. Strain the ice cream base through a fine-mesh strainer into the medium bowl. Once the base has cooled, remove it from the larger bowl, cover it, and place it in the refrigerator to chill overnight.

The next day, place the ice cream base in an ice cream maker and proceed according to the manufacturer's instructions. Once made, place the ice cream in the freezer.

To make the crumble topping, in a large bowl, use your hands to crumble together the brown sugar, confectioners' sugar, butter, almond flour, and all-purpose flour into a shaggy mass. Set aside.

To make the apple filling, in a wide medium pot over medium heat, bring the confectioners' sugar and water to a boil. Do not mix, just wait until it turns caramel in color. (It should take 5 to 8 minutes.) Keep a close eye on it; you don't want it to burn. Add the butter and mix gently with a wooden spoon. Once the butter has melted, add the apples and the vanilla bean pods and seeds. Gently stirring with a wooden spoon, cook until the apples are caramelized and completely covered in sauce, about 12 minutes. To check if they're done, insert a knife into the apple. If it slips through with no resistance, you can take them off the stove. Remove the apples from the caramel sauce and place them on a sheet pan. Set aside.

Preheat the oven to 325°F (165°C).

Place 6 apple slices into each of four ramekins roughly 1 inch (3 cm) high and 5 inches (13 cm) in diameter. Spoon 1 tablespoon (15 milliliters) of the caramel sauce (making sure to not accidentally add the vanilla bean pods) onto each, then completely cover the apples with the crumble topping. Place the ramekins on a sheet pan and bake until the topping is golden brown, about 20 minutes. Let them cool for 5 minutes before topping each with a scoop of speculoos ice cream and serving immediately.

To make the crumble topping, in a large bowl, use your hands to crumble together the brown sugar, confectioners' sugar, butter, almond flour, and all-purpose flour into a shaggy mass. Set aside.

To make the apple filling, in a wide medium pot over medium heat, bring the confectioners' sugar and water to a boil. Do not mix, just wait until it turns caramel in color. (It should take 5 to 8 minutes.) Keep a close eye on it; you don't want it to burn. Add the butter and mix gently with a wooden spoon. Once the butter has melted, add the apples and the vanilla bean pods and seeds. Gently stirring with a wooden spoon, cook until the apples are caramelized and completely covered in sauce, about 12 minutes. To check if they're done, insert a knife into the apple. If it slips through with no resistance, you can take them off the stove. Remove the apples from the caramel sauce and place them on a sheet pan. Set aside.

Preheat the oven to 325°F (165°C).

Place 6 apple slices into each of four ramekins roughly 1 inch (3 cm) high and 5 inches (13 cm) in diameter. Spoon 1 tablespoon (15 milliliters) of the caramel sauce (making sure to not accidentally add the vanilla bean pods) onto each, then completely cover the apples with the crumble topping. Place the ramekins on a sheet pan and bake until the topping is golden brown, about 20 minutes. Let them cool for 5 minutes before topping each with a scoop of speculoos ice cream and serving immediately.

Preheat the broiler.

Season the fish with salt on both sides. In a large nonstick sauté pan over medium heat, warm the remaining 1 tablespoon (15 grams) oil and the remaining 2 tablespoons (30 grams) butter. When the butter is completely melted and begins to bubble, place the fish in the pan and sear until light golden brown, 3 to 5 minutes. Place the fish with the seared side up on a sheet pan. Spoon approximately 1 tablespoon (15 milliliters) of the butter and oil mixture over each fillet. Place a rectangle of the dough on each fillet and broil until the crust is crispy and golden brown, 6 to 8 minutes.

Meanwhile, rewarm the mushroom sauce over medium heat until boiling. Using a hand blender, blend the sauce frothy. Reheat the bok choy and sautéed mushrooms.

To serve, divide the mushrooms between four plates, then place fillet on top and spoon on 2 tablespoons (30 milliliters) of the froth from the mushroom sauce (save the sauce itself for another project). Divide the bok choy between the plates. Serve immediately.

51

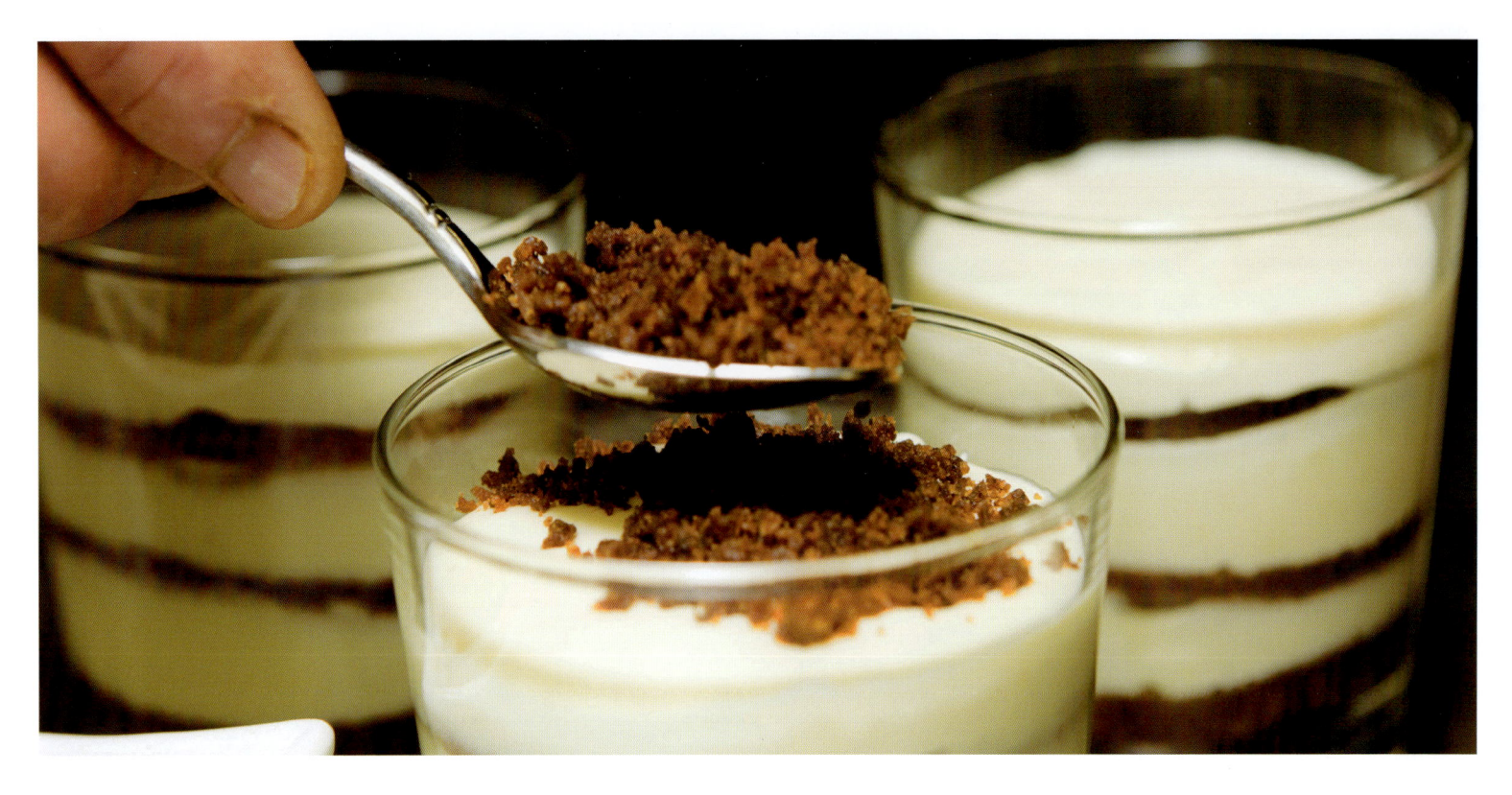

SERVES FOR
4 PEOPLE

Speculoos Tiramisu

(Step By Step)

Of course, I love tiramisu. Soon after we opened, we offered it as a special at Et Voila!, but I always felt like it wasn't true to our identity. Why were we serving an Italian dessert at a Franco-Belgian restaurant? To make it make sense, Alex and I devised a recipe that hewed to our roots featuring espresso-dipped speculoos interspersed between layers of mascarpone cream. For added crunch, there's a layer of crumbled cookies hiding at the bottom and another scattered across the top. The tiramisu must set for at least 4 hours in the refrigerator, but letting it set overnight is preferred. Once it's ready, it will keep for up to 4 days in the refrigerator. You will need four brandy snifters or similar glasses to serve the tiramisu in.

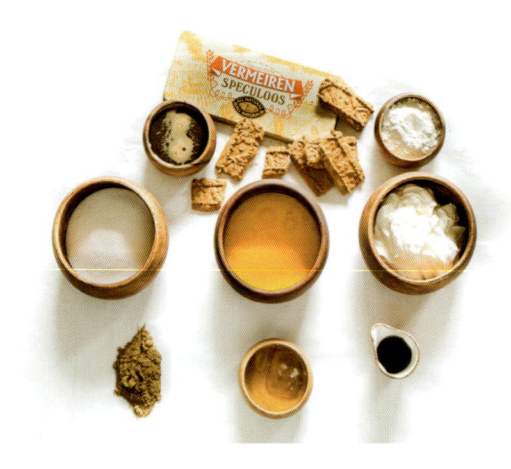

PAGE 194

INGREDIENTS

Speculoos cookies

1. 6 large egg whites (180 grams)
2. 1/2 cup + 2 tablespoons (125 grams) granulated sugar, divided
3. 9 large egg yolks (180 grams)
4. 1/2 cup + 2 tablespoons (80 grams) all-purpose flour, sifted
5. 2 tablespoons + 1/2 teaspoon (15 grams) speculoos spice mix (store-bought, or page 211)
6. 1/4 cup (28 grams) confectioners' sugar

Crumble topping

1. 4 large egg yolks (80 grams)
2. 1/2 cup (100 grams) granulated sugar
3. 1 3/4 cups (500 grams) mascarpone

Coffee syrup

1. 2 cups (500 grams) brewed coffee, room temperature
2. 1/4 cup (50 grams) granulated sugar
3. 1/2 cup (100 grams) Kahlúa or other coffee-flavored liqueur

DIRECTIONS

To make the speculoos cookies, in the bowl of a stand mixer fitted with the whisk attachment, whisk the egg whites and 1/4 cup (50 grams) granulated sugar on high speed until they form firm peaks. Set aside. [Image 1, 2 and 3]

In a medium mixing bowl, whisk together the egg yolks and the remaining 1/4 cup + 2 tablespoons (75 grams) granulated sugar until fully combined. [Image 4 though 7]

Using a spatula, gently fold the egg yolk mixture into the egg whites. Gently fold in the flour and speculoos spice mix. Set aside. [Image 8]

Spray 2 sheet pans with nonstick spray, then cover them with parchment paper. Using a spatula, fill a pastry bag fitted with a 3/4-inch (19 mm) tip with the dough. Squeeze out 2 1/2 inch (6 cm) rounds—about 12 cookies per sheet—making sure to leave 2 inches (5 cm) between them. [Image 9, 10 and 11]

Sprinkle the tops with confectioners' sugar. Let sit uncovered for at least 10 minutes and up to 1 hour.

Preheat the oven to 375°F (190°C).

Bake the cookies light golden brown, about 6 minutes. When you lift one up, you should see a slight discoloration of the parchment paper below it. Transfer the cookies to a cooling rack and let them cool completely. Crush enough cookies to make 1/2 cup (120 milliliters) powder to be used as a garnish. [Image 12]

To make the mascarpone cream, in the bowl of a stand mixer fitted with the whisk attachment, mix the egg yolks and sugar at medium speed until the mixture is fully combined. [Image 13]

Turn the speed up to medium-high, add the mascarpone, and mix until the mixture is thick and soft. Set aside. [Image 14]

To make the coffee syrup, in a medium pot over medium heat, bring the sugar, coffee, and Kahlúa to a simmer for 10 minutes. Pour the coffee syrup into a 13 by 9-inch (33 by 23 cm) baking pan. [Image 15]

Season the fish with salt on both sides. In a large nonstick sauté pan over medium heat, warm the remaining 1 tablespoon (15 grams) oil and the remaining 2 tablespoons (30 grams) butter. When the butter is completely melted and begins to bubble, place the fish in the pan and sear until light golden brown, 3 to 5 minutes. Place the fish with the seared side up on a sheet pan. Spoon approximately 1 tablespoon (15 milliliters) of the butter and oil mixture over each fillet. Place a rectangle of the dough on each fillet and broil until the crust is crispy and golden brown, 6 to 8 minutes.

Meanwhile, rewarm the mushroom sauce over medium heat until boiling. Using a hand blender, blend the sauce frothy. Reheat the bok choy and sautéed mushrooms.

To serve, divide the mushrooms between four plates, then place fillet on top and spoon on 2 tablespoons (30 milliliters) of the froth from the mushroom sauce (save the sauce itself for another project). Divide the bok choy between the plates. Serve immediately.

To assemble the speculoos tiramisu, soak each of the speculoos cookies in the coffee syrup on one side for 2 seconds at a time. Set aside on a plate.

Line up four brandy snifters. At the bottom of each one, place 1 tablespoon (15 milliliters) of the mascarpone cream. Place a cookie on top of the cream. Alternate layers of cream and cookie until you reach the top of the glass.

Sprinkle the speculoos cookie powder on top of each. Cover each glass with plastic wrap.

Refrigerate for 4 hours before serving. If you don't want to serve them right away, they will keep for up to 4 days in the refrigerator.

Stepwise Instructions

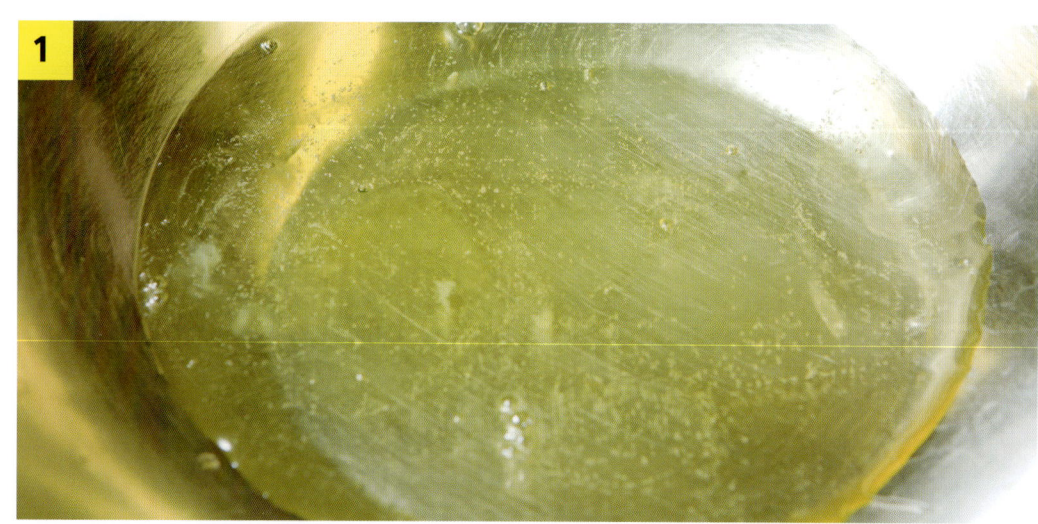

PAGE 197

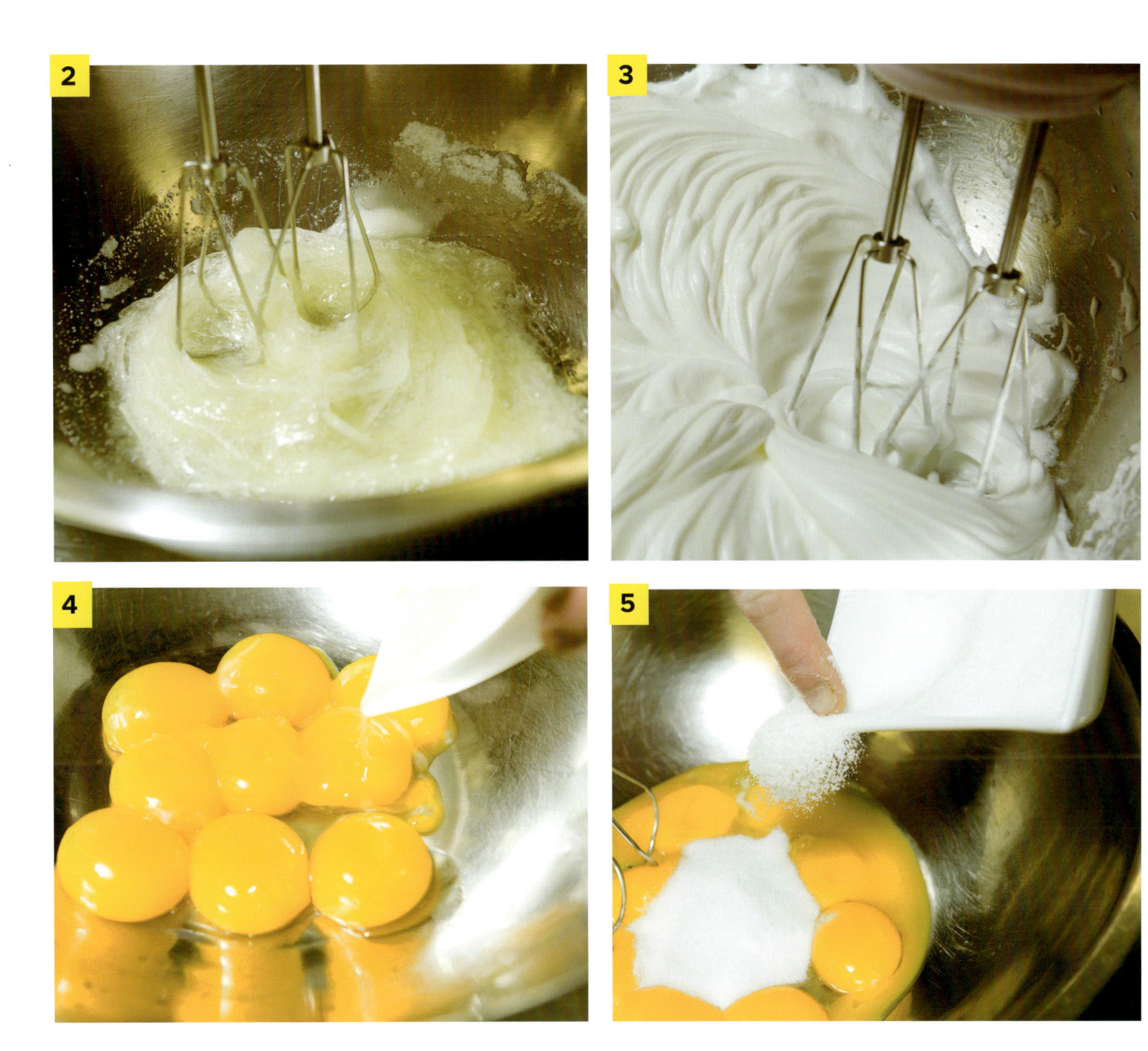

PAGE 198

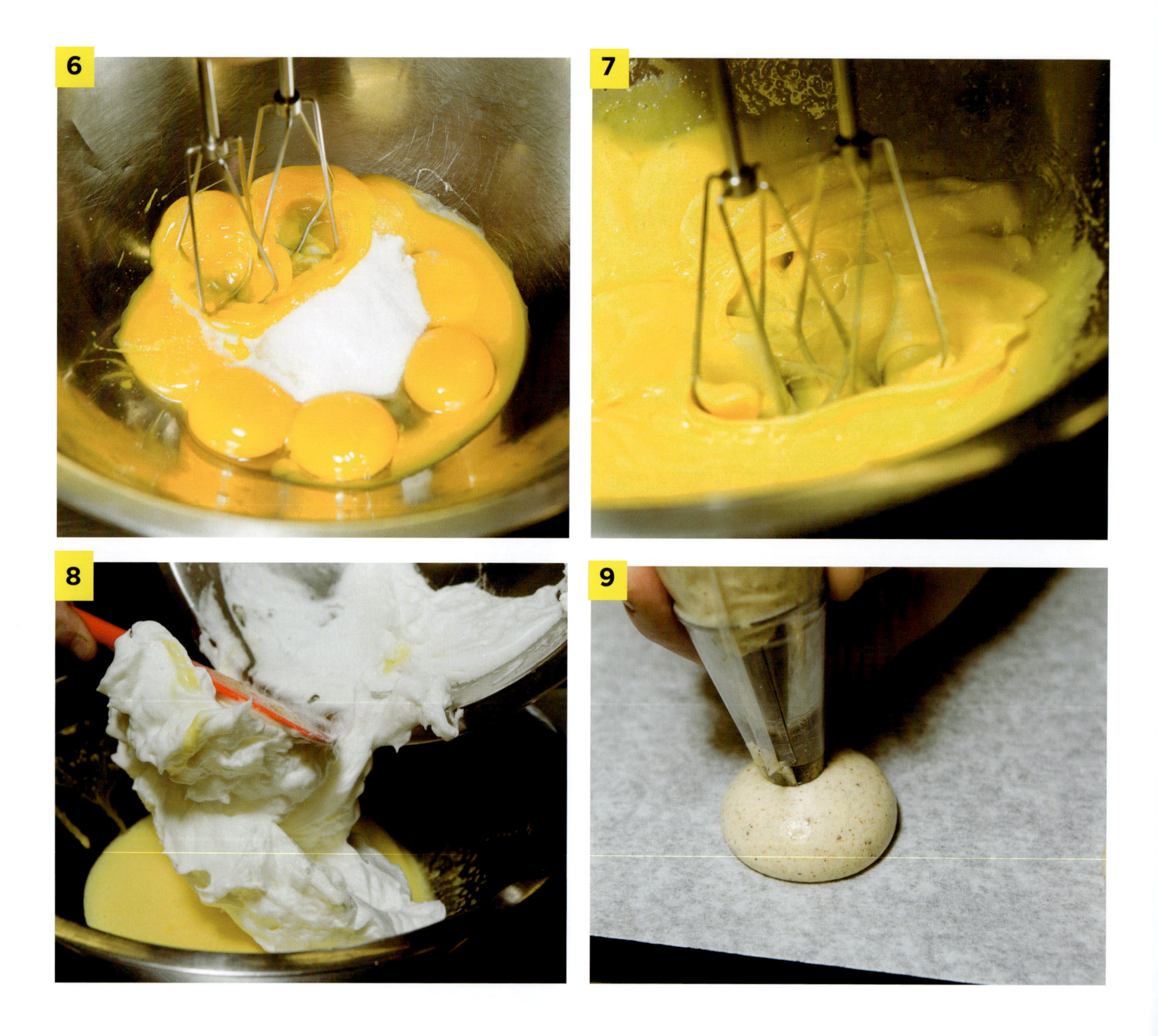

10

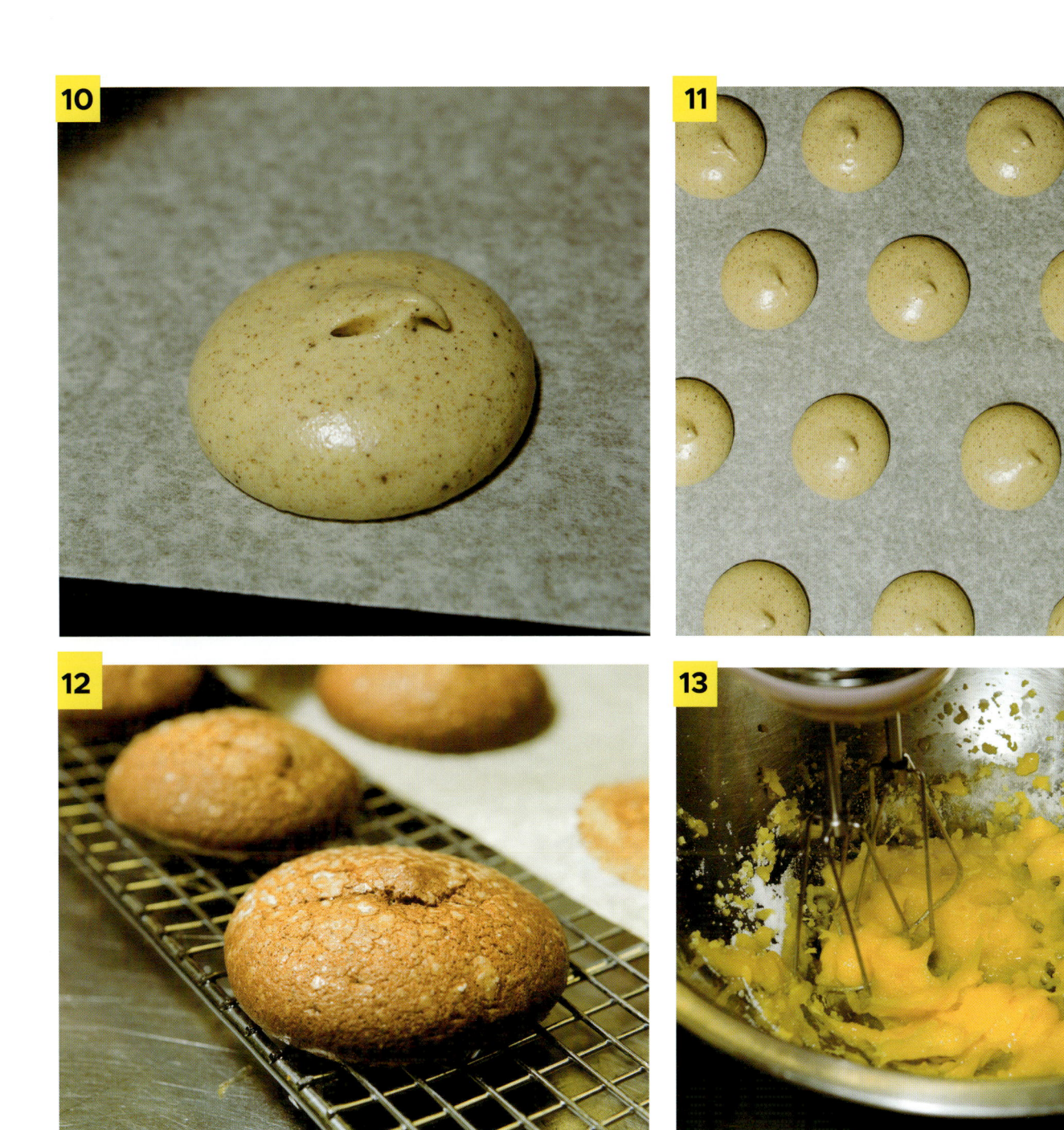

11

12

13

PAGE 200

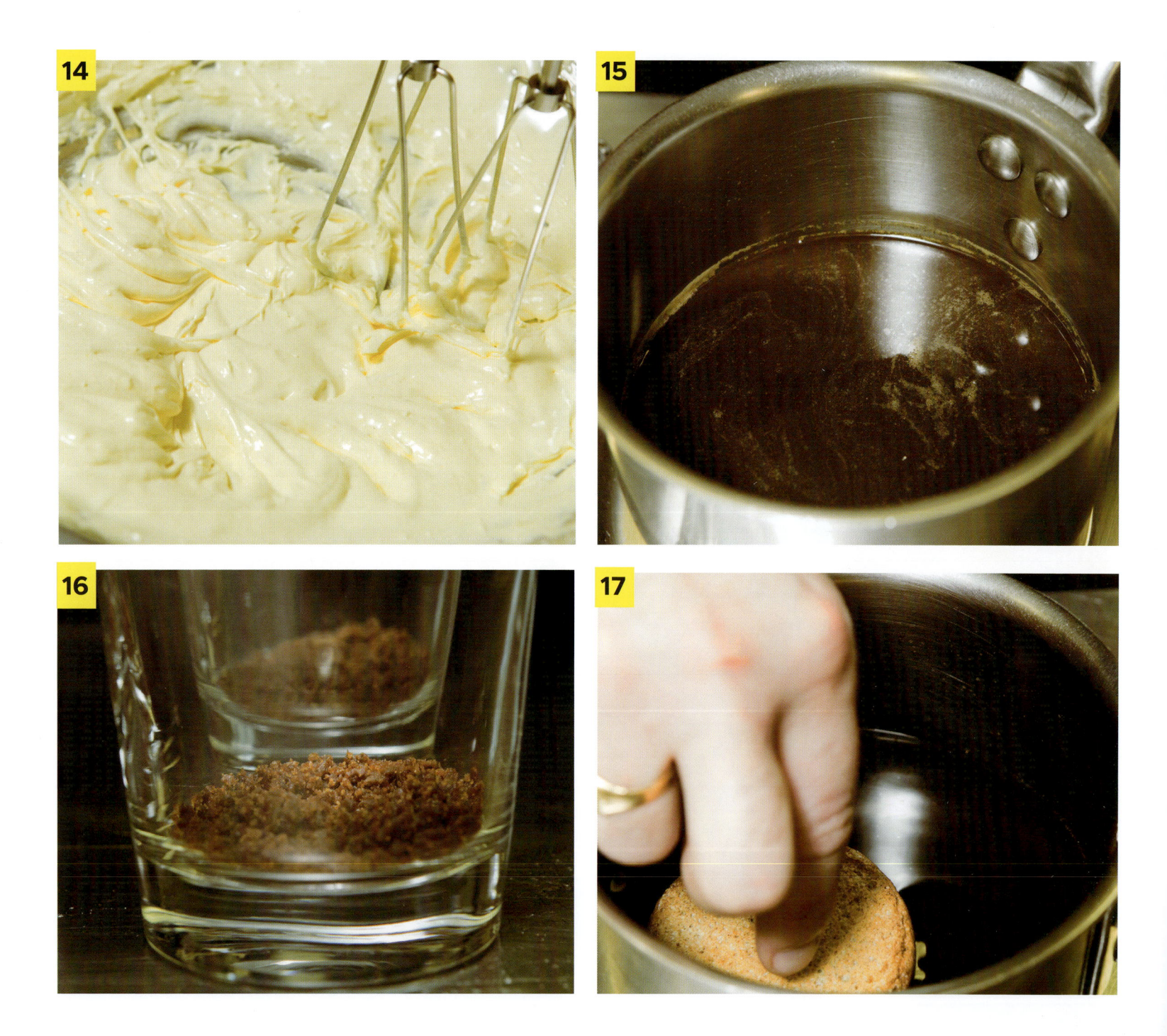

PAGE 201

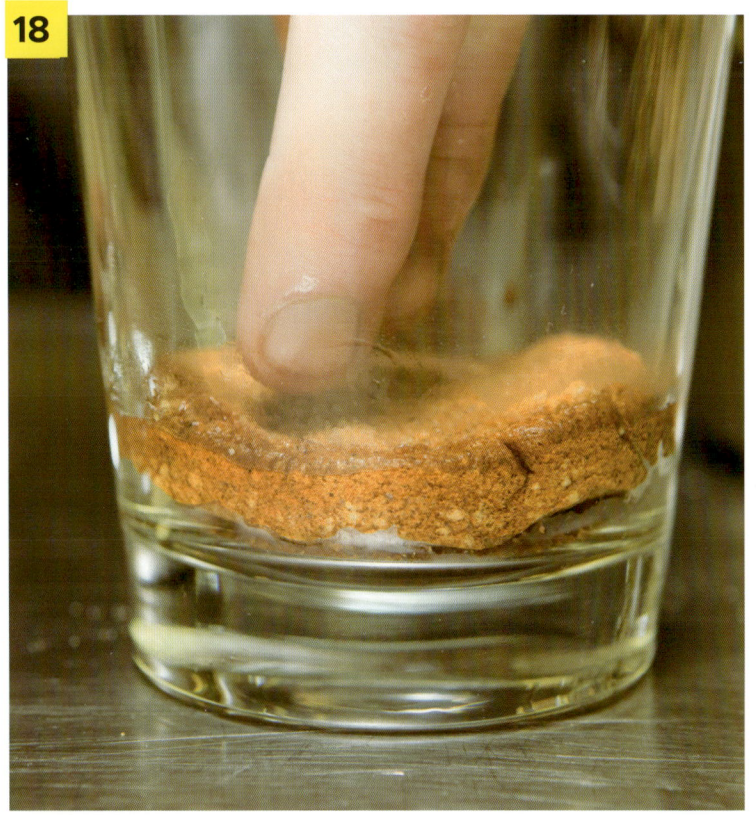

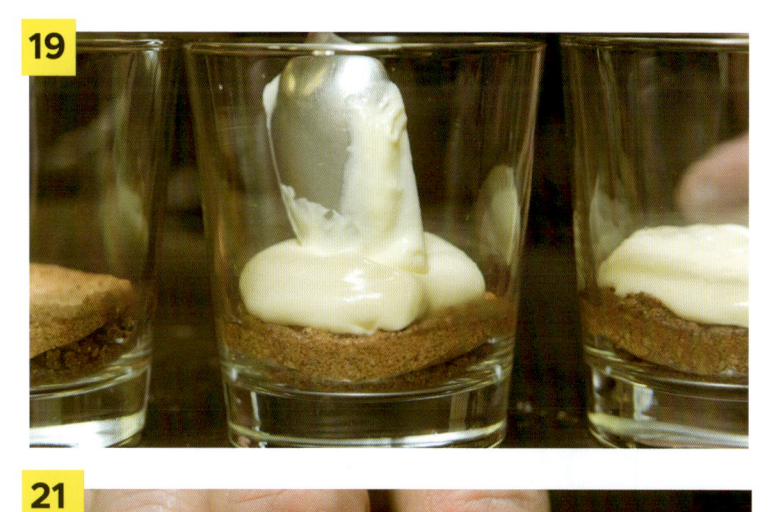

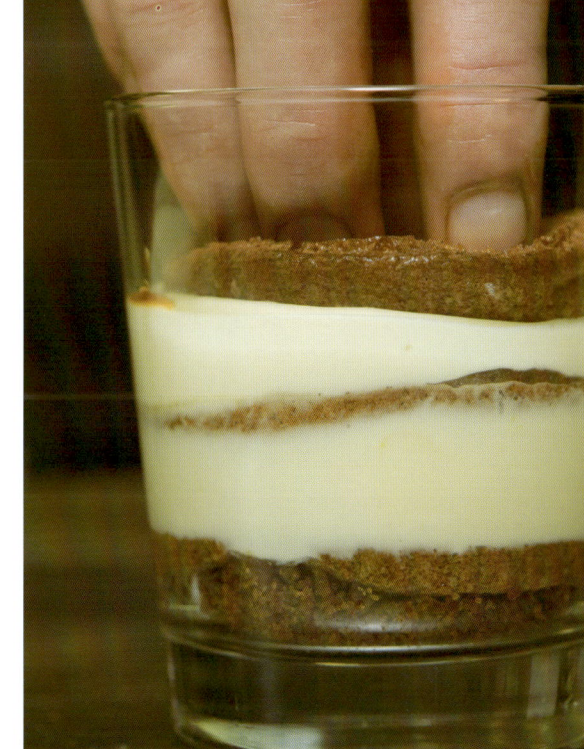

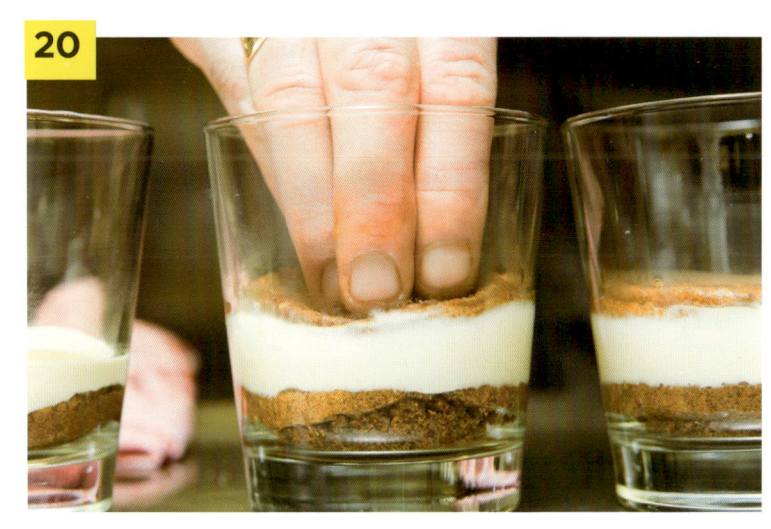

BUILDING BLOCK RECIPES

To become a good chef, you need to do the basics well. These recipes are the foundation of so many recipes in this cookbook—and beyond. Take the time to master making them, because they will elevate your dishes (and your culinary skills) to the next level.

Balsamic Dressing

INGREDIENTS

Makes 6 1/2 cups (1.5 liters)

1. 1/4 cup + 1 tablespoon (70 grams) Dijon mustard
2. 1 1/4 teaspoons (6 grams) kosher salt
3. 1 1/4 cups + 1 tablespoon (300 grams) balsamic vinegar
4. 5 cups (950 grams) canola oil

DIRECTIONS

In a medium bowl, whisk together the mustard, salt, and vinegar. Increase the whisking to a brisk pace and start adding the oil just a few drops at a time, until the liquid thickens slightly. Then pour the oil in a constant stream, whisking constantly, until it is fully incorporated. Store the vinaigrette in a bottle at room temperature; it will last for several weeks. Shake before using.

Clarified Butter

INGREDIENTS

Makes about 2 cups (about 500 milliliters/500 grams)
1. 1 1/2 pounds (6 sticks/750 grams) unsalted butter, diced into 1-inch (2.5 mm) pieces

---

DIRECTIONS

Place the butter in a medium saucepan over medium heat. Once the butter has melted, reduce the heat to maintain a low simmer. Cook until the butter reaches 212°F (100°C), is clear, the bits at the bottom are golden brown, and the foam on top is slightly browned, about 45 minutes. Line a fine-mesh strainer with four layers of cheesecloth and strain the butter into a heatproof container. Let cool completely before covering. Refrigerate, tightly covered, for up to 1 month, or freeze for 6 months or longer.

Cocktail Sauce

INGREDIENTS

Makes roughly 3 1/2 cups (740 grams)

1. 2 1/4 cups (500 grams) mayonnaise (store-bought, or page 204)
2. 1 cup (200 grams) ketchup
3. 1 tablespoon + 2 teaspoons (25 grams) brandy
4. 1 1/2 teaspoons (7 grams) Tabasco sauce
5. 1 1/2 teaspoons (7 grams) Worcestershire sauce

DIRECTIONS

In a medium mixing bowl, whisk together the mayonnaise and ketchup until well combine. Whisk in the brandy, Tabasco, and Worcestershire until fully incorporated. Store in an airtight container in the refrigerator for up to 1 week.

Mayonnaise

INGREDIENTS

Makes 3 1/2 cups (about 750 grams)

1. 2 large egg yolks (40 grams)
2. 3 tablespoons + 1 teaspoon (50 grams) Dijon mustard
3. 3/4 teaspoon (3 grams) kosher salt
4. 3 tablespoons (40 grams) white balsamic vinegar
5. 1 1/4 cups + 2 tablespoons (300 grams) vegetable oil

DIRECTIONS

In a medium bowl, whisk together the egg yolks, mustard, salt, and vinegar until fully combined and starting to get frothy. Increase whisking to a brisk pace and start adding the oil just a few drops at a time, until the liquid lightens and thickens slightly. Then pour the oil in a constant stream, whisking briskly constantly, until it is light and fluffy. Cover and refrigerate for up to 1 week.

Mussel Juice

INGREDIENTS

Makes 1 quart (1 liter)
1. 4 tablespoons (1/2 stick/60 grams) unsalted butter
2. 1/2 cup + 2 tablespoons (100 grams) diced shallots
3. 1 stalk celery, diced
4. 1 clove garlic, peeled
5. 2 pounds (900 grams) mussels, thoroughly cleaned
6. 2 sprigs fresh curly parsley
7. 3 sprigs fresh thyme
8. 1 dried bay leaf
9. 3/4 cup (200 grams) dry white wine

DIRECTIONS

In a large saucepan over medium heat, melt the butter. Add the shallots, celery, and garlic, and cook until the shallots are translucent but not golden, about 5 minutes. Add the mussels, parsley, thyme, bay leaf, and wine. Cover and let it cook until all the mussels have opened, about 10 minutes.

Strain the liquid through a fine-mesh strainer into a heatproof container. Let cool and then store the mussel juice tightly covered in the refrigerator for up to 10 days, or freeze for up to 6 months.
Though you should throw out (or, better yet, compost) the vegetable solids, don't discard the mussels—eat them, they're delicious!

Fish Stock

INGREDIENTS

Makes 5 quart (5 liter)

1. 4 tablespoons (1/2 stick/60 grams) unsalted butter
2. 1 large yellow onion, diced
3. 2 stalks celery, diced
4. 2 large leeks (white and light green parts), cut in half lengthwise
5. 4 1/2 pounds (2 kilograms) fish bones (no gills), cleaned, rinsed under cold water for about 5 minutes, and drained
6. 2 cups + 2 tablespoons (500 milliliters) dry white wine
7. 2 lemons, peeled, pith removed, and cut in half
8. 1 sprig fresh thyme
9. 4 sprigs fresh curly parsley
10. 1 tablespoon + 1 teaspoon (18 grams) kosher salt
11. 2 dried bay leaves
12. 1/2 teaspoon (2 grams) whole black peppercorns

To obtain fish bones, either save bones from your own preparations or ask to buy some from your local fishmonger or at the seafood counter of your grocery store.

DIRECTIONS

In a large stew pot over medium heat, melt the butter. Add the onions, celery, and leeks and cook until the onions are translucent but not golden, about 5 to 10 minutes. Add the fish bones and cook for 15 minutes, until the bones start to whiten. Add the wine, lemon flesh, thyme, parsley, salt, bay leaves, and peppercorns.

Simmer until the liquid is reduced by half, about 20 minutes. Add cold water until all the fish bones are covered (6 to 8 quarts/6 to 8 liters) and simmer for about 1 hour, until you can taste the fish and the vegetables.

While the stock is cooking, skim off any foam that rises to the surface.

Strain the stock through a fine-mesh strainer into a heatproof container, pressing on the solids to extract as much liquid as possible. Discard the solids. Let the stock cool, then store it, tightly covered, in the refrigerator for up to 10 days, or freeze for up to 6 months. Consider storing it in 1-quart/1-liter containers, so you can unfreeze smaller portions as needed.

Veal Stock

INGREDIENTS

Makes 1 1/2 quart (2.5 liter)

1. 3 pounds (1.35 kilograms) veal bones or shanks
2. 2 tablespoons + 1 teaspoon (30 grams) canola oil
3. 1 large carrot, diced large
4. 2 large yellow onions, diced large
5. 3 stalks celery, diced large
6. 3 tablespoons (50 grams) tomato paste
7. 2 cups + 2 tablespoons (500 milliliters) Burgundy or other dry red wine
8. 3 dried bay leaves
9. 6 sprigs fresh thyme

Veal bones or shanks are available from any butcher.

DIRECTIONS

Preheat the oven to 450°F (230°C).

Arrange the veal bones in a single layer on 2 or 3 rimmed sheet pans lined with aluminum foil. Cook until the bones brown, 1 to 1 1/2 hours.

While the bones are cooking, heat the oil in a large skillet over medium-high heat until smoking slightly. Add the carrots, onions, and celery and cook until they have softened, 5 to 10 minutes. Add the tomato paste and cook until it browns, about 10 minutes. Add the wine and cook until the liquid has reduced by half, about 30 minutes. Set aside.

When bones are finished roasting, drain off the excess fat, place them in a large stockpot, and cover them completely with cold water (10 to 12 quarts/10 to 12 liters). Over high heat, bring to a boil. Reduce the heat to a simmer and occasionally skim any foam off the top. Add the vegetables, bay leaves, and thyme, and gently simmer, uncovered, over medium-low heat for 8 to 10 hours, until the liquid is dark brown and has thickened slightly. Strain the stock into a large heatproof container through a fine-mesh strainer, pressing on the solids to extract as much liquid as possible; discard the solids.

Return the stock to the pot over medium-low heat and gently simmer until reduced by half, about 45 to 60 minutes, occasionally skimming foam off surface. Let cool, then store the stock in an airtight container in the refrigerator for up to 10 days, or freeze for up to 6 months.

Chicken Stock

INGREDIENTS

Makes 5 quart (5 liter)

1. 5 pounds (2.27 kilograms) chicken wings
2. 1 large carrot, diced medium
3. 2 large onions, diced medium
4. 1 large leek (white and light green parts), diced medium
5. 2 stalks celery, diced medium
6. 1 1/4 teaspoons (6 grams) kosher salt
7. 1 tablespoon (7 grams) freshly ground black pepper
8. 2 dried cloves
9. 2 sprigs fresh thyme
10. 2 dried bay leaves
11. 3 sprigs fresh curly parsley

DIRECTIONS

Place chicken in a large stockpot and cover completely with cold water (5 quarts/5 liters). Bring to a boil over medium-high heat, constantly skimming any foam off the top. Add the carrot, onions, leek, celery, salt, pepper, cloves, thyme, bay leaves, and parsley.

Cook until bubbling slightly, then turn the heat down to medium-low to maintain a gentle simmer. Skim the foam off surface every 15 minutes for the first hour, and every 30 minutes of the second hour. Add hot water as needed to keep chicken and vegetables submerged. Simmer uncovered for 4 to 6 hours, until the stock is pale yellow and has a mild chicken flavor.

Strain the liquid into a large container through a fine-mesh strainer, pressing on the solids to extract as much liquid as possible; discard the solids. Let cool, then cover and store in the refrigerator overnight. The next day, remove and discard the solidified fat from the top. Store the stock in an airtight container in the refrigerator for up to 10 days, or freeze for up to 6 months. Consider storing it in 1-quart/1-liter containers, so you can unfreeze smaller portions as needed.

White Mushroom Consommé

INGREDIENTS

Makes 2 cups (500 milliliters)

1. 4 pounds (1.8 kilograms) white mushrooms, cleaned and grated on a box grater
2. 2 1/2 teaspoons (12 grams) kosher salt
3. 2 sprigs fresh thyme
4. 1 dried bay leaf
5. 2 tablespoons + 1 teaspoon (18 grams) mushroom powder (preferably porcini)

DIRECTIONS

In a medium stew pot over high heat, combine 2 cups water, the mushrooms, salt, thyme, bay leaf, and mushroom powder. Bring to a boil, then reduce the heat to low. Cook uncovered until the liquid is dark and the mushrooms are gray, about 2 hours. Strain the liquid into a large container through a fine-mesh strainer, pressing on the solids to extract as much liquid as possible; discard the solids. Return the liquid to the pot over high heat and bring to a boil for 5 minutes, until dark brown and has a rich mushroom flavor. Store the consommé in an airtight container in the refrigerator for up to 10 days, or freeze it for up to 6 months.

Red Wine Sauce

INGREDIENTS

Makes 2 cups (500 milliliters)

1. 1/4 cup + 1 teaspoon (60 grams) canola oil
2. 2 medium shallots, diced
3. 1/2 medium yellow onion, diced
4. 1 large carrot, diced
5. 1/2 stalk celery, diced
6. 5 cloves garlic, roughly chopped
7. 1/4 teaspoon (1 grams) kosher salt, plus more for seasoning
8. 2 tablespoons (14 grams) freshly ground black pepper, plus more for seasoning
9. 1 quart (1 liter) dry red wine
10. 6 sprigs fresh thyme
11. 4 dried bay leaves
12. 3 3/4 cups + 2 tablespoons (900 grams) veal stock (store-bought, or page 207)
13. 8 tablespoons (1 stick/125 grams) unsalted butter, cut into 1/2-inch (1 cm) pieces

DIRECTIONS

In a large saucepan over medium-high heat, heat the oil until it smokes slightly. Add the shallots, onion, carrot, celery, and garlic and sauté until tender but not browned, about 5 minutes. Add the salt, pepper, wine, thyme, and bay leaves and let the liquid reduce by half, about 20 minutes. Turn down the heat to low, add the veal stock and let it cook until reduced by half, about 1 hour.

Strain the sauce through a fine-mesh strainer, pressing on the solids to extract as much liquid as possible; discard the solids.

Remove the sauce from the heat and store it in an airtight container in the refrigerator for up to 10 days, or freeze

Speculoos Spice Mix

INGREDIENTS

Makes about 3/4 cup (90 grams)

1. 1 tablespoon (7 grams) ground star anise
2. 1/4 cup + 3 tablespoons (56 grams) ground cinnamon
3. 1 tablespoon (7 grams) ground nutmeg
4. 2 tablespoons (14 grams) ground ginger
5. 1 1/2 teaspoons (4 grams) ground cloves
6. 1 1/2 teaspoons (4 grams) ground cardamom

DIRECTIONS

In a small bowl, whisk all the ingredients together until fully combined. Store the mix in an airtight container at room temperature for up to 6 months.

Tomato Confit

INGREDIENTS

Makes 40 tomato petals
1. 10 large Roma tomatoes
2. 1/2 cup (100 grams) extra virgin olive oil, plus more for storage
3. 2 cloves garlic, finely diced
4. 3 sprigs fresh thyme, roughly chopped
5. 1 tablespoon + 3/4 teaspoon (18 grams) kosher salt
6. 1 tablespoon (7 grams) freshly ground black pepper
7. 1 3/4 teaspoons (7 grams) granulated sugar

DIRECTIONS

Preheat the oven to 200°F (95°C).

Using a sharp paring knife, cut the cores out of the tomatoes from the stem end. Cut a small X in the skin at the other end.

Bring a large pot of water to a boil. Fill a large bowl with ice and cold water. Line a rimmed sheet pan with parchment paper.

Place the tomatoes in the boiling water for 10 seconds. Remove them with a slotted spoon and place them in the ice water.

When the tomatoes are cool, remove the skins, cut in half lengthwise, and squeeze out juices and seeds. Cut the halves in half lengthwise again. In a large bowl, gently toss tomatoes with the olive oil, garlic, thyme, salt, pepper, and sugar.

Arrange the tomatoes, cut side down, on the prepared sheet pan. Bake until very soft, about 5 hours.

Place tomatoes in an airtight container, adding olive oil to completely cover. Store in the refrigerator for up to 3 weeks.

Cooked Spinach

INGREDIENTS

Makes 1 1/2 cups (380 grams), enough for 2 side servings
1. 2 tablespoons (28 grams) extra virgin olive oil
2. 1 pound (450 grams) baby spinach, washed and dried
3. 2 cloves garlic, finely diced
4. 1 teaspoon (3 grams) finely diced shallots
5. Pinch of freshly grated nutmeg
6. 1/4 teaspoon (1 gram) kosher salt
7. Pinch of freshly ground black pepper
8. Pinch of Espelette pepper
9. 1 tablespoon (15 grams) unsalted butter

DIRECTIONS

In a large saucepan over medium heat, heat the oil until slightly smoking. Add the spinach and cook, stirring constantly with a wooden spoon, until wilted. Add the garlic, shallots, nutmeg, salt, black pepper, Espelette pepper, and butter. Stir constantly until the butter has melted. Remove the spinach from the pan and drain it in a fine-mesh strainer set in the sink. Store the spinach in an airtight container in the refrigerator for up to 3 days.

Puff Pastry

INGREDIENTS

Makes two 12 by 8-inch (30 by 20 cm) sheets, each TK ounces (TK grams)

1. 3 3/4 cups (400 grams) pastry flour, plus more for working
2. 2 1/2 teaspoons (12 grams) kosher salt
3. 1 cup (240 milliliters) ice cold water

DIRECTIONS

Sift together the flour and salt into a mixing bowl. Using a whisk, stir in water until a dough ball forms. If the dough is not coming together, add more water, 1 tablespoon (15 milliliters) at a time, making sure the dough never feels wet.

Turn the dough out onto a lightly floured surface and roll into a 12-inch (30 cm) square 1/2 inch (1 cm) thick.

Place the butter between sheets of wax paper or plastic wrap and pound with a rolling pin until it is malleable but not soft. Form the butter into a 6-inch (15 cm) square. Place the butter in the center of dough, turning so it is positioned like a diamond in the square. Fold each corner of dough over onto center of butter like the flaps of an envelope. Wrap the dough package completely with plastic wrap and place in the refrigerator to rest for 10 minutes.

Return the dough to the lightly floured work surface and roll it out lengthwise into a long, 1/2-inch-thick (1 cm) rectangle about 14 by 12 inches (35 by 30 centimeters)..). Fold the dough in thirds, like a letter. Wrap the dough again and chill for 10 minutes in refrigerator.

Repeat the process of rolling the dough lengthwise, folding into thirds, and chilling three more times. Roll out the dough into a large rectangle about 24 by 16-inch (61 by 41 centimeters) and then cut into two rectangles approximately 12 by 8-inch (30 by 20 cm).

Wrap the doughs in plastic wrap and refrigerate until needed. The puff pastry dough will last up to 3 days in the refrigerator or can be frozen for up to 3 months.

Pullman Loaf

INGREDIENTS

Makes one 13 by 4 by 4-inch (33 by 10 by 10 cm) loaf

1. 1 1/2 cups (360 grams) lukewarm water
2. 2 teaspoons (5 grams) instant dry yeast
3. 4 1/2 cups + 2 tablespoons (560 grams) high-gluten flour
4. 2 tablespoons + 2 teaspoons (40 grams) unsalted butter, room temperature
5. 2 tablespoons + 1 teaspoon (30 grams) granulated sugar
6. 2 1/2 teaspoons (12 grams) kosher salt
7. Extra virgin olive oil for greasing the pan

DIRECTIONS

Combine the water and yeast in the bowl of a stand mixer fitted with the dough hook attachment. Mix on medium speed to dissolve yeast. Add the flour, butter, sugar, and salt and mix until the dough has formed a ball and pulls away from the sides of the bowl, 10 to 15 minutes.

Transfer the dough to a medium bowl lightly greased with olive oil and cover tightly with plastic wrap. Let it rise in a warm place until it has doubled in size, about 45 minutes. Remove the dough from the bowl, stretch it out, fold it over on itself, form another ball, put it back into the bowl, and cover it again. Let it rise until it doubles again, about 45 minutes.

Oil a 13 by 4 by 4-inch (33 by 10 by 10 cm) Pullman loaf pan. Form the dough into a log and place it in the pan. Let it rise with the cover off until the dough fills the pan, about 3 hours.

Preheat the oven to 400°F (200°C).

Place the cover on the loaf pan and bake for about 1 hour,

until a cake tester inserted into the center comes out clean. Remove the cover and bake for an additional 10 minutes, until the top is golden brown. Remove from the oven and let cool in the pan on a cooling rack for 20 minutes. Remove the bread from the pan and place it on the rack to cool completely. Refrigerate in a large Ziploc bag for up to 1 week; remove from the refrigerator and let it come to room temperature before eating.

Fresh Pasta

INGREDIENTS

Makes about 2 1/2 pounds (1.5 kilograms) fresh pasta

1. 8 cups (1 kilogram) semolina flour, plus more for working
2. 8 to 10 large eggs (400 to 500 grams)
3. Pinch of kosher salt
4. 2 tablespoons + 1 teaspoon (30 grams) extra virgin olive oil

---

DIRECTIONS

Place the flour, 4 of the eggs, and the salt in a food processor fitted with the dough blade. Pulse to combine. With the machine running, gradually pour in the oil, followed by the remaining eggs, one at the time, until the mixture forms a ball. If it's still not coming together, add water 1 teaspoon at a time.

Place the dough on a lightly floured surface and form into a ball. Wrap completely with plastic wrap and place in the refrigerator for at least 1 hour, but overnight is even better.

Cut the dough into quarters and press flat. Using a stand mixer fitted with a pasta rolling attachment, or a manual pasta maker, run each piece of dough through several times until it is 1/16 to 1/8 inch (1.5 to 3 mm) thick.
Cut the dough into 8 by 6-inch (20 by 15 cm) rectangles to make lasagna noodles, 6 by 4-inch (15 by 10 cm) rectangles to make the pasta for cannelloni, and into 3/4-inch-wide (2 cm) strips to make pappardelle.

Note: If you won't be cooking the pasta immediately, sprinkle it with more semolina flour and store it in an airtight container in the refrigerator for up to 2 day, or freeze for up to 3 months. When you are ready to use it, do not thaw it first.

Leek Stoemp

INGREDIENTS

1. 24 tablespoons (3 sticks/360 grams) unsalted butter, divided
2. 3 medium yellow onions, diced
3. 2 pounds (900 grams) Yukon gold potatoes, washed, peeled, and diced
4. 5 large leeks (white and light green parts), washed and diced
5. 3 quarts (3 liters) chicken stock
6. 2 1/2 teaspoons (12 grams) sea salt, plus more for seasoning
7. 1/4 teaspoon (1 gram) freshly ground black pepper
8. 1/4 teaspoon (1 gram) ground nutmeg
9. 2 cups + 2 tablespoons (500 milliliters) heavy cream

DIRECTIONS

In a large stew pot over medium heat, melt 12 tablespoons (180 grams) of the butter. Add the onions and cook, stirring occasionally, until translucent and softened, 8 to 10 minutes. Add the potatoes and cook, stirring occasionally to ensure they don't stick to the bottom of the pot, for 5 minutes. Add the leeks and cook, stirring occasionally, for 5 minutes, until slightly softened. Add the stock, salt, pepper, and nutmeg, and cook, stirring occasionally, until the liquid is absorbed but the remaining mixture isn't sticking to the bottom of the pot. Add the heavy cream and cook for 10 minutes longer, stirring occasionally, until the liquid is mostly absorbed by the vegetables. Using a hand masher, mash the potato mixture and the remaining 12 tablespoons (180 grams) butter until the butter is fully incorporated. Season to taste with salt and pepper. Serve immediately.

Claudio's Acknowledgments

Firstly, I would like to thank my team at the restaurant, who helped me and Alex with the recipe testing, while still taking care of all their other duties. We could not have done it without you. I'm so grateful to Alex for all the time and effort he poured into this project. His hard work and inspired perspective shines on every page of this book. Many appreciations to copyeditor Suzanne Fass for her keen eye and thoughtful observations. Thanks to Jay Snap for his beautiful photographs, which bring these recipes to life. I am so glad we had the chance to collaborate together. To Nevin: You took my words and made them into stories. Many thanks for all your hard work and dedication to this project. Most of all, I want to acknowledge my wonderful wife, Mariella, and my beautiful children John and Clara. Thank you for always supporting me. My hours away from you are long, but you are always in my heart.

Nevin's Acknowledgments

My gratitude goes out to Claudio for making me a part of this unforgettable project. Many thanks to the Et Voila! team for their hospitality, help, and too many good meals and cups of espresso to count. Deep appreciations to recipe editor extraordinaire Carolyn Crow for all her hard work. A big hat tip to Jay Snap for his eye-catching photography, sunny attitude, and willingness to share his wisdom. To my wife, Indira, and my son, Zephyr: Thank you both for the infinite joy you create, the wisdom you constantly impart, and the balance you bring to my life. You two are my everything.

About the Co-Author

Nevin Martell is a DC-area based food and travel writer, parenting essayist, recipe developer, and photographer who has been published by The Washington Post, New York Times, Saveur, Men's Journal, National Geographic, Fortune, Travel + Leisure, and many other publications. He is the author of eight books, including Red Truck Bakery Cookbook: Gold-Standard Recipes from America's Favorite Rural Bakery, The Founding Farmers Cookbook: 100 Recipes for True Food & Drink, and the small-press smash Looking for Calvin and Hobbes: The Unconventional Story of Bill Watterson and His Revolutionary Comic Strip. Find him online at nevinmartell.com and on Instagram @nevinmartell.